INA MAY'S

✤ GUIDE TO ✤

CHILDBIRTH

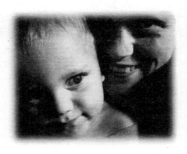

INA MAY GASKIN

Vermilion
LONDON

To the women and the doctors who helped me
become a midwife

12

Published in 2008 by Vermilion, an imprint of Ebury Publishing
First published in the USA by Bantam Dell, a division of Random House, Inc., in 2003

Ebury Publishing is a Random House Group company

Copyright © Ina May Gaskin 2003

Ina May Gaskin has asserted her right to be identified as the author of this Work
in accordance with the Copyright, Designs and Patents Act, 1988.

The Random House Group Limited Reg. No. 954009

Addresses for companies within the Random House Group can be found at
www.randomhouse.co.uk

A CIP catalogue record for this book is available from the British Library

Penguin Random House is committed to a sustainable future for
our business, our readers and our planet. This book is made from
Forest Stewardship Council® certified paper.

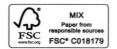

Book design by Lynn Newmark
Line art by Jackie Aher
For photograph and illustration credits, see piv
Printed and bound in Great Britain by Clays Ltd, St Ives plc

ISBN 9780091924157

Copies are available at special rates for bulk orders. Contact the sales
development team on 020 7840 8487 for more information.

To buy books by your favourite authors and register for offers, visit
www.randomhouse.co.uk

A NOTE OF THANKS

I want to thank my husband, Stephen Gaskin, for his unfailing willingness to help me during the long process of writing this book. I literally could not have done this project without him. My thanks go also to my agent, Stephany Evans; Pamela Hunt; Carol Nelson; Deborah Flowers; Joanne Santana; Sharon Wells; Pamela Maurath; John O. Williams, Jr., MD; Wendy Savage, MD; A. Mark Durand, MD; Alan Graf; Anna Meenan, MD; Joseph Bruner, MD; Marsden Wagner; Kenneth Johnson; David Frohman; Leigh Kahan; Robbie Davis-Floyd; Elise Harvey; Leslie Hunt; Dana Gaskin Wenig; Claudia Oblasser; Angelika Rodler; Michael Stohrer; Verena Schmidt; Betty Anne Daviss; and Ken Starratt. I would also like to thank my editors, Robin Michaelson and Beth Rashbaum, and their assistant, Stacie Fine.

Ina May Gaskin, CPM

ILLUSTRATION CREDITS

CONTENTS

An Invitation

Whatever your reason for picking up this book, I salute your curiosity and your desire to know more about the important work of having babies. For those who are pregnant, I kept you especially in mind as I wrote this book.

Consider this your invitation to learn about the true capacities of the female body during labor and birth. I'm not talking about a summary of current medical knowledge translated from technical to popular language. You can find plenty of that in bookstores. What I mean by *true capacities of the female body* are those that are experienced by real women, whether or not these abilities are recognized by medical authorities. The way I see it, the most trustworthy knowledge about women's bodies combines the best of what medical science has offered over the past century or two with what women have always been able to learn about themselves before birth moved into hospitals. The purpose of this book is to point you toward the best information currently available about women's real capacities in labor and birth and to show you how these can mesh with the most effective use of modern birth technology. My intention is to encourage and inform you.

I have been a community midwife for more than three decades. I live in a village in the United States in which women and girls have little or no fear of childbirth. My partners and I have attended the births of more than 2,200 babies, most of them born in their parents' homes or at our birth center. Working in this way has enabled me to learn things about women that are generally unknown in the world of medical education. It's not easy to say whether the women in my village have less fear of birth because we know that our capabilities go beyond medical understanding or that our capabilities are greater without anxiety. Actually, both are true.

The village is called The Farm, and it's located in southern Tennessee, near Summertown. My husband and I, along with several hundred others, founded it in 1971, and there we still live and work. One of the unique features of our community is that, from its beginning, the men have not interfered with the women's desire to organize our own system of birth care. At the same time, the men have always lent a good deal of support and technological expertise to make our care more readily accessible and available. They have never dictated where or how our babies would be born.

Let me be clear about what I say about fear and birth at The Farm. I don't mean that these women in my village never experienced a few moments of anxiety at the prospect of giving birth or wondered, Will I be able to accomplish this seemingly impossible act? I'm sure that many of us did wonder about this from time to time. Virtually all women do. After all, it is not immediately obvious to most people who grow up in civilized cultures—especially those in which most people live totally apart from animals—how birth can happen. When such moments of doubt occur to women in my village, they are able to fall back on the sure knowledge that their closest friends and sisters and mothers have been able to do it. This knowledge then makes it possible for them to believe that they can too—whether or not they've ever witnessed the act of birth itself. The women at The Farm have relearned and been highly successful at kinds of female behavior that modern women in civilized cultures aren't known to be good at—those that go *beyond* the common medical understanding of women's bodies and birth.

My experiences as a midwife have taught me that women's bodies still work. Here is your chance to be exposed to a new understanding of an ancient system of knowledge that you can add to your general understanding of what birth means. Wherever and however you intend to give birth, your experience will impact your emotions, your mind, your body, and your spirit for the rest of your life.

The women in my village* expect to give birth vaginally, for that is the way all but one or two out of every hundred have their babies. Yes, we do sometimes have to transport a woman to the hospital for a cesarean or instrumental delivery, but such interventions are compara-

---

*I want you to understand that this village includes a school, a clinic, a water system, a soy foods production plant, and several businesses, including a small factory that manufactures and markets a personal radiation detector that was invented in our village.

tively rare for the women who give birth at The Farm. (Our cesarean rate up to the year 2000 was 1.4 percent; our forceps- and vacuum-extraction rate was 0.05 percent. The U.S. national cesarean rate for 2001 was 31.1 percent, and the instrumental delivery rate was about 10 percent.) Women at The Farm know that labor can be painful, but many of them know as well that labor and birth can be ecstatic—even orgasmic. Above all, whether or not they experienced labor as painful, to a woman, they found labor and birth a tremendously empowering passage.

Have you never heard anyone speak positively about labor and birth before? If so, you are not alone. One of the best-kept secrets in North American culture is that birth can be ecstatic and strengthening. Ecstatic birth gives inner power and wisdom to the woman who experiences it, as you will learn from many of the birth stories told here. Even when women in my village experience pain in labor, they understand that there are ways of making the sensations of labor and birth tolerable that do not involve numbing the senses with drugs. They know that it is better to keep their senses alive if they are to experience the true wisdom and power that labor and birth have to offer.

In Part I of this book, you will hear the voices of these women as they tell their birth stories. Some of the stories are told by the pioneering generation that collectively created the birth culture of our village; others are told by their daughters and daughters-in-law, who grew up within this culture or whose partner did. A few are told by women who were born at home and grew up within our birth culture, who gave birth with other midwives. Other stories are those of women who decided to partake of our successful birth culture by having their babies at our birth center. If you are pregnant or plan a pregnancy in the near future, you may want to return to these birth stories again and again to strengthen your own spirit in preparation for giving birth.

My first book, *Spiritual Midwifery,* was one of the first North American books about midwifery and birth when its first edition was published in 1975. It quickly sold more than half a million copies and was translated into several languages, introducing me not only to a generation of childbearing women and their partners but to a surprising number of doctors and other birth professionals as well. In some countries, the book was made part of the curriculum of midwifery schools. In several, doctors told me that they read it in order to recover from some of the more frightening aspects of their training in obstetrics. I began to meet a breed of doctors who called themselves *MDs* (Midwives in Disguise). Because of the book and the birth statistics published in it, I was invited to travel all over the world and to share the results of my colleagues' and my work with birth professionals and women from many different countries and cultures. This kind of cross-cultural experience has let me look at birth and maternity care with a broad perspective and compare how certain obstetrical practices and habits that become entrenched in certain countries actually work against the most efficient functioning of women's bodies. My experience has also taught me how necessary the midwife's role is in any given society and how important it is that the profession of midwifery stand on its own—independent of obstetrics but always able to work with obstetricians in the comparatively rare instances when the need arises.

Not long ago an obstetrician acquaintance remarked, "The two most interesting pages in *Spiritual Midwifery* were the last two." He meant the pages devoted to reporting our birth outcomes at The Farm. He said, "You need to explain *how* you were able to accomplish what you did, so that we who work in hospitals may incorporate your work into what we do." Part II of this book is for him and for everyone who wants to understand why the birth culture of The Farm has been such a success. I discuss the guiding principles that surround and define our work and recommend techniques that can be transposed from home birth to hospital birth.

In Part II, I discuss in detail why there is so much mystery surrounding the functioning of women's bodies in birth and how we at The Farm were able to remove much of that mystery and turn it into working knowledge available to virtually everyone in our community. I explain why there is such a wide range of women's experiences in birth and why there can be such divergent interpretations of what is safe or unsafe in birth-giving. There *is* a logical explanation for all of this. The same goes for pain in labor: In Part II, I delve into how it is that birth can be experienced as painless—even orgasmic—or, more commonly in civilized cultures, as the most intense kind of pain. You'll learn that a woman's uterus in labor can close as well as open and about the conditions that are likely to make labor stall or go backward. You'll read about some practical ways to make the sexuality of birth work for you, not against you.

In addition, Part II includes an overview of the practices and treatments you are likely to encounter in a North American hospital, along with a guide to those that are based upon solid scientific evidence and those that are not.

Birthing is so integral with life—so common—that choices surrounding it often get relegated to chance. We tend to go along with what everyone else is doing, assuming that must be for the best. Living in a technological society, we tend to think that the best of everything is the most expensive kind available. This is generally true, whether we are talking about cell phones, cameras, cars, or computers. When it comes to birth, it ain't necessarily so.

—*Ina May Gaskin*

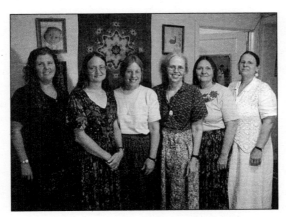

My partners and I. *Left to right:* Joanne Santana, CPM; Deborah Flowers, CPM; Pamela Hunt, CPM; Ina May Gaskin, CPM; Carol Nelson, CPM; and Sharon Wells, CPM

I

BIRTH STORIES

Introduction to the Birth Stories

There is extraordinary psychological benefit in belonging to a group of women who have positive stories to tell about their birth experiences. This phenomenon is exactly what developed within our village. So many horror stories circulate about birth—especially in the United States—that it can be difficult for women to believe that labor and birth can be a beneficial experience. If you have been pregnant for a while, it's probable that you've already heard some scary birth stories from friends or relatives. This is especially true if you live in the United States, where telling pregnant women gory stories has been a national pastime for at least a century. Now that birth has become a favorite subject of television dramas and situation comedies, this trend has been even more pronounced. No one has explained the situation more succinctly than Stephen King in his novella "The Breathing

Method."* Commenting on the fear many women have of birth, his fictional character observes, "Believe me: if you are told that some experience is going to hurt, it will hurt. Most pain is in the mind, and when a woman absorbs the idea that the act of giving birth is excruciatingly painful—when she gets this information from her mother, her sisters, her married friends, and her physician—that woman has been mentally prepared to feel great agony." King, you may not know, is the father of several children born at home.

The best way I know to counter the effects of frightening stories is to hear or read empowering ones. I mean stories that change you because you read or heard them, because the teller of the story taught you something you didn't know before or helped you look at things from a different angle than you ever had before. For this reason, Part I of this book is largely devoted to stories told by women who planned to have home or birth-center births with me and my midwife partners. You may find this part of the book to be the one you want to read the most during pregnancy. At The Farm, the only horror stories we shared were those of previous births in which the care had been radically different from that given by Farm midwives. As women began to have positive experiences giving birth, their stories helped to calm the fears and worries of those who had not yet had babies. The confidence that these women gained from one another was a significant factor in why the midwifery care at The Farm has produced such good results.

Stories teach us in ways we can remember. They teach us that each woman responds to birth in her unique way and how very wide-ranging that way can be. Sometimes they teach us about silly practices once widely held that were finally discarded. They teach us the occasional difference between accepted medical knowledge and the real bodily experiences that women have—including those that are never reported in medical textbooks nor admitted as possibilities in the medical world. They also demonstrate the mind/body connection in a way that medical studies cannot. Birth stories told by women who were active participants in giving birth often express a good deal of practical wisdom, inspiration, and information for other women. Positive stories shared by women who have had wonderful childbirth

*Read it after you've had your baby, as it is a frightening story, even though the scary part isn't about the birth process.

experiences are an irreplaceable way to transmit knowledge of a woman's true capacities in pregnancy and birth.

✣ James's Birth—November 16, 1986
By Karen Lovell

Huntsville, Alabama—Rocket City, U.S.A., where "the sky is not the limit." My husband, Ron, had gone to work for the maker of the world's fastest supercomputers and was stationed at the NASA Marshall Space Flight Center. For all intents and purposes, it appeared that we were people geared toward state-of-the-art technology, people who would accept the latest and greatest, even when it came to childbirth. So why The Farm?

That answer begins with the birth of my first son, Christopher. I had just completed working for teacher certification. My plan was to get a job teaching that fall, but before that could happen, I realized I was pregnant. Here I was, fresh out of school with a lot of science courses under my belt, and I felt I didn't know *anything* about childbirth. Yes, I knew the mechanics, how the body responded, what happened, but I was totally ignorant as to how hospitals and medical professionals responded to childbirth. Learning something about what options I had started me on my search for alternatives.

My first visit with a highly recommended obstetrician in town was pretty unpleasant. The first thing I was told was the temperature in the delivery room could not be adjusted, although the lights could. When I asked to not have an episiotomy, he skirted the issue entirely by asking me what kind of episiotomy I meant, never once saying whether he would or would not give me one. This bothered me, but I knew this was about as magnanimous as he was going to get, so I let it slide. For the time being, I was getting good prenatal care. I could change later. However, as time went on, I was less and less sure of this doctor. In fact, I grew to distrust him. All along, there were little hints that he and I were in different head spaces. The biggest came during the sixth month of pregnancy, when I was sent a certified letter that made no sense whatsoever, unless one read it *do it my way or else*. Finally, in the seventh month, the doctor said there could be no Leboyer birth,* after leading

---

*The Leboyer method of birth, described by Dr. Frederick Leboyer in *Birth Without Violence*, calls for dim lights, soft voices, and the placement of the newborn baby in a body-temperature bath.

me to believe all these months there would be. It was at that point that I knew I didn't want this man touching me—and internal exams were to begin in two weeks. I knew I had to find someone else.

A nurse who practiced as an underground midwife suggested a doctor from a nearby town who would provide more considerate care. Under his care I was able to have a Leboyer birth experience, but the hospital gowns and masks meant to create a more "sterile" environment were just that—sterile, cold, and intimidating. Also I had to labor on my back because of the monitor and ended up with a big episiotomy and forceps delivery.

One of the pregnant women, who became my friend after the birth of my son, used an original copy of *Spiritual Midwifery* as her bible, and even tore out pictures and pages and pasted them on her wall. Her daughter's birth, which took place at home, had a profound effect on me. In the back of my mind I thought that, perhaps someday, I would have a child whose passage into this world would be really loving and spiritual.

My second pregnancy was hardly noticeable. It seemed that the baby sort of slipped in and was no problem. The only indications of my pregnancy were that I missed my March and April periods and my clothes were a little tight around my waist. I wasted no time in finding the most "lenient" obstetrician in town. I had no problems with him and found he was very honest with me. He flatly told me he insisted on an I.V. and that the hospital required an internal fetal monitor, although I could sign a legal waiver and not have the monitor. I had resigned myself to this type of birth if necessary but decided to investigate further. I finally obtained a copy of *Spiritual Midwifery* from a health-food store in Nashville, where I grew up. Several weeks later I wrote to The Farm, and Deborah Flowers responded.

I immediately felt as if a deep-seated prayer had been answered and prayed that if The Farm was right for me I'd end up there. When I told Ron about hearing from The Farm, I think he was worried. After all, I had seemed so content this time and the hospital was only ten minutes away. Why did I want to go up to The Farm, which was about seventy miles away?

Ron and I had a continuing dialogue about childbirth at The Farm. Finally, we both decided to go visit with an open mind (although I must admit I wasn't quite as open-minded as Ron; I simply knew I wanted to be at The Farm). When we arrived, we met Deborah Flowers and Pamela Hunt, who showed us the facilities and checked me. Deborah said I was one centimeter dilated and loose, which I attribute to her absolute gentleness and the strong rapport I felt with her.

Ron was impressed that the birth cottage had hospital equipment to stabilize an infant in an emergency. He was also impressed with the fact that the midwives were emergency medical technicians and very qualified in their work. He decided to go along with a birthing at The Farm if our insurance would cover it. We found out in a few days that it would.

Because Deborah was my main midwife, I would bare my soul to her. I just knew things would go well. The Farm had it all: "in tune" midwives, a birthing house, a clinic with a holistic outlook, and doctor/hospital backup if necessary. I also liked subtle nuances such as helping the baby's head stretch the mother out without tearing, not relying on cold machines such as ultrasound and internal fetal monitors, knowing how to deliver breech babies, and having faith in the universe.

When I went into labor back in Huntsville, I didn't believe it at first and continued my project of cleaning all the carpets in the house. Intermittently, I rested on the bed to reduce the contractions until 4:00 P.M., when I realized I could no longer clean rugs. I waited a while to make sure of what I was feeling, then at 5:00 I called Ron to come home. He showed up, took things to the car, and we took off down the road after calling the midwives.

Contractions were steady and strong. Ron clocked them at seven minutes apart. Because I sat as still as possible, they remained unchanged. My back hurt with each contraction, which surprised me. Our drive was a little over two hours, and I was grateful for almost no traffic. Once at The Farm, Ron called Deborah, who came to let us in. I crawled onto the bed, where Deborah checked me. Ron brought things in while Deborah helped me through my labor. Chris had fallen asleep on a nearby fold-down chair. Ron sat down on the bed to help me with my back, which really hurt. Deborah grabbed my thigh while Ron pushed my back. It helped, and I told them so.

I could feel the baby moving down. I remembered Kim, this young woman giving birth on a video that Deborah had shown me. She had been really calm and didn't have a husband to rely on. What a chicken I was, groaning, "Oh, my back!"

Just at transition,* I wailed, "My back is killing me." Then, and it was truly a prayer, "Oh, God, help me." Just then I felt my whole bottom bulge. The midwives commented on how stretchy I was. I pushed, and they could see the head. I pushed again and out came the head. Such a relief. The rest of the body seemed like nothing. Ron got to cut the umbilical cord after it was clamped, and Chris awoke in time to see the cut. A few minutes later I was easily able to push the squishy blob (the placenta) out of me.

I had a beautiful baby boy, born around 11:50 P.M. with hardly any head molding. He wanted to relax before nursing. We looked him over, then gave him to Joanne to weigh and dress while Deborah and Pamela gave me two stitches for a small tear.

I was grateful to have had such an easy pregnancy and that the birth itself was not just a psychosocial event but spiritual as well. I was thankful to have such loving, caring midwives and such a loving, thoughtful husband. I knew that this was the right way to have a baby. I enjoyed how the midwives paid attention to every detail and looked at things intuitively as well as on the surface.

The next day I felt so good. I looked at the clear blue November sky and the brown oak leaves left on the trees and basked in the warmth of the sun. I realized that I was truly blessed, that there really were some things on which technology could not improve—one of those was the billion-year-old evolutionary process of human childbirth. To some it may have seemed primitive; to me it was perfect.

❧ Harley's Birth—October 19, 1995
By Celeste Kuklinski

Around five o'clock I started feeling unusual cramps. Not wanting to give a false alarm, I didn't say anything. I had my General Education Development (GED) class that night, and I didn't really feel like going. Playing "truant officer," Donna, my mentor and friend, drove me to class. Mary, the teacher, said I was probably just having those fake, practice cramps (Braxton-Hicks). I went home early, unable to concentrate.

The cramps were getting stronger, and I was feeling warm and ex-

---

*Transition refers to the time of full dilation just before the urge to push is felt by the mother.

cited. I still didn't want to call these cramps "contractions" in case it wasn't really happening. I timed them and they were about four minutes apart. Donna asked if I wanted to go see a midwife, but I decided to hold off until I was sure I wasn't getting excited over nothing.

Finally, in the middle of a *Star Trek* rerun, while my body was positioning itself in contorted ways all over the chair I was trying to sit in, I concluded that I had better see a midwife. Donna and I drove over to Pamela's. She checked me and informed me that I was three centimeters dilated and that I would probably give birth that same night. Surprised and happy, we went home to prepare.

Finally, the moment had come. Pamela soon arrived, followed by Ina May and Deborah. By this time, my ability to converse had deteriorated. I was just trying to deal with what was happening to my body. Things were happening quickly. I didn't try to hold any of the contractions back. I just let them come as fast as they wanted to, knowing that would help the birth happen without delay. It all felt very natural. I just "went with it." I went with taking a bath too, which was very helpful and relaxing. Ina May and my mother gave me support in the bathtub. Ina May showed me how to breathe deeply and slowly.

I tried it, and just then one of the strongest contractions yet overwhelmed me. I had to stand up. Some bloody, gray stuff dribbled and plopped into the bathwater. About this time, I started saying, "Oh, God!" I came out of the bathroom and did what I had to do, whether it was squat, bend over, walk around, say, "Oh, my God," or dance like a whooping crane. The contractions were getting very intense. I hardly had time between them to rest.

I remember looking at all the ladies there, who had done this quite a few times, and thinking they had been nuts!

I got on the bed and kind of writhed around. My mother said something about letting gravity do its thing; I could really feel it working. Watching the baby move downward in my belly, I tried to breathe effectively and let the birthing happen as best it could.

The time came when I felt the need to push. I instinctively massaged my gates of life to help them open. Then I felt the baby's head crowning, ready to come out. The contractions were so heavy, I just wanted them to be over with. So I gathered all my might and, with a big push and some loud primal grunts and yells, I finally oozed the baby's head out. Then, with another push, out slid the rest of the body. What a relief!

Even though I hadn't been able to say much other than, "Oh, my God," and "Oh, baby," I was about to utter, "Get the camera!"

When I look at Harley, my heart overflows with love. I'm taken by his pure presence, his innocence, his so adorably cute noises and expressions, and his wonderful, sweet sleeping face. Even though having him was painful, I wouldn't call it that; I'd call it INTENSELY NATURAL.

Pamela's labor with her first baby seemed endless to me (as well as to her, I'm sure). After I had been with her for twenty-four hours or so, I got the idea of calling in our mutual friend, Mary, who had given birth a few days earlier. Most of the women of our community were in awe of Mary's birth-giving abilities, since she had a history of having her babies either without knowing that she was in labor or before we midwives could get there.

❧ A Story of Sisterhood—February 13, 1972
By Mary Shelton

I had given birth to my second son a week or two before I got the call to see if I could assist Pamela with her rather difficult, long-lasting birth process. My son's birth had been smooth, energizing, and delightful, so Ina May thought maybe I could help Pamela.

On the afternoon before my son, Jon, was born, I was reading Ram Dass's book *Be Here Now* and feeling very centered and high with it. I remember I fastened on a particular word and meaning: *surrender*. I began having contractions and feeling big waves of energy moving. I visualized my yoni as a big, open cave beneath the surface of the ocean, with huge, surging currents sweeping in and out. As the wave of water rushed into my cave, my contraction would grow and swell and fill, reach a full peak, then ebb smoothly back out. I surrendered over and over to the great oceanic, engulfing waves. It was really delightful—very orgasmic and invigorating. Michael, my husband, was lying with me, and we experienced the wonderful rushing together for some time.

Finally, when it came time to call the midwives, the phone didn't work, so Michael delivered Jon himself. It all went very smoothly, and Michael and I were clear, focused, and very high.

When I went to Pamela's birth, I was still quite full of the invigorating energy from my son's birth. Pamela had been working very hard at dilating for hours, and she was tired and afraid. I sensed that she was frightened that she wasn't going to be able to pull off getting this baby out. I wanted to connect deeply with her and share my recent experience to help her relax and open. Pamela was naked, propped up on pillows on the bed, holding on to her knees. I took my clothes off (except for my underpants and pad since I was still bleeding from Jon's birth) and crawled up on the bed with her. I laid next to her—head to head, breast to breast, womb to womb. I told her about my cave and ocean and the great rushing, swelling, and opening. I told her about surrendering over and over and letting go. We began experiencing her contractions together. We held each other and rushed and soared together. My womb, though empty, was swelling and contracting too. I could feel blood rushing out with the contractions, but not too much—I knew it was okay.

As Pamela relaxed and shared her wondrous birthing energy with me, she began to open and dilate smoothly. Before long, she gave birth to a beautiful, serene little boy. What a glorious experience!

ꙮ Ramez's Birth Story—
May 30, 2003
By Njeri Emanuel

When I was pregnant, I thought I would probably want an epidural, because I heard that labor was going to be excruciatingly painful. They talked a lot about pain in my labor class. At first, I thought I might want a C-section, because then I wouldn't have to push, and I had heard that pushing was the hardest part. But when I thought about it more, I knew I didn't want a C-section, because it would take a long time to heal. (My mom used

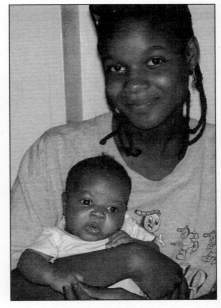

Njeri and Ramez

to go to births with The Farm midwives during the five years we lived on The Farm, so I knew a little about natural birth.)

When my labor actually started, I got into the shower for a while, but that didn't help my back labor as much as walking did. My midwife at the hospital kept asking if I wanted to lie back down in bed, but I said, "No, I like walking." My aunt Carolyn stayed with me and applied pressure to my back during contractions.

Pushing turned out to be the easiest part—a big relief. Someone held a mirror so I could see my progress while I was pushing. They told me to expect burning, but there wasn't any. I didn't have an episiotomy or a tear, and my mom says that my son, Ramez, was born with his eyes wide open. After he was born, I was more happy than tired. My total labor took eight hours. Ramez is six weeks old now, and he's good at breastfeeding. He has gained five pounds since his birth.

Brianna Joy's Birth—June 20, 1995
By Bernadette Bartelt

I was thirty-eight and pregnant with my first child. I was so excited. I had a fairly easy pregnancy, with no morning sickness or any other complication. I worked out regularly at Jazzercise, doing the low-impact

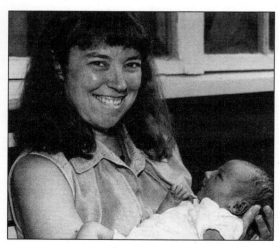
Brianna Joy

exercises recommended by my obstetrician. I planned to have my baby in Nashville, where I had been living for more than a decade. I had an ultrasound at four months but was scared to look at the pictures because of all the talk about the risk of being over thirty-five.

Late in my pregnancy, concerned that my doctor was so busy that my husband, Rick, and I didn't get much time with her, I decided to visit the midwives at The Farm in March. I had lived at The Farm when I was in my early twenties, having moved there with my father and siblings. The way the midwives checked me made me feel comfortable. Their clinic was not as modern as the doctor's office had been, but I sensed a friendlier feeling about the place. After doing some research and asking lots of questions, I decided that I wanted the midwives to attend my birth. I realized that if my labor lasted longer than twelve hours, my obstetrician was more likely to get scared of my being almost thirty-nine than the midwives were, and that increases the chance of a cesarean.

I was hoping that Ina May could attend my birth, but there was a problem with this plan. She had to speak at a midwifery conference and wouldn't be back until June 19. Carol checked me on June 12 and said I was dilated one centimeter. I went for a long walk the next day. My uterus contracted a lot throughout the next two days. On the night of the 15th, I had a hard time getting any sleep because of contractions that came every ten minutes. Carol came over to check me the next morning and said that my cervix was thinning and was open to three centimeters. She advised me to continue walking, so I did. I went to bed that night but had another hard time sleeping, because of contractions. This time they were much more intense. Rick and I walked down to the creek, where I sat with my feet in the water for a while. It felt so cool and relaxing. That night I had part of a wine cooler to help me sleep, but it didn't work. I paced the floor for part of the night. The next time Carol checked me, though, she gave me good news. I was open to five centimeters.

By the morning of June 18, Carol apparently thought that my labor needed a boost, because she came over with some castor oil. I was close to six centimeters open, but I could eat, sleep (short naps between contractions, that is), walk, and continue functioning. I went to a potluck meal at the house of one of the midwives. That night Carol stayed with me and helped me get through the contractions, since there was no way I could sleep at all. I tried a lot of positions. I sat on a birthing chair for a while. I knelt beside the bed and hung over a pillow. I pulled on a rope that was hanging from the ceiling. It was hard to stay relaxed. I tried to focus on my breathing instead of the incredible amount of back labor I was having. At this stage, I could really understand why women might resort to the use of some pain relief. I was about seven centimeters open. I appreciated the help I was getting from Carol, and that kept me from worrying about future pain. I should also add that I know a lot of women who have had home births, and I thought that if they could do it, so could I.

On June 19, the midwives encouraged me to eat some breakfast. I had some toast and jelly. I was a little nervous, but somehow I knew that I was in such good hands that everything was going to be all right. I ate some soup around noon, and Carol came back with some energy-replenishing drink to bring up my strength for the labor ahead of me. Rick went upstairs and slept for a while, because he hadn't gotten much sleep from trying to make me comfortable for the last few nights. Ina May called me from the airport and said she would see me in about two hours. She came right over and said she would stay until my baby was born.

She encouraged me right away to try to get some rest. I slept a little, and Rick rubbed my feet. I got nauseous and vomited, which made me feel a little better. I began having stronger contractions down lower and some burning pain. The next time someone checked me, I was eight centimeters open. I tried many other positions and took a shower. Ina May heard me making some sounds and helped me focus on slowing and deepening my breathing. That helped me relax, since I needed to focus on something besides my back labor. When she checked me again, I was at nine centimeters—big progress. Then I thought I needed to go to the bathroom, but I was starting to push the baby down. I moved from the toilet to the birthing stool, and very soon the head was crowning. I felt that I had to lean on someone, so Rick sat behind me. I kept concentrating on breathing slowly in between urges to push. The midwives were talking about how strong I was, because I wasn't complaining or fighting the feeling. Actually, I felt relieved to be pushing and *liked* this part of the labor. I hadn't thought I would, but now I remember this part as the most fun. It went the quickest, and I knew that I would soon see my baby.

Someone held up a mirror, and I could see the baby's hair. The head was scrunched up so it didn't really look like a head to me. The most intense part was when the baby's head came through. I felt a burning pain and was told not to hurry through this part. I pushed for about forty-five minutes. It was easier after the baby's head was out. Actually, her hand had come out with her head. The rest of her came out real quick and smooth.

She cried right away, and they immediately put her on my stomach. She was so beautiful. She weighed eight pounds thirteen ounces and was in perfect condition. I felt so much relief after the birthing was over. Deborah made some breakfast for me. It felt so good to eat again. Brianna Joy was the 1,937th baby born on The Farm. I was too excited and having too much fun to go to sleep for a while.

ஃ Abigail Rosalee's Birth—April 21, 2000
By Katie Hurgeton

My husband, George, was born in The Farm Birthing House almost twenty-three years before we found out that I was pregnant, and as an outspoken advocate of natural and home birth, he was adamant that our baby would be born in that same house. It didn't take too much arm-twisting to convince me that this was the best method of birth for my baby as well as for myself.

I expected my mother to be excited and pleased that we had decided on a home birth and would be taken care of by the most renowned midwives in the country. She was neither excited nor pleased. Instead, she and my father joined forces in telling me that I was endangering not only myself but their unborn grandchild as well. Every time I spoke with my mother, she had another birthing horror story that ended with "...and if she hadn't been at the hospital, she would have died." After she had exhausted those stories, she expounded on my choosing not to have an epidural.

"You're going to need one," she'd say and smile sweetly. George and I finally had to tell my parents that we knew what their opinion was, that we were going to do this our way, and that the topic was not open for further discussion. We also let them know that if they continued to attack or question our decision on this matter, we would simply have to stop coming over. They stopped bringing it up—with us. My mother proceeded to call my pediatrician, my physician, her best friend—who is a registered nurse at Vanderbilt Hospital in the labor and delivery ward—and my former obstetrician/gynecologist to check up on the midwives' credentials. She eventually came back and told me that all of these people had told her The Farm midwives were the most knowledgeable and experienced midwives to be had anywhere, that they knew what they were doing, and that my mother should RELAX!

This was still only the beginning.

At my next prenatal visit Ina May and Pamela went down a checklist, asking me if I had been exposed to any of these various diseases since I'd been pregnant. When they got to rubella, I stopped them. "The first month I was pregnant, I got a rubella vaccination that was required for me to be admitted to college." They froze and looked at me with half smiles of disbelief. Ina May said, "But they're supposed to make sure that you're not pregnant before they give you that shot."

"Well, they asked me," I explained, "but I was on birth control and my period hadn't been late yet so they gave me the shot." Neither of them said anything. I started to get nervous. "Maybe I'm wrong. I'll call my doctor tomorrow and find out."

"Yes," Ina May said, still half disbelieving, "do that and then call us."

I didn't ask any questions, but when George and I got home I looked up rubella in my copy of *What to Expect When You're Expecting* and cried for the rest of the night. The question in the book read something like, "Should I have an abortion if I've been exposed to rubella in my first three months of pregnancy?" And the answer began, "Not necessarily." The book also warned that rubella could cause congenital heart deformities. I was shocked and grief-stricken. When I called my doctor the next day, he informed me that the shot had merely been a booster and he didn't think it would have any adverse effect on the baby. An ultrasound at twenty-two weeks indicated that mine was still a low-risk pregnancy and could be handled at the Birthing House.

Our second trip to the hospital came quite unexpectedly. We were visiting the midwives for what would be one of the last times before the actual birth. They took my blood pressure, as usual, and began running down the list of standard questions.

"Any headaches?"

"Yes." It was really the first bad headache I'd had since I'd become pregnant.

"When?"

"This morning."

"Did you take anything for it?"

"Yes, some Tylenol. But it didn't do anything."

"I'm going to take your blood pressure again. It's high."

I didn't really think anything of it. The midwives left the room to talk. When they came back in, Ina May approached the table where I was still reclining and said, "We feel that you have enough of the signs that we would like for you to—" And here George and I were both holding our breath. We were positive that Ina May was about to tell us that they wanted me to go ahead and move into the Birthing House because they thought I'd be going into labor soon. Our joy at this thought was short-lived. "—go to the hospital to have some tests run. You are showing symptoms of pregnancy-induced hypertension." George and I both deflated. The hospital? Pregnancy-induced hypertension? After they had explained to us what PIH was and some of the risks associated with it, we drove, heavyhearted, to meet them at the hospital. If I had PIH, the midwives would not handle my birth on The Farm and I would have to have my baby in a hospital.

At the hospital I was given a room and a gown and was hooked up to heart and blood-pressure monitors. After about an hour of observation and my doctor's comment that "Maybe your high blood pressure is due to your being nervous about having your baby on The Farm" (my blood pressure was normal at the hospital), I was issued a clean bill of health. (Doctors call what I had "white coat hypertension.")

This little run-in, however, made my already nervous parents even more so. My mother provided me with a portable blood-pressure cuff so that I could intermittently monitor my blood pressure at home. It was a couple of days after my visit to the hospital that I got an alarmingly high blood-pressure reading. My husband was on a conference call at work, so I called my mother, who immediately suggested that I go to the hospital. Unfortunately, the hospital that my primary-care physician worked for was at least two hours from our apartment. And because my mother would've been enormously relieved if I had to have my baby at a hospital, I decided to call her friend, Anne, the Vanderbilt labor and delivery nurse who had been incredibly supportive of my decision from the start and had an amazingly calming effect on my mom. On this point, however, she agreed with my mother. She thought that I had enough symptoms and found my blood-pressure readings way too high. At my last hospital visit they had done no blood work. Anne was not happy about that and was insistent that I have blood work done. In order to do this, my primary-care physician would have to call in a referral. The doctor was none too happy to do that. After a rather frigid conversation in which she again stated that she thought my high blood pressure was due to being nervous about having my baby on The Farm and added that she was going to suggest to Ina May that I have my baby in a hospital because of that, she called in the requested referral to the doctor whom Anne had picked out for me. She promised to pick someone who would not be induction-happy.

My husband left work and we drove to Vanderbilt Hospital, where I was seen by a physician, admitted to the labor and delivery ward, and given a room. Again I was hooked up to the fetal heart monitor and blood-pressure machines. They took some blood and we waited for the test results.

We had both called our families and told them to be on alert in case the doctor decided to induce. When the results came back, I was not found to be hypertensive. We were sent home with the reassuring words that "the midwives can, by all means, deliver this baby safely." My parents didn't know whether to be relieved or more nervous still.

My water broke at 4:00 A.M. on the morning of April 21, the day of my grandfather's funeral. He had been my last living grandparent. We called Ina May and asked if we should leave immediately. She advised us to try and relax for a couple of hours and then to make our way down.

My first contraction came at 4:22 A.M. We left about two hours later on some advice from my mother, who'd told me, "Contractions are not fun. But contractions in a moving vehicle are even less fun." We grabbed our things from the apartment and took off. Other than the fact that throwing up in a car is harder to manage than in a bathroom, I don't remember there being that much difference in the feel of my contractions.

We arrived at the Birthing House a little after seven. It was a cold day but the midwives had come by hours earlier and turned the heat on, so inside the house was cozy and inviting. Ina May and Pamela arrived shortly after and checked my dilation. "It's a good thing you decided to go ahead and come," Ina May said. "You're already eight centimeters."

While I was in labor I tried to keep an eye on the clock so that I could remember how long everything took to happen and record it accurately later. However, other than the time of my first contraction and the time that Abigail was born, I don't recall much of the time frame. When I recorded the story in my journal later, I wrote that the contractions had lasted for about four hours and the pushing for about two. Ina May told me that some women like the contractions better and some the pushing. I liked the pushing best. It seemed to me the most clearly effective means to the end.

After approximately two hours of pushing and after having crowned for only one push, Abigail Rosalee was born. Her recorded birth time was 10:22 A.M., exactly six hours after my first contraction. She was taken by Ina May and Pamela, who cleaned her up, weighed her in at eight pounds thirteen ounces, and dressed her in her snuggest layette.

We called my parents from the Birthing House and they answered their cell phone right as they were stepping out of the car at the funeral home. They announced to all of the friends and relatives there that they were proud grandparents. (This was their first grandbaby.) They said that people kept coming up and shaking their hands, saying, "Congratulations!" and then immediately, "We're so sorry." My mother said that for her it was a powerful reminder of the circle of life and death and that God is holding us all in His hands.

✺ Autumn Apple Windseed's Birth—November 11, 1970
By Kim Trainor

The birth of my first child in Manhattan was a standard-procedure hospital birth. I was first put in a room by myself, left to my own fears, and had my amniotic sac ruptured by an attendant. Then I was stuffed in a ward of screaming and yelling women in labor. Most of them did not speak any English. The attending physicians were all Chinese, and they spoke very little English or Spanish.

They proceeded to give me oxytocin to step up my labor. (Oxytocin—called Pitocin in the United States or Syntocin in the United Kingdom—is a powerful synthetic hormone given to women in order to start or to stimulate labor.) I was told to stay still. Because I sat up once, I was strapped on my back to the bed and scolded by the nurse on call, who said, "Stop trying to squat!"

A fluorescent light was set up to glare on me so the attendants could see when they came in. Because there was an air of assembly-line birth in that hospital, they left the light on and then left me alone to labor, strapped to the bed. After what seemed like days (it was fifteen hours), I felt the baby's head between my legs. I called to the nurse that I thought I was ready to deliver. I was whisked off to the delivery room, had my feet put in stirrups and stockings, and given a standard-procedure episiotomy—twelve stitches. The baby literally shot out of me, screaming and red, and was taken away before I could see what gender baby I had. Then they knocked me out with ether to sew up the unnecessary episiotomy. When I awoke, I was told, finally, that I had a healthy girl, weighing eight pounds nine ounces.

I tried then to breastfeed her but was given only twenty minutes in which to do this. I was having difficulty, so I asked for some help. An irate nurse reluctantly tried to show me how to breastfeed. She squeezed my breasts roughly and declared that I wasn't the kind of woman who could breastfeed. When they took my baby down the hall to the neonatal nursery after this unsuccessful attempt, I ran after my crying babe. I caught up with the nurse and grabbed my daughter in order to comfort her. At this point, I was hauled off by a couple of ward attendants. They took me away from my baby, brought me to my room, and gave me a powerful sedative that kept me awake but unable to move. This was an incredibly traumatic experience. I came away from birth bruised and battered, drugged and ripped off of my nurturing instincts and sense of confidence. After such a trauma, I knew I would never again give birth under such inhumane conditions.

Lily Rose Heart's Birth—November 20, 1976
By Kim Trainor

It was six years later before I was to give birth again. I knew I would definitely have a home birth with a midwife, but I didn't know how to go about it. A friend of mine told me about The Farm and its offer to women who didn't want an abortion but who had no support. I knew I wanted to have this child. The father wasn't there for us, so I felt I should at least have my baby in a place that encouraged natural birth.

I arrived four months before the birth of the baby and lived in an old Army tent with a wood frame, a sort of combination house and tent. I was integrated into living in the Tennessee woods, with many other birth parents and extended families. We were a community of about four hundred when I arrived in 1973. I was always employed in some form of community service, and my five-year-old daughter was involved in the community with the kid group and got to take care of horses and play in the woods and be cared for by other mothers when I was working. Along with about four other mothers, I took care of a group of kids when I wasn't working at something else.

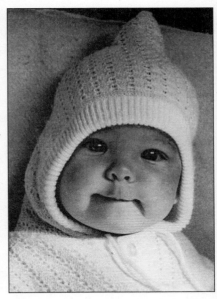

Lily

When I was ready to give birth, I was already familiar with the women who would be my midwives. I felt whole and healthy on the completely vegetarian diet of The Farm. My daughter, my unborn baby, and I were indeed thriving.

When my water broke, I called Leslie, one of the midwives on call, to let her know that I was about to start my labor. She hurried over to check my dilation. It all felt relaxed and loving. My daughter wandered in and out of the room for a while, but she had one of the women to look after her while I was in labor. The birth rushes were strong and steady. I was surrounded by five wonderful women, who all had had their babies at home and knew what I was feeling. They encouraged, rubbed, joked with me, and kissed me. I felt like I was a precious person giving birth to a precious baby.

When I was in transition, I gasped and thought I could not go on. At this point, the woman behind me said, "What you need is this," and gave me a kiss. That made me laugh. Then I began pushing, which I thought was a great sensation. It felt so good. I moaned very deeply, almost sounding like a cow. It began to get dark and cold, so we lit the kerosene lamp and stoked the fire in the woodstove.

The ecstasy of birth was so wonderful. My daughter slipped out, a long and graceful baby—all nine pounds ten ounces of her, without a tear. We all laughed. Such a feeling of elation. The midwives put Lily on my chest, and we all admired and adored her. I thanked the midwives and they thanked me for being so easy to help in birth.

I bonded naturally with my baby. She nursed easily and happily, and I felt strong and powerful. I thought, if I could do this, I could do anything. This community of hardworking and honest people showed me how to be who I really was. I decided to stay and live with them and have them be my tribe and family.

Otis Francisco's Birth—July 2, 1980
By Kim Trainor

The summer Mount St. Helens blew up was one of the hottest I can remember, and I was beginning to feel my baby wanting to be born. I started to rush steadily at five in the morning. The sun was just coming up, but the heat was already strong. I had slept downstairs the night before because it was so hot and I was restless. I got up and started to prepare for a long, hot birthing.

A few hours later the rest of the household was up, and I told everyone that I was going to have a baby soon. The midwives came by to check on me and found that my cervix was about five centimeters dilated. My water did not break as it had in my other two labors. The midwives suggested that I take a hike in the woods with my husband, so that gravity would help to open me up more. We walked for about an hour or two, and I felt in a timeless sort of space in which every sound, scent, and color was illuminated and heightened. I could feel my baby move me open, and when the intensity of the rushes increased, I just leaned on a tree. The rushes grew more intense and came more often. I decided to head back up the hill to my bed.

When we got back, I was almost eight centimeters dilated, but the water bag was still intact. I paced back and forth beside my bed for a while. When my water bag broke near full dilation, incredible amounts of water poured out of me. That's when I felt the baby's head press directly against my cervix, and I immediately felt the urge to push.

It felt so good to push. The baby's head soon crowned and was born. Ina May told me to stop pushing and she swiftly removed the umbilical cord, which was around the baby's neck three times—*bloop! bloop! bloop*! Out came the rest of him, all dark purple, almost black-looking. It was amazing. Otis had the longest umbilical cord the midwives had seen. It was about four feet long and had a knot in it. Otis was so happy to be out. The midwives placed him on my chest immediately. He was born hungry and weighed ten pounds two ounces.

Not long after the birth, I decided to walk downstairs. It was very hot, and the sky was dark purple, like my son had been at first. I remember the way the wind blew up the stairwell as I walked down with my beautiful son. Then the thunder and lightning began, and it started to pour rain, making everything cool and comfortable. I was grateful to have my baby among friends and family. He was welcomed and adored by the rest of the household.

✤ The Joy of Delivering Grace—April 30, 2000
By Kathryn B. Van de Castle

You might think that I would be an unlikely candidate for a birth at a rural Tennessee birth center. I am a typical upper middle-class American female who doesn't like to experience pain. I grew up knowing that my mother had an extremely difficult time birthing me. I get light-headed when I hear words like *phlebotomy*. Now add to this that I married Keith (who is a doctor) at the age of thirty-seven after an eight-month-long courtship, and we conceived our child two weeks later. Obviously, we were still getting to know each other throughout our pregnancy. Keith

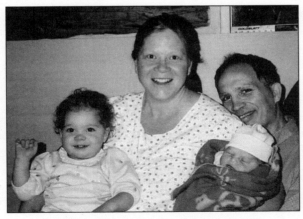

Grace, her baby sister Faith, Kathryn and Keith, her parents

was an incredibly wonderful partner throughout a pregnancy that was sometimes difficult because of prolonged nausea and a death in the family. He shopped for foods that appealed to me when I was so nauseous that I could not even enter a grocery store, helped me with diet when my Virginia doctor decided I had gestational diabetes, and kept my spirits up.

My sister, who is an ob/gyn nurse, gave me some good advice. "Don't read a bunch of books," she said. "And don't write a birth plan. The more you write down exactly how you want it to be, the less likely it is that you will get it that way." She explained that too much reading could interfere with the ability to flow with what your body is telling you. I was convinced and never picked up a birth-preparation book.

As for choice of birthplace, I knew instinctively that the bustle and routines of a hospital would be hard for me to deal with. I could see myself shutting down with the constant comings and goings of the hospital staff. And although Keith is a doctor, he has an unusual familiarity with home birth, since he lived for fifteen years on The Farm before going to medical school. He trusted The Farm midwives, and I trusted him.

We traveled to The Farm a month before I gave birth. That gave me the opportunity to relax, walk for hours each day, and eat well. As we walked I would talk to Grace and ask her to help me in the birth process and promised her I would deliver her safely. She obliged me by positioning herself head-down three months before birth. My contractions started about four-thirty in the morning eleven days before my estimated due date. I decided not to wake Keith, as they were still ten minutes apart. He woke later, and we watched a movie and took a walk before going to our midwife's house for lunch. Once there, I took one bite of potpie and threw up. My contractions got stronger.

Ina May tried to help me relax by massaging my thighs, but I needed something more. Keith reminded me that I had planned to relax in a tub. When I stepped into the warm tub I was dilated one centimeter, and when I emerged seven hours later I was fully dilated. Throughout that time, I asked for reassurance many times, because I felt scared to feel so much power in my body.

Keith told me a thousand times that I was okay and helped me breathe so that the contractions were bearable. My friend Cynthia had told me a few days earlier that she felt labor was like surfing. I kept thinking of that during the hours in the bathtub. Keith helped me over and over again to get on top of the wave. As he helped me breathe slowly and deeply, I kept focusing on the drawing of a purple flower on the wall above his head. I began repeating to myself, "I am a flower opening up." With all this help, I was able to remain strong. I did not let the contractions overwhelm me.

Ina May, Pamela, and Pamela's daughter Stephanie helped reassure me throughout labor that I was okay and let me know what to expect next. I became aware that I had a choice to think about negative things or the joys of my life. I learned to discipline myself to come back to the present and breathe with Keith and affirm that I was okay and listen to the others saying that I was doing a great job.

The cycle of my labor followed this pattern: Keith would notice a contraction coming and he would start slow, deep breathing, and I would keep that pace with him. I would peer at the flower above his head and either go to positive or negative thoughts and listen to people saying I was all right or would repeat that to myself. Between contractions, I would rest and relax. Then the cycle would begin again.

I noticed that when I tried to look at things, it put me more in a thinking mode, but when I was listening, I was more in a feeling/instinctive mode. For instance, hearing that I was all right really made me feel better. If it had been written down and I was reading it, it would not have made me feel as good. Thinking was scary. Feeling wasn't. When I was in feeling mode, things didn't seem so overwhelming.

When I was fully dilated, Keith helped me walk to the bed. These were the longest ten steps of my life. I was dearly hoping I would not have a contraction in the middle of the hall. I sat on the bed for a few moments but felt uncomfortable there and didn't know how to relieve that feeling. Keith reminded me that I had been interested in trying a birth stool. The midwives brought it over; I sat on it and began pushing with all my might.

Pushing was absolutely exhilarating. I loved it. I began making incredibly deep, loud cries that helped me move Grace down. I was ecstatic as I pushed Grace out.

Through the process of natural childbirth, I gained a lot of confidence in myself. I left my comfort zone and the culture I had grown up with. I learned that I can work through scary and painful situations and be strong and present when I need to be. My fear of not knowing how to be a good mother has disappeared as my confidence in my intuition of how to love Grace has increased. I have felt incredible energy and life force through my body, and I have really been reborn a happier, healthier, and more confident person. I have learned I can choose to focus on the darker side or the lighter side of all that is around me. I choose the lighter side and have the discipline to keep it up.

❧ Shannah's Birth—May 22, 1985
By Mary Ann Curran

The major catalyst in deciding to leave our obstetricians was our Bradley natural-childbirth classes,* which we began taking during the last half of my pregnancy. It was through these classes that we learned of some dangerous practices that are standard procedures at the hospital we were going to use: routine electronic fetal monitoring and intravenous lines delivering Pitocin to intensify labor. The Bradley classes really opened our eyes and also made me realize how many important things I was compromising by doing things the way the doctors wanted. My original hopes for a birth with midwives in a regular bed began to sound better and better. Then we tried to change our hospital-admittance consent form, on the advice of our Bradley instructor. Little did we know what a fracas that would cause!

It wasn't until the next day that I was ready to break ties with the medical world. I had a visit with one of my obstetricians, who had heard from the hospital about our trying to change the consent form. I think it's safe to say he was outraged. His internal exam was noticeably rougher, and he spent forty-five minutes afterward lecturing me about the doctor–patient trust relationship. On the verge of tears, I tried repeatedly to explain our feelings to him, but I don't think I got through. By the time I got home, I knew that if I were to go into labor that night, to The Farm I would go!

In spite of all this, my husband, Jim, and I thought it safe to retain our obstetricians "in case of emergency." But at the next and last visit to the obstetrician, the doctor started talking about a cesarean section because I was "overdue." How could I be overdue when the visit fell on

---

*The Bradley method of natural childbirth stems from the work of Dr. Robert Bradley, an early follower of Grantly Dick-Read's method. Bradley, influenced by his wife's reading of Dick-Read's book *Childbirth Without Fear* while he was in his obstetrical training, wrote *Husband-Coached Childbirth*. His work is carried on by Marjie and Jay Hathaway, who founded the American Academy of Husband-Coached Childbirth (P.O. Box 5224, Sherman Oaks, CA 91413).

the date my obstetrician had estimated that I would be due? This got us pretty upset, and after calling a cesarean prevention hotline, we decided to break ties completely. We had my medical records transferred to The Farm Midwifery Center and never looked back.

We left Alabama for The Farm the night I began having labor. It was pouring rain when we arrived, and it rained all night. Joanne and Deborah, my midwives, told me to try and get some sleep to have strength for the birth. I tried to sleep, but the contractions made it very difficult. They were two minutes apart, and I was trying too hard to relax, making them worse. I finally realized what I was doing and that I could sleep between contractions, although at first sleep in two-minute intervals didn't seem very restful. I did the breathing and relaxation exercises we learned from our Bradley lessons. They helped, but there was still pain, which I wasn't expecting. I thought that doing the exercises and breathing would eliminate or keep pain to a minimum, but it doesn't work that way for everyone.

Through my off-and-on semiconsciousness, I watched morning come, and Jim and my midwives woke and were getting ready. Joanne had checked my dilation a couple of times during the night and checked me again first thing in the morning. I was a little discouraged, having stayed at four centimeters since 10:00 P.M. At 10:00 A.M., Joanne checked me and said I was five centimeters. Not long after that, I was nearly fully dilated, and Joanne broke the water bag.

Very soon after that, my contractions became much stronger. The stage I was entering is called transition, and if you've ever been through it, you'll understand why. I felt as if I was in another world, totally out of touch with the regular everyday world. The world I was in was called Labor, and my only purpose in life was Birth. It was a time of intense concentration, and I felt pretty shaky. Jim and my midwives were all there to support me, yet I was afraid to look into their eyes. I was afraid they would have worried looks! Finally, I looked into Jim's eyes and saw that he didn't look at all worried, just very calm. I didn't have the concentration to turn around and look at my midwives—the contractions were too frequent and intense—but I could feel Joanne squeezing my foot at the peak of each contraction, letting me know that she was going through it with me. Meanwhile, my uterus and baby were working intently, bringing on the birth. My sign that a contraction was beginning was feeling Shannah's feet pushing up toward the top of my uterus, her head turning back and forth at the cervix, the uterine muscles closing step by step—like a hand closing into a fist—and climaxing at the clench point. Then, in the same graduated process, the contraction would undo itself.

Finally, Joanne checked my dilation and, to my great relief, I was fully dilated. "You came through transition beautifully," Joanne told me.

"Oh, was that transition?" I asked. That's how much in another world I was.

So there I was, half-reclining on Jim's chest and really geared up to push away. This is the good part, I was thinking. And it surely was. Pushing was HARD work. Don't get me wrong: It was so rewarding and fulfilling, I can't explain it. It seemed like slow going until the head crowned, and I had to concentrate so hard, I couldn't even look up at the mirror Deborah was holding. After the crowning, a little more s-t-r-e-t-c-h-i-n-g and pushing, Shannah's head was born.

After Shannah's head was born, the rest of her came out in one push, and there she was in all her glory! Of course, we got to hold her immediately.

I felt accomplishment, wonder, thrill, and relief.

Barbara's Reflections
By Barbara Wolcott

I guess the most important thing I figured out was that your attitude and how you approach your birth is of the upmost importance. In other words, it is important to face each birth like a bull, with full force, no fear or hesitation, with the attitude that you can do this and you aren't going to hold back. This is your opportunity to remember your power as a woman, inhibitions not allowed. Those contractions are power surges, and each one gets that baby closer to birth. Your baby feels your strength and also your fears. The midwives helped me so much with this and kept reminding me of my strength.

I attended Sara Jean's birth in 1971. A Farm resident during her early years, Sara Jean grew up in a culture in which women expected to have unmedicated births in their own homes, attended by midwives they knew well. When she became pregnant for the first time, she lived in another state, where her insurance coverage would not allow for a home birth. She chose midwifery care in a hospital.

⚘ Sara Jean's Story—December 5, 1999
By Sara Jean Schweitzer

I was due in three days and felt impatient. Gerrie Sue, a former Farm midwife and close family friend, agreed to be at my birth to support me. She told me that it was important to try to have this baby a little early rather than late. Because I'm small, she didn't want me to have a big baby. I tried all sorts of methods to help trigger labor. Every day I hiked in the hills, asked my husband, Richard, to make love to me and nurse my nipples. I even tried having the pressure points on my feet massaged. I didn't want fear to prevent the baby from coming, so I tried not to dwell on thinking about the birth experience. I thought, If I have to jump off a cliff, why think about how I'm going to do it? Just jump.

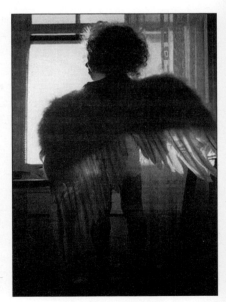

Luca with angel wings

Staying active was important to me and seemed to help. The day before Luca was born, I went on a hike in the hills with friends. I walked ahead of them all the way, thinking that if I moved strong and fast, the baby might be shaken up from his serene little world and come out.

When we got home, my sister was upstairs in my mother's apartment, crying over a personal issue. I went to console her, but it made me feel like I was putting my baby and everything I needed to do to get him out on hold. I knew my baby could arrive any hour, but I really needed to talk to my sister. I felt her pain as if it were my own. Throughout my pregnancy, all the emotions/vibes that I was exposed to felt as if they were being fed directly into my baby. That night I stayed up until about 2:00 A.M. talking with my sister, the whole time feeling anxious about the baby.

When I finally fell asleep, I dreamed I was having period cramps. By morning the cramps woke me up. I called my mother, who told me to call Gerrie Sue. I didn't want to wake her up, so I waited about forty-five minutes while Richard and I monitored my cramps. I told her that the cramps persisted and were getting stronger and closer together. She thought I was in labor and that I needed to call my midwife. My midwife told me to go about my day as usual and to maybe take a walk. She said that I might have the baby in about a day to a week. When I told Gerrie Sue what my midwife had told me, she said, "I really think you're going to have the baby today, so I'll be there soon." She also pointed out that Farm women seem to go into labor quickly. While I was in the shower, my mucus plug came out of my vagina. Richard was on the computer, keeping track of my contractions as I moaned them out to him.

My mother came down to my apartment with eager friends and family. As soon as she looked me in the eyes, she knew I was seriously in labor because of my tears and the intense look on my face. As soon as Gerrie Sue arrived, she gave me a pelvic exam. She found me dilated enough to say, "We have to get her to the hospital now and call her midwife."

Everyone scurried around, gathering everything and loading up cars. Richard and I rode in Gerrie Sue's car, with me sitting on a plastic bag in case my water broke. The ride to the hospital was an exciting one. My heart was beating fast and I was thinking about how we were about to have a totally new life with our little baby in just a few hours. I was having very strong contractions, which were intensified by the car ride.

We arrived at the hospital around 12:00 P.M. I signed some papers and went straight to a birthing room. An I.V. was hooked up to my wrist and I was given a hospital gown to wear. More information was collected. I felt that I could barely deal with more questions and red tape.

Gerrie Sue told me to make deep low-pitched moans with my contractions to stay calm. This really helped. She also suggested that I take a warm shower to relax my muscles. I stayed in the shower for at least two hours, while Richard massaged my back; it felt so nice. When I got out, I vomited what seemed like gallons of juice. (My midwife had recommended that I stock up on juices for energy during labor. I didn't feel like eating at all, so with slightly lowered blood sugar, I really needed the nourishment.) I was told that vomiting was a sign that the baby was about to come and that pushing would begin soon.

I lay down on the delivery bed so my midwife could check my dilation. Six centimeters, more than half open. Later on she broke my bag of water, I contracted some more, and was told I could start pushing. Still later I had a real strong urge to push, which felt like I was going to have the biggest bowel movement ever. In retrospect, I think I should have started to push at *that* point, rather than earlier, to avoid wasting my limited energy. I pushed again and again for maybe forty-five minutes without progress. I moved into several different positions, including squatting on the floor, dangling from a bar above the delivery bed, and standing up while leaning against the bed, and still no progress. I started to get really tired, thirsty, and hot, so I was given ice to chew on and a cold cloth for my head. I thought things could drag on and on this way.

I pushed for another twenty minutes or so. The nurse put a fetal monitor on me. We heard the baby's heart rate drop slower and slower every time I pushed. My heart sank. My midwife told me that his cord was probably being compressed by his head squeezing through my small frame. I knew this was serious and that if I panicked I would waste precious energy, making the situation worse. I realized then that I alone couldn't push my baby out and that my energy was fading. All I focused on was strength and the life of my baby. I asked if there was a way I could get an energy boost, and the nurse put in the sugar-water I.V. My midwife quickly called in a doctor. The baby's head was showing, but I didn't have the oomph to push him out on my own.

The doctor came in and immediately put me on oxygen. He demanded action from just about everyone in the room and told me to do absolutely everything as he instructed. Of course, I more than agreed. The energy felt intense and rushed. My mother was crying in the corner, and the room quickly filled up with additional hospital staff and interns. Richard sat behind me for support, as I leaned back with my legs apart and pulled my knees up toward me. There was a very hot bright light shining on me. The doctor tried pulling the baby out with a vacuum extractor, which looked like a toilet plunger. I gave my strongest push—he pulled with all his might and still the baby didn't budge. We tried again and again—still nothing. His heart rate was frighteningly slow now—it seemed as if there was only a slow beat every few seconds. There was a feeling of panic in the room. I felt as if I had to reverse that feeling for my baby's life, so I concentrated on staying calm, positive, and focused. I blocked out everyone in the room and only heard what the doctor was telling me to do.

He decided that an episiotomy would speed the birth. I was given a local anesthetic and sliced so fast that I didn't even know it had happened! The doctor told me to give a final extremely hard push. I pushed again so hard that I thought my eyes were going to pop out and my face explode. *Aaghh*, the baby finally came out!

It was 5:14 P.M. The doctor practically threw the baby to the nurse, saying, "He's your baby," and then quickly continued to work with me, telling me to push again for the placenta. The birth took about eight hours from my first contraction. The baby's vital signs were checked and all good. He weighed eight pounds two ounces! No wonder it was such a struggle to have him. I bathed and had my hair brushed. I wished that I could have seen my baby the way he looked immediately after birth—before he was cleaned up.

After the placenta came out, the doctor told me not to touch anything near or below my belly while he carefully stitched many deep layers of muscle and skin. That took about an hour. I looked over at my baby on the table nearby, but I could barely see him because my eyes were so swollen and blurred from pushing. I asked Richard to go look at him and tell me what he looked like. He was absolutely perfect, healthy and beautiful even through blurred eyes.

He had platinum blond curls all over his head, with a pinkish-orange color to his skin. I immediately fell in love with him. He seemed so familiar. I couldn't wait to touch him, but I felt like I had been hit by a truck on a foggy night and had just barely made it alive. I was also bound to the table as I was being stitched. My mother started escorting a few people from the crowd in the waiting room to see our baby. I didn't want everyone to come in, because I was overwhelmed, my legs were still spread, and I was sure I looked like hell. I was anxious for the medical procedures to end so I could hang out with my new family, but they dragged on. After I was stitched up, I got to hold our sweet little baby and nurse him. He latched right on to my breast. It felt like such a natural way to love and nurture him.

Later, I tried to urinate and couldn't. My insides were in shock, and I was bloated from juice, so I had to be catheterized. I was given some strong painkillers and then wheeled to our recovery room, where we could sleep with our baby. I thought I could finally spend some time with our baby now, but his body temperature was slightly low, so he was taken away and put under a heat lamp for about an hour. Richard followed to make sure he was in good hands, which he was. When they returned him to me, I nursed him again and told him how proud I was of his bravery and strength during the birth. I let him know that I was so happy he had made it through our journey.

That night in our room I realized what an amazing gift our new baby was, but I also felt sadness and a sense of loss within myself. I knew this was the beginning of his new life and the end of my selfishness and the part of me that was holding on to still being a child myself. My life was no longer my own. This was still the happiest and most spiritual day of my life. I felt so grateful to have Luca.

In my early days as a midwife, I felt free to change some of the language surrounding birth as a way to help women cope with labor pain. I have a master's degree in English and was aware of how language can condition our response to a physical/emotional/spiritual process such as labor. I began to use the word rush *instead of* contraction. *Why use a word that suggests tightness and hard muscles when successful labor will require expansion of the cervix, I thought. Many of the women at The Farm adopted this change in language. Rosey's mother, Janet, gave birth to her on The Farm in 1974, and I was her midwife.*

✷ Rosey's Story—September 20, 1994
by Rosemary Larson

I had an arrangement to have my baby with midwives on the California coast, which is about an hour and a half away from my home. There were not many choices of midwives in my area. There was one nurse–midwife, but she attended hospital-only births. There were rumors of home-birth midwives, but they couldn't take insurance and they were hard to locate. I was intent on having my baby at home, if at all possible. I had read and heard too many horror stories of hospital births, and I felt much more confident having my baby at home. I was a home-birth baby myself, born at The Farm, and my two sisters were also born at home.

My pregnancy was normal, although there were some worries about my blood pressure rising too high. I wasn't worried, and I knew the baby was coming sooner than my due date. I had a couple of false starts, which left me about three centimeters dilated and fully prepared for my trip to the coast. (This happened just before I reached thirty-six weeks' gestation.) I was slightly worried about the drive over. The road is long and winding. The plan was to have the baby in a cabin that was available to women who lived too far away to have the midwives come to their home.

At thirty-seven weeks, on the night of the full moon, I woke at about 3:00 A.M. and had to pee. I remember being disappointed that I hadn't felt any contractions. I had been sure this would be the night. As I was peeing, I heard a popping sound and felt a big gush of warm liquid. I stood up to see if it was my waters breaking or if it was my imagination. Sure enough, water dripped down my legs. The moon was still high and bright in the sky. I ran into my bedroom and excitedly told my husband, Aaron, that my waters had broken. He sleepily said, "They did?" I was laughing and getting a towel for myself. We called Suzan, one of my midwives. She told me to go back to bed until my contractions started and became strong and regular. Go back to bed? I thought, how crazy! But I did lie down and soon after I felt my first contraction. It felt much more intense than the previous Braxton-Hicks contractions I'd felt before. Amazingly, I was able to sleep for a while. When I wasn't sleeping I was very relaxed. Looking back now, I realize that I didn't think about anything "extra" the whole time. I didn't think about how the birth would be, or about the fact that I would soon have a newborn in my arms. I knew it, but I didn't think about it then.

I called my mother, Janet, around 6:30 A.M. to tell her I was in labor and to arrange for her to pick us up. She really wanted to be there for the birth, her car was smoother and bigger, and she'd offered to drive to the coast. I thought it would make her day, her life, if I invited her to be there. I was a little worried about my husband being totally comfortable sharing the birth with my mother, but as it turned out, things went wonderfully between them. My contractions were getting stronger and stronger, but I was handling them fine by myself and was able to prepare for the trip. I had a mug of raspberry-leaf tea and I ate a banana and my prenatal vitamins. I wasn't hungry. I just thought it would be good to fortify my body for the work ahead. The drive over was better than usual, even though the contractions were steadily becoming more intense. I had a towel between my legs, because amniotic fluid would gush every little while. As my husband and mother continued ordinary conversation in the front of the car, I was feeling slightly neglected in the back as I concentrated on my contractions. My mom, perhaps sensing my isolation, asked if I was even having any contractions because she thought I wasn't acting like I was in labor. I assured her, emphatically, that I was. After that I decided not to feel sorry for myself or weird at all, because this was going to be a fun experience if I let it be.

We had left around 8:00 A.M., and it was close to 10:00 as we neared the cabin. My contractions really picked up as we drove the last five miles parallel to the ocean. They were coming every two or three minutes apart. I let everyone know this and they could tell by my behavior that I was serious. As soon as we got to the cabin, my mother raced to the phone and told the midwives she thought I was close. Suzan was surprised to hear all this because she hadn't heard anything since 3:00 A.M. when my waters had broken. She arrived within ten minutes. When she checked me, I was seven centimeters open. Everyone was surprised except me. I still felt relaxed and clear. The contractions were strong enough that I began using Aaron to help me through them. I hung on his shoulders and leaned forward into his neck. I bounced lightly during the peaks and tried to keep my mouth relaxed. Suzan commented that I wasn't acting like I was seven centimeters dilated. She said that she was always really grumpy at this point. I didn't see any reason to be grumpy. In fact, the thought seemed ridiculous. Being grumpy would have ruined it.

Suzan was busy preparing things and calling for the other midwife and her assistant, Dawn. As a midwife, Suzan was very steady and dependable. She would check the baby's heartbeat and then back off and allow me to rely on my instincts to handle the labor. I found that the toilet was the most comfortable place to be. I was peeing a lot anyway. After a while, I felt like going back into the bedroom. I had been feeling really hot, then really cold, and nauseous. (All signs of transition, but at the time I didn't even notice.) I was completely inside my body. I didn't feel like a "me" at all. I wasn't looking around or checking out what other people were doing. I knew peripherally that my mom was taking pictures and Suzan was sterilizing her equipment. I moved to the bed. All of a sudden, I knew I was going to throw up. I quietly told Aaron, and they quickly got a pan. Just as Dawn, the assistant, arrived I threw up all over the bed. I laughed and told her that she had quite the sense of timing. There I was sitting on the bed with a big mess. I felt much better after throwing up.

The contractions got to a point of leaving me with no relief. The teeny space between each one, if there was any, was still so intensely intense that the thought occurred to me that I should try to push. I told Suzan, and she told Dawn to check me to see if I was fully dilated. Dawn reported that all she could feel was the baby's head—the cervix was all the way back. From talking to other women, I had the idea that the pushing part would be fairly easy and a relief from the intensity of the contractions. In fact, it was extremely hard work and the most intense part of the whole experience. I never physically felt like pushing, I just continued to have the thought in my mind that I should do it.

Everything around me was extraordinarily clear and sparkling. It was around noon, and the sun was beaming in through the window above the bed, all golden and holy. Everyone's energy in the room clicked and it felt very mellow. Everyone had a job to do. My mother was taking photographs and Dawn was warming up olive oil and hot washcloths. The warm washcloths proved to be one of the nicest things I've felt. They actually managed to feel *good*, even though I was at a point where it felt like nothing could bring me relief. Suzan continued to monitor the baby's heartbeat, which was fine. She also provided me with instructions on how to push and when, which were so in tune with what I was doing that I almost thought she could feel it. She was my rock, my stability, grounding me when my body was overwhelmed with contractions. Aaron was on the other side of Suzan, on the bed, comforting me, massaging me and supporting me when I squatted. That was funny because Suzan and Dawn suggested that I try squatting and I said, "No, that sounds too intense," and they said in unison with my mom, "That's what you want! You have to go into it." So I did. I squatted and pushed and then would lie back down when the contraction was over. They asked if I wanted to see the baby's head, and I couldn't believe that it was far enough down to see since I hadn't pushed very much. A hand mirror magically appeared, and I saw the purple-gray, squashed little quarter of my baby's head. The mirror helped me focus. I would look down as I squatted and pushed and would be so involved that the pain seemed far away. The midwives asked Aaron if he wanted to feel the head and when he did, he was totally amazed.

As the delivery approached, Dawn began to take charge, handling the washcloths and warm oil. She coached me through some particularly strong pushes and I yelled that it hurt. It was said in a factual way, not as a complaint. I just needed a release. Then I mentioned that it hurt right above and below my birth canal. They checked it out and saw that I was tearing in both places. But what was there to do but go on? I knew I had no choice but to keep pushing. It was hard. As the head was crowning, I was pretty tired. It was just so intense. I gave a final push, and the baby's head was out, all purple and squashed and facing my right thigh. Seeing his head brought a smile to my face. I really couldn't push anymore, so Dawn helped pull the baby out and placed him on my tummy. All the pain and force that I had been feeling a moment before was completely gone. I knew my baby as soon as I saw him. I checked to see if he was a boy or a girl; he was definitely a boy! He was crying pretty loudly, saying, "I'm here!" I told him he could stop crying by saying, "Hi, Baby," and talking to him. He was all pink and fat and healthy. He immediately made eye contact with me and consoled himself by sticking his fist in his mouth. I tried to pull him up to my breast, but Dawn stopped me because the umbilical cord wasn't long enough for him to reach that far. My placenta came quickly after the cord stopped pulsing, and Aaron cut it. I pulled the baby to my breast and he began nursing like he'd already done it before. Aaron curled up next to me and met our new child. I had torn enough for a few stitches but my attention was fully on our baby and I couldn't have cared less. It was a little after one o'clock in the afternoon.

After about an hour of hanging out with the baby we weighed him and discovered he was eight pounds exactly. A little while later, we had the most delicious meal of my life. All that work had left me with quite the appetite. I followed the meal with an unsteady shower, assisted by Aaron, as my mother held the baby. The midwives were pleased with how well things had gone and joked about how they didn't even have to stay out late.

❧ The Most Painful, Most Wonderful, Most Beautiful Experience: A Birth on The Farm—May 17, 1997
By Tracey Sobel

On Thursday I was in the garden all day and running around doing things. I didn't have the huge burst of energy that everyone talks about, but I had a little burst of energy. I had a feeling that the baby was coming the next day. (He didn't. I was in labor for forty-one hours.)

I didn't get to sleep Thursday night until about 2:00 A.M. Then I woke at 4:00 A.M. and went to the bathroom. There was blood. I didn't feel any contractions, although that might have been why I woke up. I woke Dan and told him we might be about to have this baby, but I decided not to call the midwives and to lie in bed a little longer. I wanted to wait for at least an hour, because during the last two weeks I had had a lot of "practice" labor that lasted for about an hour and then stopped. This time, the contractions kept coming every four to eight minutes and didn't stop.

About 6:00 A.M., I called Pamela. She said she would come right over. When she checked me, I was 2.5 centimeters dilated. "Yes, you're in labor," she said. She thought from the way my contractions were coming on that my labor was going to go quickly. She stayed for a while, set up her supplies and equipment, cleaned up a little, and made some food,

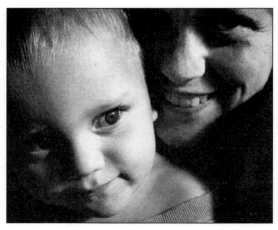

Tracey and Jed

but my labor didn't get any stronger. Pamela decided then to leave Dan and me alone, saying that we should call if there was any change. Hours and hours later, Pamela returned and checked me. I was only at three centimeters!

By this time I was really tired, so we lay down to take a nap. I would fall asleep for a couple of minutes, then wake up with every contraction. It hurt more when I was lying down than when I was sitting or standing. All I wanted was to sleep, and I kept waking up in pain.

Most of Friday passed. When the midwives came by again, I was still at three centimeters. It felt like the contractions were getting stronger, even though not much was happening. I got into the tub about 9:00 P.M. The bath eased the contractions a lot. When I came out an hour later, Dan's mom, Mary, was here. The plan was for her to catch the baby.

"Lie down and rest," the midwives said. I did fall asleep between contractions for a couple of minutes, but each time another came, I woke up. I remember asking whoever was with me, "How long was I sleeping?" It would feel like an hour, but they would say, "Four minutes."

Ina May came over to check me around 5:00 A.M. This time I had made some progress: 4.5 centimeters. The contractions kept getting stronger. At 6:00 A.M., I was at 6.5 centimeters. Ina May thought that things might move more quickly, so she called Dan's mother and Pamela. Everyone rushed over, and I spent the whole day in the bath. Ina May and Pamela took turns massaging me, which helped. Someone was always sitting with me, which was a good thing, because I slept between contractions while I was in the bathtub. I even ate in the water, because it felt so good to be there.

"Imagine a flower blooming," said Pamela, while I was in the bath. "As the flower blooms, the baby is being pushed out." I was reminded of the story of Thumbelina. That image clicked strongly for me and really helped. From then on, even when I was in strong labor, I kept thinking of that image—a huge, beautiful flower opening, and the baby coming out.

All of a sudden, in the afternoon, I couldn't sit anymore. The contractions were so strong that I had to stand up and lean over the bed to deal with them. Every time I peed, they came up even harder. I became scared to pee, because they hurt even more when I was sitting down. I had to be on the move.

All three midwives had the same opinion: "You might want to go for a walk." I couldn't imagine doing that, but I couldn't sit either. Instead of pacing around the house, Dan and I went walking in the woods. Every time I had a contraction, I grabbed on to him so I wouldn't fall. I had to bend my knees during the peak of each contraction; otherwise, it would have hurt worse. I couldn't have kept from bending my knees if I'd wanted to. My body was just doing what had to be done.

When we were out in the woods, the trees and flowers and plants were very vivid and alive. It was the most real experience I've ever been through—so in-the-moment and so bright.

We stopped walking and sat for a little while. We were trying to kiss, but every time I had a contraction, we would realize that it wasn't working. Ina May had said that kissing might help the baby come quicker, but as soon as I sat down and felt the first contraction, I said, "This is not happening." Dan had to help me back up, and we went walking around some more. I didn't want to go back yet. We walked through a little field of flowers at the edge of the woods and through the horse pasture. We saw a horse that was pregnant. Just a week before, I had gone out to the pasture; the horse and I had touched bellies and had our picture taken.

When we got back to the house, I walked around and around in it. Every time I felt a contraction begin, I would look for something or someone to grab on to. And someone—either Dan or one of the midwives—would push on my back. That eased it so much. Without someone massaging my back, it was too much.

Every contraction had a definite end. There were no two ways about it. It would be so strong, then all of a sudden it would be gone. That was the best feeling in the world. Once it was done, I was euphoric. Right after a contraction was when things would be the most vivid. I would feel so good.

I kept walking around. Every time I tried to sit, it felt like the baby's head was already halfway out and I was sitting on it. (His head was nowhere near out, but that was how it felt.) For a while nothing happened. I was just dealing with the contractions. When Ina May checked me next, I was 8.5 centimeters. Pamela suggested that I get on all fours, which I did, and the contractions got even stronger. She kept saying to me, "Breathe between contractions." When I did have a contraction, she would say, "Breathe it out, breathe it out." I had started screaming. Ina

May came in, and she was telling me to go, "Pfffff" like a horse blowing out its lips, between contractions. I did and each time it would make me laugh, which helped me relax.

But I was starting to think, Oh, my goodness! How can I stop this? I felt like I was on a roller coaster: The whole ride is kind of scary, up and down, up and down; you get to the very highest peak and you're about to go down the steepest part—and you think, I'm going to die. I want to get off. That's how I felt, but I kept saying to myself, There is no way to stop this. I'm stuck in this now. I'm here. A couple of times, I thought, No wonder people just go to a hospital to get some kind of painkiller. I wouldn't have wanted to do it that way, but when I was in the crazy part, I kept thinking, No wonder people do it.

I had no clue who was in the room. I knew Dan was on the right side of me. I was squeezing his hand, and sometimes I grabbed on to him. Once during a contraction, I reached over and bit his chest! Another time, I was leaning on Pamela's shoulder and I almost bit her! I stopped myself when I realized what I was about to do. It was just a reaction. There were times I was thinking to myself, I can't do this, it's too much, I can't do it. A few times, Pamela put her face a couple of inches away from mine, gently pulled back my hair, and said "You're doing fine. You are having this sweet baby. Keep breathing." This helped.

For a while I stood on my knees with my body upright during contractions. Between them I rested on all fours with my head down on the bed. Then the baby's head moved further down, making that position painful rather than comfortable. Suddenly I couldn't kneel on all fours anymore. I had to be upright. I could feel he was coming. My body started pushing down. I thought the baby was coming out my butt. The midwives assured me he wasn't. "I know he is, I can feel it," I said. I thought something was wrong, and I was scared to push.

Pamela was right in front of me, and Dan was right next to me. I was squeezing on to him for dear life, and Pamela kept pulling my hair back out of my face and talking me through it. It started burning badly, and I screamed. I heard these noises come from myself that didn't sound human. They sounded beastly, primitive. My whole body was coming down and trying to get the baby out.

Eventually, I thought I might be able to lie back. When I did, the midwives saw I was crowning. They kept wiping my face with a washcloth, and I was thinking, Can't you just pour a bucket of water on me?

But I couldn't get the words out. They sprayed oil on me and the baby's head came right out. (I watched the video that was made, and it actually took a couple of minutes, but I thought it happened instantly.)

Dan's mom was in position to deliver, and her touch felt good. I felt my baby's head push through. The rest of his body shot out. It felt different from the head, but it felt so good. I was so relieved. I lay back and just breathed for what seemed like the first time in a year.

When I was pushing, I was thinking, Never again. I'll never do this again. But as soon as he came out—the second they laid him on me—I thought. Wow, look at you! For you it was worth it. You are so beautiful.

Then they started talking about the placenta coming out, and I thought, Oh, no, there's more! I asked if it was going to be anything like pushing him out, and they told me it was a lot easier.

I had never wanted to have a kid. The two or three times I had held a baby in my life, I felt really awkward. When I got pregnant, I was okay with it, but I was still worried. I knew I would love him, but I hoped I would adore him. The second he came out, it was as if he had always been with me, he was meant to be with me. Nothing felt weird about it at all. It felt so natural and so perfect. I just held him, and I looked at him, and I thought, You're what was missing in my life.

Early in my career, I attended a birth and learned from it an important technique for lessening labor pain for women for whom it is culturally appropriate.

⚘ Who Knew?
By Anonymous

The midwives came and helped me breathe deeply through the contractions. This deep breathing did make the pains less. Then the contractions became even more intense, and I was not sure I could stand any more. Seeing that I was scared, Ina May suggested that I kiss my husband during the next contraction. This was the furthest thing from my mind, but I did what she said. I should say here that my relationship had been rather rocky around this time, and the way we kissed each other had never been very satisfying to me. Anyway, while kissing, the contractions continued to be strong. Ina May was sitting on the end of the bed, and she advised me to open my mouth enough to surround my husband's. It was at this point that I became more aroused than I had ever been in my life! There was no pain—only the most extreme sexual pleasure and complete openness. It was orgasmic. I'm sure that all of this happened within just a few seconds, but I passed through transition, and before I knew it, I was starting to push the baby out. I could not have been more surprised. Not only did I have a new son, but I now had a brand-new feeling about my husband. What astonished me the most was that the latter part of labor was not just pain-free, but really good. My husband and I have been married more than thirty years now and have two grandchildren. I tell my kids about my son's birth, because I know that this birth experience helped me through the years with my marriage—it confirmed the trust in such a vulnerable and sacred place.

✿ Galen's Birth—September 16, 1972
By Anita Staengl

On the morning of my son's birth, I started getting what felt like cramps. Luke, my husband, waited awhile and then called the midwives. It was a beautiful sunny day, and I spent most of it walking around outside.

Contractions started getting heavier. My water broke. "I feel scared," I said.

Ina May got right up into my face and asked, "Of what?"

I thought it was obvious. I was afraid of this incredible pain that felt like a lightning bolt going through me.

During the next contraction I realized that I was indulging in self-pity. Then I thought, No, I'm supposed to be having a baby here, not thinking of myself! I began to follow Ina May's instructions of taking deep breaths with each contraction. I felt like I was turning myself inside out with each push. Sitting up helped me use up all of the energy of the contraction so that I didn't really feel pain.

Galen was born with a few pushes, one and a half hours after my water broke. When he came out, he was a bright reddish-purple. I thought an organ of my body was slipping out when he began to appear. He lay perfectly still, like a blue Aztec statue. We all held our breath, and slowly pink spread over his body. One of the midwives cleaned his nose, and he started crying and alternately clenching his fists and spreading out his fingers.

He immediately took to my breast.

We slept. The next day Luke looked beautiful to me, his hair and skin tinted golden by the sun. He was singing, "That's the way God made it, because that's the way He wanted it to be."

Galen had a wonderful fragrance emanating from his little head. It lingered for days, filling our room. I have since heard that sweet smell is a sign of the presence of angels. I believe they were present.

☙ Samuel's Birth Story—July 18, 1979
By Patricia Lapidus

By evening I knew I was not going to go to bed for a normal sleep. I wasn't rushing much yet. I was just tending to float away—and I had an amazing feeling of energy that I was ready to use in a big way! We decided to go to bed and snooze while we could.

Some time during the timeless hours, Mary Louise, one of the midwives, brushed my hair in a very soothing way. She was so thoughtful that she understood I had to spit the ice out during each rush and have it back to suck on between rushes. Things like that became important and I hardly had to explain.

Whenever I felt a rush begin, I would look at Don and say, "Ready, babe?" and he would grin. I would look into his eyes and we would laugh. Everyone laughed with us. I realized it was up to me as the laboring woman to set the tone. When I decided to have a good time, we could all have a good time. The rushes felt like riding giant ocean waves. I'm from the coast of Maine, so I know waves. The image of waves washing over me helped me allow the universe to do its work. The waves pounded the granite shores of my flesh. I was beyond choice, beyond mind.

Leslie, my midwife, managed my labor very thoughtfully. She suggested I sit on the edge of the bed and lean on Don, allowing gravity to assist in opening. He was wonderful, so steady and present and patient with his strong, unchanging body. I hung on to him just to be grounded in physical reality. I thought it was magical of him to be able to hold his body still. Now he became the granite shore and I became the waves. A huge rush would take me, all of me—every muscle, not only the ones in my uterus around the baby—every muscle all the way to my scalp. The rushes were so intense now that they took my neck muscles into their rhythm and then let go, leaving my neck flaccid and my head lolling against Don's chest.

Each time a wave crashed through, the midwives cheered, no longer concerned with creating a quiet atmosphere. "Good one!" they encouraged. I had the thought that I was supposed to be able to hold my head up—although there was no longer any way of controlling my muscles. As Leslie and the others cheered my progress, I realized whatever was happening must be just right. I could be rowdy if I liked.

In position for the birth, I made some cow noises. Leslie told me that an open, relaxed mouth helped open my bottom.

Then they managed a lovely surprise. As I was getting ready to push, my dear friend Kay Marie (who was also a midwife) came into the room. She lived in Washington, D.C., and was present on The Farm only because of a midwife conference taking place. Knowing that she had not been present to catch my older son, the midwives had invited her to catch Samuel. Leslie, who had done so much for me during all the hours, moved over with a smile, as pleased as I was with Kay Marie's being there. She had no ego investment after all those hours. I was so grateful.

A few pushes and Samuel appeared, headfirst, then shoulders, with a little help from Kay Marie, who supported him gently. He seemed to slip out easily after all the effort.

She put the baby on my belly. "Look at him, honey!" I exclaimed to Don, and we began to study our child the way parents do. His eyes were open. He seemed to see us. He was an old soul, only temporarily small, come to us for his own inscrutable purposes. He inspired respect and devotion.

Angelika and Viktor are German nationals who became pregnant while traveling in North America.

⚘ Angelika's Story—June 18, 1991
By Angelika and Viktor Engelmann

We were married for fifteen years before getting pregnant. The pregnancy was a surprise to us, since we had been together so long and had never used birth control. Having no kids made it easy for us to travel around different parts of the world in our camper. My birth story begins

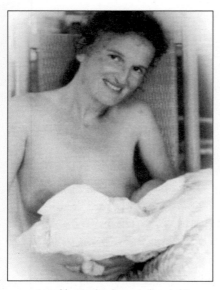

Angelika and Felix, one hour old

when we were working in Washington State in a fish-processing plant for a few weeks to earn money. One day we were processing a kind of fish that has a double penis. Some of the Native Americans who worked there were making jokes about how their people believed that handling this fish increased people's fertility. I guess that in Viktor's and my case, it turned out to be true.

Viktor: Angelika said to me, "Stand behind me and feel these breasts!" Sure enough, they were different. We had been talking about the possibility of pregnancy, and we knew that her period was really later than usual. Her periods had already been irregular, but the swollen breasts were what convinced me. I had made a lot of plans during earlier times when we'd thought Angelika might be pregnant—for instance, once when we were in Crete and her period was pretty late. I had thought we would have to make something like a nest and settle down. But by the time we were in Arizona, and we were really faced with pregnancy, she had convinced me that we would not have to settle down, that we could have the baby and still go on traveling.

Angelika: I decided early in my pregnancy that I didn't want to tell anyone at home in Germany about the news. I knew there was a possibility of miscarriage at my age, and I didn't want to worry anyone. Besides, I didn't want all the "good advice" that would come from home. We would have been advised to come home immediately. They would have told me of all the dangers and difficulties of being pregnant at the age of thirty-eight. Besides that, we would have heard endlessly about the unsuitability of our lifestyle for pregnancy and having a baby.

In January I began to feel the baby kicking. We were around Ciudad Valles, Mexico, by this time. We began to dream about the future. I was knitting a sweater for Viktor while he read stories from Boccaccio's

Decameron. We spent four weeks staying with a friend in Texas. There we met a woman who was pregnant and due one month before me.

After stopping in Louisiana, Mississippi, and Alabama, we reached The Farm in Tennessee late in March. One day later I had my first prenatal checkup at the clinic. The baby was to be born in early June. What a good feeling it was to have this prenatal care and to learn that everything was okay. Viktor listened to the heartbeat of the baby. It was a pleasure to be around the midwives. They weren't worried about me having my first baby at the age of thirty-eight. That made us look forward to the birthing. After a few weeks more of traveling, Viktor and I decided that we would go back to The Farm to give birth.

My rushes began at midnight six days after my due date and came every thirty minutes. The intervals between them got shorter. Viktor called Pamela at about 5:00 A.M. She and Ina May arrived soon after his call. They found that my cervix was only one centimeter open, and the rushes seemed to melt away. The atmosphere at dawn, with the birds singing and first light, should be experienced more often. But I realized that in the future I would probably be seeing it more often than I would really like. I felt good, especially because I had no rushes for a while.

I had rushes off and on throughout the day, but they weren't very strong yet. I had a sleepless night that night. Between lying in bed,

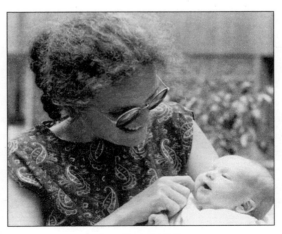

Angelika and Felix

sitting in the rocking chair, and going to the toilet, I emptied myself. I was happy that after every contraction, I had a nice rest during which I could relax and try new ways to deal with the next one. I felt sorry for Viktor, because he didn't get any sleep either and had to wake up for each rush. He put a pillow and sleeping bag in the rocking chair, and he rubbed my back. Although we slept a little while in the morning, we were pretty exhausted. I was too tired to get much out of what Pamela was saying the next morning. I was a bit afraid when she said something about women getting too tired and having to go to the hospital. Viktor and I both felt pretty down around that time. When Pamela checked me, my cervix hadn't changed much. I knew I had to change my attitude and loosen up.

The midwives left us alone all that day, as my cervix hadn't yet begun to dilate. I didn't waste my time by looking at the clock. My rushes continued anyway, and I enjoyed being alone with Viktor. The pleasant atmosphere, a short visit from Ina May, and even the Scrabble game were enjoyable. Viktor was distracted during the game, which he says is why I won.

A couple of days passed. I had the feeling that the event was approaching, but I couldn't imagine what it would be like. I was so glad that Viktor was with me and that he didn't lose patience waiting for the baby to come. He spoiled me and let me know that he loved me. In the afternoon, I knitted for a while and thought about whether the baby would be healthy. I came to these thoughts because I suspected that my water bag was broken. Pamela did a test to see if it was. (It wasn't.) I wondered about how many women attempting home births had such a test done, and what was likely to be done with someone older than thirty-five who thought she had already been in labor for a couple of days. I was very glad that we were once again in the right spot at the right time. I couldn't imagine being more comfortable than being in the forest with the birds singing around us and the dogs visiting at our door in the evening, because of the presentiment that there was something special happening. Even the deer came up to the porch. Because everything here was treated so naturally, my fears that the baby might be abnormal vanished very quickly, and I believed the prophecy that I would have a good, healthy baby soon. But when was "soon," I wondered.

Ina May: *I visited Angelika and Viktor several times during the days*

when we were waiting for her labor to get going strong. At one point she told me that while they rarely quarreled with each other, they usually did argue after a Scrabble game. "Now, what is there about Scrabble that gets you into an argument?" I asked, surprised at what I was hearing.

"Well, for one thing," Angelika said, "playing a game of Scrabble in German sometimes takes a couple of days, because some of our words are so long."

"Oh," I said, still not understanding.

"The other thing is that the winner gets all the chocolate."

For that I did have a solution. "Why don't you just let the winner have the satisfaction of winning and then share the chocolate?" I said.

"Oh, you Americans," Angelika said. "You have so many ideas about how to change things!"

I can't remember now which of my partners made this observation, but whoever it was told me of the exchange she had with Viktor and Angelika. We all had commented to each other how much they seemed to love each other and how lucky this baby would be to come into this family. At the same time, she noticed that whenever one of them wanted a favor from the other, they didn't have a very pleasant way of saying that to each other. It came out sounding like an order, which made the other less happy about doing whatever it was. At that point, she made a suggestion as to how they could resolve this little communication problem: "Why don't you ask each other in a sweet way for a favor so the other will be happier to do it?"

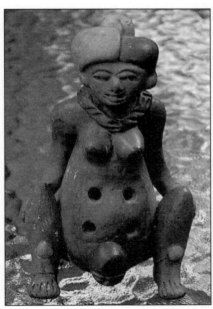

Mexican ocarina

Viktor and Angelika looked at each other and laughed. "You Americans have such good ideas about how to change things!"

Angelika: Then the rushes began to get more intense. After each one, I had to waddle instead of walk. I felt more and more like the gorilla mother we saw on the Discovery channel, bent forward and looking for something to hold in my hands. Ina May, Pamela, and the midwife assistant sat with me. I didn't think it could take much longer, but then time disappeared somehow. The jokes could no longer distract me from the rushes, which were getting frequent and strong. I loved the massage of my back, neck, and legs. I remembered the night before when I couldn't stand anything touching me. I had pushed off the sheets, blankets, and Viktor's hands. Now I couldn't bear the midwives massaging me counterclockwise on my belly, so I told them. My cervix was four centimeters open, and because it was so thin, Ina May stretched it open to five centimeters. I couldn't feel it. Sometimes I only saw Viktor at my feet or beside me. I looked in his eyes, squeezed his hand, and was happy that there was a rest in between the rushes.

Ina May had brought several Mexican objects with her. There was an ocarina in the form of a woman giving birth with the baby's head already born, and a Huichol mask with deer that protect children. There was also a beautiful rain stick in the form of Quetzalcoatl, the feathered serpent, carved in dark wood. It rained in the room, but outside they said the night was very clear and that Jupiter, Venus, and Mars were all visible, with the moon half full. It was exactly the way I had wished for the date of birth.

Then I wondered if all this would really help me bear the hours to come. Every time I felt I was at the doorway of life and death, I sent a little prayer upward. I asked Viktor to light our last two candles, and while I was sitting in the rocking chair, I looked into the lights without my glasses and thought that I would soon know what the baby would look like. I was getting anxious to know whether it was a girl or a boy.

At about 11:00, Ina May broke the water bag with an instrument that looked like a crochet hook, and the warm water flowed out. Now the baby's head, which pushed like a rock against the cervix, would open it the rest of the way. The waves were strong and I had to use a different breathing technique to manage them. While breathing deeply and exhaling through my lips with the sound horses make, I began to feel like pushing. When I pushed, ancient sounds came out of me. I wondered if I was too loud or whether someone outside could hear me. I had these thoughts between pushes, but then I kept hearing, "Good, right, these are good birthing sounds," "You look so pretty," and so on.

The baby's heartbeat stayed in the normal range, between 120 and 140, and I lay in the bed with some cushions behind me. With every wave I brought my legs closer to my body. It was timeless. I tried pushing in the all-fours position, pressing my head into the pillows. The urge to push came from inside, but I didn't get off a good one. Something was missing. It was Ina May, who typed something in her computer; that distracted me. I looked over my shoulder, and she came over to me promptly. I tried another position, sitting on Viktor's lap. I felt his thighs trembling. This was a totally unstable-feeling position, and we moved into another position on the other side of the bed, where I could pull on the rope that was threaded through the pair of horseshoes fixed to the beam above the bed. If this doesn't bring luck, I thought . . . I was cold, so I put on my long socks, the ones I had worn at the fishery.

Ina May lay on the bed, and I envied her. I wanted to just lie there and sleep. That would be marvelous. The ropes gave me a better grip, but even so, I didn't make much progress while pulling on them. I was afraid that I would bleed on the carpet, and I also worried about that when I was in bed without the pad under me. Therefore, we went into the tiny bathroom, where I sat on the pot. I had the feeling that I could let go, and after I heard someone mention the word *vacuum* for some reason, I knew that I had to succeed in bringing the baby down. Viktor stood in front of me, and I put my arms around his neck and pulled him down. Everything inside gave a mighty push. The heartbeat dropped to around ninety beats, and they gave me some oxygen.

Very slowly the head worked farther down, and with every contraction I felt more of a burning sensation. They began to see the head, and they suggested that I go back to the bed. That was nearly impossible, as I could already feel the head between my legs, and it was burning like fire. I hung on to Viktor. I don't know who supported me on the other side. I climbed into the bed and got into the all-fours position—on my knees and elbows. Everything went very quickly from here. Because of the burning, I put one hand down and felt what was there. Then I recognized that it was the baby's head and not Ina May's hand that was causing this feeling.

I didn't want to tear. That was a feeling I had that sat really deep. I tried to do everything I was told. I had to pant like a dog, and Ina May assured me that I have a "good German butt." I felt the head be born, then how one shoulder came after the other, and how the rest of the body glided out. I made it! Everything seemed to be in slow motion. Viktor and I hugged each other, and then we looked to see who Ina May had in her hands. We were sure that he was a girl. Then we saw the cord and something more: We realized he was a boy. What a big surprise for us! I was happy that Viktor, after so many women in his life during our time together, had his male companion at last.

Felix lay on my belly and immediately started sucking. We had eyes only for this little one.

Pamela began cleaning up; they weighed Felix and dressed him and measured his huge head. Thirty-eight centimeters. I lay on the bed and waited for the placenta. It came half an hour after Felix. Viktor buried it in the forest the next day, because we were not keen on a stew à la Kitzinger. Viktor washed me, and they put everything away. Our little family lay in bed and looked at one another.

The midwives were all tired and said good-bye with a kiss and a hug. After two hours we decided that it was time to let our relatives at home know that we had a baby. Since this was their first news of our pregnancy, they had a hard time believing what we were telling them.

Ina May: When I handed the ocarina to Angelika, she took it and held it and turned it this way and that. I told her that I thought this flute was a Mexican way of telling women that it is possible to give birth. I made sure to tell her that it wasn't just brown-skinned women who can give birth, because I wanted her to know that fair-skinned women work perfectly well too. When she finally handed the ocarina back to me, she looked different—a little more relaxed.

Many hours later, when Angelika was on her hands and knees pushing and the baby's head was about to be born, she looked back at me and quickly asked, "Am I going to tear?"

"Not with your good German butt!" was what came out of my mouth. Angelika laughed at that reply—as if out of surprise. But the beautiful thing was how that laughter just at the most intense moment of crowning relaxed Angelika's perineum enough that, despite the burning sensation she was feeling, she gave birth to that thirty-eight-centimeter head without a scratch. Felix's birth felt like such a triumph over fear.

✢ Evan's Birth—January 24, 1998

By Diana Janopaul

When I was seventeen, I found a copy of *Spiritual Midwifery* in a bookstore on Eighth Street in New York City. I'm not sure that I even knew what a midwife was prior to that, but through this book, the allure and beauty of birth reached out and grabbed me. Since then I have been fascinated with birth and have long held a desire to become a midwife myself.

It was many years later, when I was thirty years old, that I prepared for the birth of my first child. I trusted that my body would function as intended and that the birth would go well. I chose to work with a nurse–midwife who had been highly recommended to me by several friends. I knew the hospital I would be in had a thirty-three percent cesarean-section rate, but I never imagined that it would apply to me.

My membranes ruptured at home one evening, one week past my due date. I stayed at home all night, trying to sleep and hoping that contractions would begin soon. We went to the hospital the next morning. I was having mild contractions and was only one centimeter dilated. The midwife recommended Pitocin augmentation, and we agreed. What happened after that was a series of interventions I had never planned on: constant fetal monitoring, a narcotic called Stadol, intravenous antibiotics to fight the infection I had developed, and finally an epidural. I made very slow progress, even with the intense contractions brought on by the Pitocin in the intravenous fluids, and felt totally out of control and defeated. My midwife was in the room with me for a total of about thirty minutes during the eighteen hours I was there. She was busy with other births and even left the hospital for a period of time. I felt totally deserted. My husband and family could do nothing to help. I remember tears running down my husband's face. This was not what we had planned!

The midwife came in around midnight and told me I was completely dilated and could start pushing. We turned off the epidural, but I still had no control over my legs and never felt a pushing urge. (I found out later that epidurals often interfere with laboring women's ability to push.) After a few pushes, the midwife left again and I pushed for over two hours with the help of my family and a kind nurse. When the midwife finally came back, she checked me and told me there was no progress. Also, she discovered that I had been pushing on an anterior lip of cervix that had never been noticed. In other words, I wasn't really completely dilated during that two hours of hard pushing. No wonder all that pushing amounted to nothing. We began to see worrisome signs in the baby's heart rate. Lucas was delivered by cesarean section shortly thereafter. He weighed ten pounds seven ounces. The midwife said he was just too big.

The feelings I experienced after this ranged from inadequacy to failure to anger. I found myself apologetically explaining my cesarean to complete strangers. "You have such a big baby!" they would say.

"Well, he was a C-section," I would answer.

When I found out that I was pregnant again, I wanted to try for a vaginal birth after cesarean—a VBAC. I chose a different nurse–midwife and a different hospital. I wanted an out-of-hospital birth, but because of the first section, there was no one in my area who could help me. The home birth midwives in my area were not attending VBAC's out of hospital because of lack of physician backup. I went two weeks over my due date. I knew I was growing another big baby, but I didn't want to go on Pitocin again.

I finally went into labor, with contractions never much closer together than five to six minutes apart. I was making progress, however, and felt things were going well. I was five centimeters dilated when I got to the hospital. The baby's head was moveable, and immediately I understood that my caregivers took this as a sign that this baby wasn't going to fit. I labored to about seven centimeters before agreeing to a cesarean. Kenna weighed eleven pounds six ounces, with a 15¼-inch (38 centimeter) head. I was told by an obstetrician during this labor that I have an "adequate pelvis for an average-size baby." (The same obstetrician later told me that white women couldn't have eleven-pound babies!) I remember thinking that I would never grow an "average-size baby" and therefore was pretty much excluded from ever having a normal birth.

After Kenna's birth, my midwife suggested that if I were ever to become pregnant again, I should schedule a cesarean. But I just couldn't help feeling that, if given the support I needed and if able to avoid the interventions that occur so routinely in the hospital, I could give birth to my children. When I became pregnant again, I decided that if I wanted a different outcome, I needed to drastically change my approach. I called The Farm and spoke with Pamela. She told me that she could not guarantee me a vaginal birth. I told her I didn't expect a guarantee but wanted a fair chance.

I received prenatal care from a wonderful home-birth midwife in my area. We arrived at The Farm about two weeks before my due date. One week before my due date, my membranes ruptured. Pamela checked me and found me one and a half centimeters dilated. My contractions began immediately, although they were not very close together. Pamela checked me again the next morning, and I was three and a half centimeters. Pamela hung out with me at the birth cabin, and I really enjoyed getting to know her during that time. Ina May came by early in the afternoon and sent my husband, Steve, and me out to walk the roads. We strolled about for a couple of hours, with me hanging on Steve's shoulders during contractions or squatting to make them stronger. At four o'clock, Pamela checked me again and I was still at three and a half. I was feeling discouraged by the lack of progress, even though Pamela assured me that my cervix was thinning and the baby's head had dropped more. I was really questioning my ability to handle a long labor. (One of my issues about my past births was that I had "chickened out" and asked for pain relief.)

Carol, another of the midwives, suggested that Steve and I kiss during the contractions—she said it really helped her during her births. We did. It was definitely a welcome distraction that helped me feel really connected to my wonderful husband! I progressed from three and a half centimeters to nine and a half centimeters in about five hours. The hardest part of my labor was getting "hung up" at nine and a half centimeters for over three hours. I felt I couldn't handle it and was again discouraged with the lack of progress. However, the midwives were so supportive and encouraging that I knew I could go on. Finally, Pamela checked me once again and pushed the cervix up over the baby's head. I was complete!

Pushing was a whole new adventure, since I had never really had the urge to push with my other labors. At first I used the birthing stool, which really helped me bring the baby down quickly. It was a padded wooden chair with legs short enough that my knees were flexed as I sat in it. The portion of the seat near my crotch was cut away to give room for the baby to emerge. I pushed with all the strength I could muster. I could hear myself roaring like a lion. It sounded like it was coming from someone else, but it felt great. After a little more than an hour of pushing, I reached down and felt my baby's head crowning. Within moments I gave birth to my son Evan Alexander. I looked down and saw him on the bed between my legs and held his little feet in my hands while the midwives got him going. I held him close and put him to the breast right away—all the things I was never able to do with my other children. Carol had to go get another scale, since the one in the cabin only went up to ten pounds! Evan weighed ten pounds ten ounces and had a fifteen-inch head—bigger than my first baby, who was, according to the midwife, "just too big!" A small tear required a few stitches.

I have learned so much from Evan's birth. I am a lot stronger than I ever imagined—I felt so powerful pushing that big baby out! I also learned how influenced we are by others' perceptions and beliefs. The Farm midwives trusted me and my body completely. There were none of the frowns or worried looks that I had experienced before. They didn't think I was going too slowly. I think they had more faith in me than anyone ever has, including myself. I also learned that my "adequate" pelvis is more than adequate for an "average-size" baby. It's just that *my* average-size babies weigh more than ten pounds. I found out that I am perfectly designed to give birth to them.

Not a day goes by that I don't think about it in one way or another. I think the insights that I have gleaned since Evan was born are as powerful as the birth itself. The first thing I noticed was that the pervasive sadness and grief I felt surrounding my other births disappeared. I don't feel the overwhelming desire to cry when I think about those births now. In that way, Evan's birth was truly a healing experience.

The most amazing change I have noticed is how much stronger I feel as a person. A friend told me once that after the birth of her son, she felt as if she could have climbed a mountain. I thought she meant how she felt *physically*, but now I realize that she meant much more than that. She was empowered. I have always been told and have always told others that birth is empowering. But I never had the chance to experience how true that really is. My first two births were not at all empowering. I felt defeated, dejected, and discouraged afterward, and the disappointment was almost unbearable.

After Evan's birth, I was physically sore and tired. But I felt so victorious and strong inside. My husband and I were watching the winter Olympics one evening shortly after Evan's birth, and I found myself talking to the athletes as I watched them luge, ski jump, and figure skate.

"Hmph!" I scoffed. "That's nothing. I could do that. Try pushing out a ten-pound ten-ounce baby, and then we'll talk!" Funny words from a woman who had stitches in her perineum and hemorrhoids galore. I couldn't have ski jumped at that moment if my life had depended on it. But I felt so *powerful!*

How many women will never feel that power? Maybe the true price of an unnecessary cesarean is not the scar or disappointment or pain of recovery. Maybe it is the loss of that empowerment. There is a picture of me holding Evan shortly after the birth. I am exhausted and worn out, but there is a look. It's the look I have seen on other women's faces as they reach for their newborn babies. Finally, it is reflected in my face. Joy, accomplishment, strength, and serenity. So beautiful!

Many people fail to realize how many ways babies may be positioned and still be born vaginally.

✤ It's a Nose!—December 22, 1982
By Valerie Gramm

I was thirty-three years old and about to have my third baby on The Farm. Since we had two girls previously born on The Farm, we were kind of hoping for a boy. The pregnancy went well, and I was in for my nine-month checkup at the clinic. Ina May, our midwife and good friend, checked me. I could tell after several minutes of checking that maybe something was wrong, especially when they called in the doctor who lived on The Farm.

They had felt a bulge or bump that surely was not the normal, smooth surface of the crown of the head. Not being sure, Ina May called the obstetrician in town to tell him we were coming in. I felt in good hands because Ina May and my husband, David, were going with me. When she came to pick me up, I told her that I thought my labor had started.

We went flying over the old potholes on the dusty roads of The Farm. I still knew it was all right, since Ina May was in the front seat and had assured me that she had delivered a baby in a car before. Besides, she had attended my last birthing. I trusted her. No problem.

We arrived at the doctor's office, and of course I had to wait and

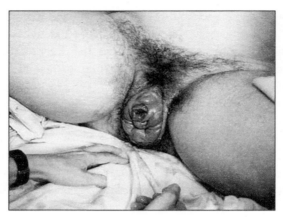

Jerome faces the world

wait... but, hey, what more could I ask for? I just wanted to make sure my baby was all right, since I was a little worried. Finally the doctor checked me and chuckled. "It's a *nose*," he said. Most doctors may be able to say, "It's a boy," or "It's a girl," but he had to say, "It's a nose." I was so relieved that the bump they had felt had turned out to be a little nose headed in the direction of delivery. We went back home to prepare for the birth. (Ina May: *It was the obstetrician who told us that we could safely take Valerie back to The Farm to give birth.*)

Ina May wanted us to give birth at our birth clinic rather than at

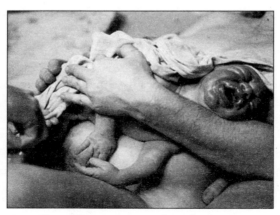

The swelling was gone within a few hours

home, to be closer to backup care if it was needed. Later on, my rushes became a little stronger. This labor was slower than my two others but not different from them in any other way. I was surrounded by loving midwives and my children's father. I was so glad to be there and not in the sterile environment of a hospital. I knew I wouldn't have a cesarean, because Ina May was very good at her job.

Several hours later it finally started happening. It took a lot of strength, but the love for our baby overpowered the hurt. Sure enough, here came that nose first, stuck up in the air and on its way out. With a final push, our dream came through: a boy! He was a little bruised, but this disappeared by the end of the next day. My son was healthy, strong, and beautiful!

✄ Heaven Morgaine's Birth—December 22, 1990
By Beth Colton

Mark and I were starting our first quarter in college when we found out I was pregnant. After reading the results of our home pregnancy test, we immediately went to an obstetrician. There were mixed feelings about the whole thing. I figured everything would work out, until I talked to my doctor's accountant. We were shocked about how much a normal, vaginal birth cost at our local hospital. I tried explaining that we were just starting college and no way were we going to have that kind of money, then or in three months. Mark and I walked out of the office even more mixed up than when we went in. We both knew that we wanted to keep this child, but we saw no way we could afford it.

We weren't sure what to do, until a girlfriend of mine from college told us she had heard of a place called The Farm, where they have a birthing center. About a month later, we went to The Farm for my first prenatal visit. Pamela talked with us for a while and mentioned that this was going to be natural childbirth. I had always assumed that drugs were a required part of delivery and had never considered delivering any other way, so I was quite shocked when I found out there would be no drugs involved. They didn't have any. Pamela gave us *Spiritual Midwifery* to read, and I was able to read quite a lot of it on our five-hour drive back to Atlanta.

I was amazed. I never thought the birth of a child could be so wonderful. Some of the stories I read were very touching. I was relieved to find that some of the things that were policy in hospitals were not policies at The Farm. The more I read, the more I realized that drugs were not necessary and were worth doing without.

As my due date approached, we decided to spend the Christmas holidays with some relatives in Decatur, Alabama, which is only an hour and a half away from The Farm. When I went into labor one morning, we were all excited, except for Mark's brother, who was concerned. It had been raining for three days straight, and the roads had started flooding out. Mark's brother started hinting that I should maybe think about going to a hospital. I had already packed and was just waiting to leave for The Farm, not a hospital. I had read that a lot of times women can make themselves regress in labor, so I wasn't too concerned about making it to The Farm on time.

By two in the afternoon we were ready to leave. The rain was really coming down, but the sound of it beating on the car was soothing, and I was glad that it was raining. The rushes were definitely getting stronger, and my mind was doing some really crazy things. Before we left Alabama, I had been playing a computer game. Every time I would start a rush, my mind would really focus in on this game, giving me new strategies for playing it, and the background music of the game would race loudly through my brain. It was wild, and I don't know if I can explain enough for someone else to understand its intensity. I really believe now that you don't need drugs during labor, because your body makes its own.

We reached The Farm by 4:00 P.M., and my rushes were about four minutes apart. We got settled at the Birthing House. Ina May checked me, and while she was examining me I opened up to three centimeters.

After a while Ina May suggested that I take a hot bath. That was the best news I had heard in hours. I'll never forget that tub. It was the biggest, best tub I had ever seen. I could stretch straight out and still not be long enough to reach both ends. I stayed in the tub a long time. Mark was great. He washed my back and kept me company. At some point I submerged myself completely; the only thing not covered was my face. Then my mind really let loose, things got real floaty, and I didn't feel like me. I felt like a cloud.

We went back upstairs and Ina May checked me again. I was now seven and a half centimeters. Ina May suggested that I get into a comfortable position. Mark was behind me, and I was lying in his lap. When things got painful, I would stretch my arms out and grip real tight on his leg and arms. By this time I had started making some pretty bizarre sounds.

As I approached full dilation, I lost my mind. I just did not think I was going to make it. I kept saying, "I can't do this anymore!" I started to panic, and it was really scary, but Ina May talked me down and reminded me that this was all normal and that the more I said I couldn't do it, the more I was doing it.

The room was warm, and the lights were dim. I appreciate that now. Hospitals are so bright and cold. There was no way I could have dealt with the intensity of a hospital in that mental state. At some point, I changed the sounds I was making from low and breathy, throaty sounds to a high-pitched almost-scream. I could really feel the difference. Keeping my sounds low-pitched kept me loose, and screaming was like someone running their nails down a chalkboard, very unnerving and tight.

It was really beautiful to start pushing. I felt safe and loved. This was definitely the kind of environment I wanted my child to be born into. It's true when they say it feels like shitting out a bowling ball—not so much in a painful way, although it is kind of painful. I used to always wonder how, when you were pushing, you could stop and just pant. I always thought that once I started pushing, there was no way I was going to stop halfway through it, especially when the head was out. I thought, Forget it, I'm going all the way. But it wasn't that hard to stop. In fact, it was necessary. I was getting pretty tired and needed to take periodic rests.

I remember saying to Ina May, "It really hurts right now," and she asked, "Does it sting?"

I said, "Yes," and she said, "That's because the baby's head is out." A couple more pushes, and I felt a slithering sensation. The next thing I knew I had a baby on my stomach, staring at me with huge blue eyes.

When they told Mark we had a girl, I wasn't surprised. I had known for the last month from mother's intuition. About five minutes later, Ina May informed me that I still had to deliver the placenta. I told her I just couldn't push anymore, and she said, "Oh, that's the easy part. It doesn't have any bones."

I thought that was funny, and she was right. She and her assistant cleaned me and the baby up, then put away the birthing kit, showed me how to breastfeed, made sure that I was all right, and left Mark and me with our new child.

Tom and Suzi Mitchell came to The Farm for a vaginal birth after a previous cesarean.

✳ The Birth of Dylan Zade—March 1, 1991
By Suzi Mitchell

Thursday night was the full moon. I could hardly believe I was having rushes, so I made sure they were lasting. I didn't say anything to anyone in the birth cottage where we were staying. I soon started chanting through the rushes, and Kirk (our friend) and my husband Tom started timing them. As they got closer together, Tom called Ina May, and we quickly changed beds. Kirk moved upstairs with JoJo, our son, and Tom and I moved downstairs to the birthing bed.

I remember looking at the clock. It was almost midnight, and things were moving fast. When Ina May arrived, she checked me, and I was seven centimeters dilated. I was chanting through my rushes, "Ommmm, Ommmm," a releasing, open-throat sound. Deborah suggested that I take a deep breath and then "blow raspberries" through my lips. Ina May said this was a good idea, because there was no way my cervix could stay tight while I was doing this. (Ina May: *See Chapter 4 for my explanation of why this is true.*) That sounded really good, so that's what Tom and I did. After that, I rested for a while. It seemed that I was more relaxed at this point than earlier.

The rushes started getting stronger then, and Deborah suggested that it might be a good idea to look into somebody's eyes. I remembered reading this in *Spiritual Midwifery* and was glad to try looking into Deborah's eyes. They seemed to give the strength I needed during a rush. After a rush, I could connect with Tom again.

By 6:00 A.M., I had begun to get frantic. I couldn't keep still through the rushes anymore. I started throwing up, and everyone said this was good because it meant that I was getting ready to have the baby. "You can't fool me. My body is violently reacting to pain!" I said. I wanted to take a shower, but I knew I was doing this so I could get away.

As I showered, the rushes were really strong and connected. This was the hardest part of labor for me. I wasn't getting any break, and I desperately wanted one. My chanting kept getting louder. I kept hoping someone would rescue me, and Deborah did. She came into the bathroom and stood near the shower, getting sprinkled with water as she talked to me. She told me that mine hadn't been a real long labor, and I knew what she was talking about, since my labor with Joey had been very long. I realized that I was actually having a great labor and that things were going fantastically well. I had been thinking that I could go to the hospital, where they would give me some magic potion that would take the pain all away. I wondered if I knew this because of my previous cesarean. For a while I forgot that not only do they take the pain away, they take all the feelings away, and ultimately they take the baby away. Deborah said that all I had to do was decide what I wanted and I could have it.

I listened to her for a while and then asked her to send Tom in. I knew I could plead with Tom, and he would help me make the right decision. He came in and said he knew I could do it and that going to the hospital wasn't really what I wanted. He also said the midwives said I was doing great, which was certainly more than my midwives had said during Joey's birth.

I got out of the shower and tried harder. I didn't do so well with the first rush. About that time, Pamela came in and told me about her first birth. It was comforting to hear her tell about her experiences. She then reminded me about *The Little Engine That Could*. Little did she know I had just read Joey that story when I put him to bed. It is one of his favorites. I started saying, "I think I can," and then I started saying, "I know I can." (Ina May: *Just after Suzi tried saying, "I think I can," her words turned into a pushing roar, and the baby's head was through her cervix. It was pretty dramatic.*) After two rushes, Tom and I felt relaxed enough to smooch. Our kisses were so blissful, I'll never forget them and will draw on them for the rest of my life.

After that I started pushing. It wasn't a conscious effort. My body just took over. Pushing made the contractions much more comfortable.

The baby began to come out, and I felt like I was in a warm womb, floating and drifting, and all my needs were being met. The midwives kept saying they saw a dark head. I wanted to see and hear more. After a couple more pushes, Tom showed me the baby's head with a mirror. I felt like a horse. I started feeling a burning sensation, and Ina May squirted oil on my perineum, which eased it. When the baby began crowning, I wasn't really sure I wanted him to come out, but he did anyway. First a head, then his shoulders, and then he was on my belly! Oh! Thank you! I had no episiotomy or tear, and I had my vaginal birth after cesarean and my perfectly born son. I was ecstatic.

𝕏 Felicia's Birth—November 21, 1973
By Susan Levinson

My kids are so much a part of my life, yet so separate. I saw them every day for two decades. Now they've been on their own for some years. I'm so proud of their independence, and yet I'm thrilled when they ask for advice. I don't think I've gotten in their way too much. I fulfilled a major goal of parenthood: We like each other.

When Ralph and I arrived in Tennessee in 1972, we had recently been married in West Virginia. We had already been living together for two and a half years. My previous experience with child care was baby-sitting sleeping kids. I looked at the job only as a great chance to chalk up some phone time. Somehow, though, when I got to The Farm and saw all the families, I felt I wanted that too. I got pregnant quickly. It all looked rather effortless, and I was blissfully unaware of details on what the next nine months—or, for that matter, the next several decades—would entail. My pregnancy was easy and delightful. I don't think I was even aware that it could be otherwise. I had very few demands on my life and adapted readily to all the changes.

Until labor. Then I thought, Never mind. I changed my mind. Let's go on to something else. I did have a lot of time to get used to the idea, as labor lasted a full two days. I felt more like an observer than a participant during much of that time. I knew a lot was going to be expected of me—but not yet. The midwives were very attentive and confident. Things just went slowly, and I was in no particular rush. (Don't panic until you have to.) There were four other labors going on at the same time. I could wait, and I did.

But things did move along, then seemed to plateau. Ina May kept popping in and finally decided it was time to break my water. That really jump-started things, and detachment was getting harder. There was kind of a formula for labor that I was not following all that well. Get naked—in front of all these people? Make out with your husband—now? I'm busy. Any subconscious holding things back—nah. What did make me go to full dilation was Ina May checking me and declaring that if I didn't, we might need to go to the hospital and finish this off.

In full swing now, the midwives were rubbing me with oil. I thought I knew what the word *push* meant, but I had it all wrong. Finally I got it right, and Felicia crowned and was quickly born. It took us days to name her. She was so new that it was hard to think of something as permanent and unchanging as a name.

I was really proud of myself for giving birth the way I did, and I look at my children's births as major highlights of my life. I have not suffered any health problems from natural childbirth, and I've always been grateful to The Farm for showing me what raising children was like and giving me the confidence to have my own.

Occasionally (once or twice in a hundred births) we midwives need to transport a baby to the hospital for further care. Lorrell and Tomm Friend's son, Jake, was a Farm-born baby who took his first car ride soon after his birth.

Lorrell and Tomm raise horses and race them. Between babies, Lorrell is sometimes a jockey.

Jake's Birthing Tale—May 31, 1989
By Lorrell Friend

Tasha, the children's mare, was having eye trouble. When our vet, "Doc," came to treat her, he scanned my belly and asked, "When is your due date?" I told him. Years of life experience twinkled in his eyes as he shook his head from side to side. "You think she's going to wait that long, Tomm?" he asked my husband.

By the next morning we were packed and on our way to Tennessee. We decided to have Jake at The Farm after having five children at home. I could tell that Jake was a much bigger baby than our previous children had been. I had also been quite sick through the second trimester with flulike symptoms I couldn't shake.

At The Farm, Tomm and I set up housekeeping in the birthing cabin on Tower Road. We hiked along the Natchez Trace. We saw a herd of deer at the river's edge in Davy Crockett State Park. We climbed the fire tower on the road to Hohenwald. On the second tier of metal steps, we saw a perfect nest in which a robin had laid three perfect blue eggs.

This exercise paid off on the evening of May 30, when my water broke. I called our midwife, Deborah, who was happy for me and said I might want to catch some sleep before labor began. I was concerned that I wasn't having any rushes yet and couldn't sleep. A couple of hours later, labor began in earnest. In about four hours, I was completely dilated.

Now I'm a good pusher, but it was downright difficult to move this baby down. We made slow progress. His head came out all right, but he got stuck at the shoulders. The midwives consulted and Deborah asked me if I wanted to try something new. They had me flip over onto my hands and knees. I was most happy to oblige. The new position seemed to change the pressure I was feeling. With a bit of fancy handwork (it's nice if your midwife has slender hands), Jake was out. A big, beautiful boy, but he was barely breathing. The midwives used a suction device to clear his passages but he was still having considerable difficulty. Margaret placed a call to Maury Regional Hospital so they would know that Jake was on his way. Deborah stayed with me while I delivered the placenta.

As the Volvo made its way to Columbia, Pamela held Jake. She meditated with him. They breathed slowly and rhythmically in unison, for it seemed that one hiccup or sneeze and Jake would be gone.

The emergency room staff knew Ina May and Pamela and that the situation was serious. The head of the hospital had come in to meet us. He got things rolling very quickly. Jake was put on a ventilator and injected with ampicillin and Gentamicin. A chest X ray revealed fluid around his lungs. The doctor handed Tomm a medical encyclopedia opened to the page on Group B strep, which indicated a fifty to eighty percent mortality. The doctor then called the Angel One unit from Vanderbilt University Hospital in Nashville. Jake was whisked off to Vanderbilt before I reached Maury Regional. What a different experience this was from the births of our other children.

When we got to Vanderbilt, we were playing the waiting game. Finally, Tomm explained to the attending doctor that Jake and I needed to see each other.

Jake was lying in a clear plastic box. He was a forbidding sight: blood-spattered and slightly yellow. I hesitated, but when I touched him, there was a surge of energy between us. He jolted as if from recognition and then lay calm.

Later, we found out that Jake's nurse, Andrew, was a Farm alumnus and his wife had given birth at The Farm. He assured us that he would keep an eye on Jake.

We drove back to The Farm and both fell into a deep sleep. Early next morning, we drove up the Natchez Trace toward Nashville and stopped beside the side of the road where the Old Trace comes close to the Parkway. There we walked under the trees and prayed.

When we got to Vanderbilt, we were informed that Jake was all right. He was no longer sick. There was no negative response to the antibiotics. It would be six long days before he got his first square meal, but he was out of danger.

The respect with which both hospitals regarded Ina May, Pamela, and the other midwives made an incalculable difference when it came down to our ability to withstand this trying experience. There is a high percentage of negative outcomes when it comes to shoulder dystocia deliveries. Our midwives refused to panic. Their quiet competence and the ingenuity of the Gaskin Maneuver has made Jake our miracle baby. (See page 98.)

When we were finally able to take Jake home, he was eight days old. He was not too sure about the world he'd been born into. He cried as we placed him in the carseat between us. As we headed down the road, I pushed a well-worn reggae cassette into the player, the one we'd been bopping to on our journey to The Farm. Bob Marley's "Comin' in from the Cold" came on. Suddenly from Jake, silence. A look of pure recognition on his face as if to say, "They found me." Then he fell into his first deep sleep.

✤ Joel's Birth Story—July 6, 1973
By Kathleen Rosemary

We expected a July 4th baby and actually did start labor that day. David was almost finished sanding the floor on our new little house. We cleaned up and called the midwives, but they said the contractions weren't close enough yet. I was surprised when they said it was best for me to just keep moving around doing my household activities. I had a mental image that everyone was going to start fussing over me just because my uterus was flexing. I had compost to bury and flowers to tend and meals to cook, but my attention was certainly on my belly. Finally, by the next evening, we got some action, and Pamela and one of the other midwives started to ask me if I had anything to discuss, to get out in the open. Now, that was a shock. What did they mean?

When I started scratching around in my inner feelings and thoughts, I eventually came up with something. Deep inside I had hidden some fears about my new role as a mother and about David's willingness and emotional ability to support this new family. I had to verbalize these feelings, evidently, in order to free up my body to allow this baby to come out. Throughout the next few hours David and I were coached on how to talk to each other in a better way, and I felt that he made a shift. I learned for myself that complaining was counterproductive and that it created a different feeling in the energy than just stating my feelings and needs without blaming anyone.

I felt lots of uncomfortable sensations, such as being chilly in the cool summer evening, having my legs suddenly jerk now and then, and, of course, the pressure from the contractions. It felt like I was in boot camp, supposed to perform but struggling with my emotions and my body not cooperating. If I whined or moaned, my midwives lovingly encouraged me to change my attitude and try to experience the contractions as rushes of energy. At this time in my life, I had little awareness of energy and was mostly caught up in my belief that I really was uncomfortable and that I was supposed to complain like they do in the movies! To top it off, I felt bad that I wasn't having a rollicking grand time, like other Farm women had told me it would be.

This birthing turned out to be my first major proof that mind and body are one. As I felt David's shift and I worked on my own attitude, I was able to muster up some positive, loving statements to him about how much he and this baby meant to me. About the time my mouth opened and let out positively charged words, my cervix opened a lot more than before. We kept this up, in between paying attention to the contractions as "rushes" and the breathing as a way to ride the waves of energy. Now I knew what they meant by energy! It really did feel like waves coming over and through me, and I knew what a blessed event this was in my life. I experienced gratitude in a new way—for the midwives, for David, and for God to let me have a healthy baby.

Joel came out crying angrily, as if he was saying, "It's about time!" and we all laughed. I loved everyone in the room and started nursing right away.

Looking back twenty-three years to this event, I see that this experience taught me how very important our thoughts are in manifesting the reality we experience as "material." I had a new tool to use in observing the world, which I continue to use. In fact, my vocation is to teach people how to become aware of their thoughts, so they, too, can be the creators of their reality. I gave up complaining, because I saw how it caused me to be angry and blaming. Instead, I try to pay close attention to my thoughts through mindfulness practices. I insert positive, affirming, and grateful thoughts into the stream, and ride them like a raft on the white water of a turbulent mind.

The Magic of Life—March 13, 1990
By Tazio Qubeck

My stepmother, Nancy, is a doctor. She was working in Nashville three to four days a week when she was pregnant with my brother. She had to commute to work two hours away from our home in Waynesboro. Our family worked out a schedule where either my dad or I would drive her in to work, since she was way too pregnant to drive or travel by herself. The hectic lifestyle was beginning to wear on all of us when we got to the point where we had only one more week before she planned to begin her maternity leave.

It was my turn to go to Nashville with Nancy, and I was thinking about what would happen if she went into labor while I was with her. We had planned that she would beep me on her beeper if she started, and I would drive her to our home two hours away, where she wanted to have a home birth. Coincidentally, our excursion took place over the full moon, and I thought that might influence her to go into labor. I definitely felt that something big was about to happen. Luckily, we made it home all right, and everything seemed peaceful.

Steve, my dad, and Theron, my brother, had the kerosene lamps going and a wonderful trout and catfish dinner prepared from their fishing trip earlier that day. Everything seemed very comfortable and mellow, enhanced by the still-magical moon shining through the windows. I felt safe, finally, from the possibility of having to deal with the birth. On the way home, Nancy said that every bump we hit had caused a contraction. As I fell asleep that night, though, the birth was the last thing on my mind.

At six in the morning, I stirred from a deep sleep to hear commotion coming from downstairs. My aunt and cousin were running about, and I heard someone mention "the midwives from The Farm." Immediately, I knew what was going on. My mom was going into labor three weeks early. For at least five minutes I just lay in my bed and tried to come to grips with what was becoming reality. I had not yet come to terms with the idea of a baby in the house, much less watching the delivery. When I went downstairs, everything seemed like a dream, and I was absorbed in the preparations for the birth. The next thing I knew, Nancy was on her bed about to have the baby.

Although I felt a little nervous about seeing my first birth, I knew I would enjoy the whole thing. My job was to take pictures of the birth, so naturally I was very close during the delivery. At first, I had a hard time getting into the spirit of the birth and felt uncomfortable, but that feeling passed as time went on. I began to relax and feel more comfortable behind the lens. Everything seemed to be going smoothly, and I could see Nancy's belly metamorphosing in front of me. The baby was almost ready to come out.

This is when one of the most incredible experiences of my life occurred. I was standing at the foot of the bed when her water bag broke and soaked me from my belly down. Talk about a shock! I was so surprised, I didn't know what to do for a second. The feeling of hot and wet body fluid all over me could have made me sick, I suppose, but it didn't really bother me. I changed my clothes in a flash and went back to see the rest of the birth.

I don't imagine that too many people have been hit by the water bag breaking, but that is not why the experience is important to me. I feel that the energy that bonds parents and children touched me, creating a spiritual aspect to the whole occurrence between Nancy, the baby, and me. For a moment, I was caught up in the magic of life, and I am still in a state of euphoria three days later. Someone at the birth compared being soaked in the breaking water to being baptized, and it is definitely comparable. Being at a birth is a very magical experience. It brings life into a wonderful, realistic view. My unusual experience has stunned me and created something I can always look back upon to remember the intense life energy I felt. I'm not totally sure how this will affect me, but right now I feel thankful for my brother's health and our family's intensified closeness.

In 1974, in The Farm's first published book, Hey, Beatnik! This Is The Farm Book, *we midwives offered that women considering abortions could come to The Farm to give birth if they were interested in an alternative that included free care and the chance to either keep the baby or to leave it with foster parents. I did not feel that abortion should be illegal, but I suspected that some women would prefer another choice if it were available. Nearly three hundred women responded to our offer during the years when we were able to keep it open, including a number of women who weren't considering abortion but were in need of financial and/or emotional support. Rita, who tells her story below, was among this latter group.*

Harry's Birth—August 2, 1976

By Rita Winningham

I phoned The Farm in 1974 to ask one of the midwives if I could come there to have my baby. In a moment, I heard Mary Louise's kind voice telling me to come on down. It didn't take much encouragement. There I was in New York City, feeling very seduced and abandoned. Any song with a refrain of "He's gone and left me" would have me in tears. The other side of the story might be that I was just plain dumb.

Friends saw me moping around, not knowing where to go or what to do about delivering the baby, and suggested The Farm. Their description of it sounded like the answer to my prayers. Quickly, I got rid of silk dresses and high heels, overdue library books and cats. A friend drove me down to Tennessee.

Suddenly, there we were in deep country—the real thing. No Greenwich Village, no sidewalks and skyscrapers. Only trees and fields. I was quickly whisked from the gatehouse to a relatively small household (for The Farm at that time) known as "The Hutch." It housed three couples, seven small children, and one single mother. All of them were fun and friendly, honest, witty, and wise. I spent the first weeks learning how to bake rolls, biscuits, and corn bread, not to mention how to roll tortillas.

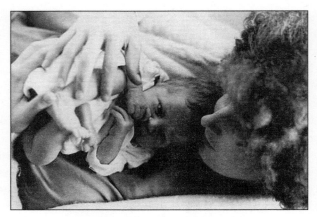

Rita and newborn Harry

Most important, I went to the prenatal clinic and was seen by the midwives. I was too ignorant of what I had gotten myself into to even know to be apprehensive about childbirth. I hadn't paid much attention to the stories that said it hurt. I totally accepted the Farm attitude that birth was a strengthening rite of passage for women. It made sense to me. The midwives, unafraid of confrontation, looked at me point-blank and told me that I had never done anything difficult in my life and that now I was in for it. That was all right. It was what I was there for.

The birthing stories in the early edition of *Spiritual Midwifery* created my concept of what would happen during the birthing process. I was especially moved by the tales in which a selfish, inconsiderate mate was transformed into a loving husband through seeing his wife in labor. It may seem naive, but I sent a copy of the book to my absent partner-in-crime, hoping to turn him into that sensitive prince. It didn't work. Nonetheless, the moving accounts of strong, brave women seemed worthy of emulation.

The people I lived with were endlessly kind, endlessly patient. What I deeply appreciated was that the married women freely let me chat with their husbands. Not to flirt, not to take anything away from them, but they allowed me the male companionship and attention that a woman like me requires. I thought then and I know now that it was incredibly generous of them.

One Sunday afternoon in early August, after I had gone on a long walk with one of the children to retrieve some cat food, Susan, a perceptive midwife, told me that my hour had come. Dilation had started but was not real advanced, and Susan and Mary Louise decided I could take a bath. It was while I was lounging in the warm water that the moment of truth came. It started to hurt—not any worse than strong gas pains, but it wasn't easy. I said to myself, "They didn't let you come here and feed you all these soybeans for you to make a conniption fit scene now. Get it together." And I did.

Just then I got a long-distance phone call from two friends back in New York. They gave me their blessings, and that helped immensely. Then I was brought to what would be my birth bed. It was dim and peaceful in the tiny loft. Four strong, kind women were in there with me, encouraging, gently laughing and teasing. Mary Louise said the magic words that made all the difference to me in labor: "You are being so good to this baby."

She meant that a reasonably calm deportment made for a better delivery, but with those words she erased a lot of the doubt and worry that a single mother can feel.

I bobbed up and down on the contraction waves. During the ebb tides, I would fall asleep for a few seconds, and in those brief spaces of time I was able to work through a lot of my feelings of attachment to the baby's father. I got to a stage when I felt totally unmoored from all that I had known, spinning in the cosmos. I said, "When do I get to the time when I'm supposed to throw up and get angry?"—which is how transition had been described to me. The midwives laughed and said, "You are in it now."

Then I got to the true labor part of the whole business—the pushing. Normally not at a loss for words, I found myself grunting out, "Me no talk now me push." Mary Louise's liberal use of anointing oil and deft massage made it all easy. I kept thinking, She's doing all the work. Then Harry, my boy, my angel, eased into the world gently, slowly, graciously. Greeted with enthusiasm and approval, he looked with fully alert, conscious eyes at his world. I basked in approval. My housemates—who had fully expected me to freak out and cause many a scene throughout labor, because I had been such a nervous, speedy critter coming into this new world in the woods—were amazed at what a mellow baby producer I turned out to be. Supported by so much loving, kind attention, I could not allow myself to be anything else.

I am convinced that due to all of the goodness and warmth that supported and nourished me throughout this time, my boy, Harry, was born into a real state of grace. It shaped his character from the very beginning. I am so grateful for that community ethos.

Jeanne Madrid is a Florida licensed midwife.

✗ Mulci's Birth—October 13, 1974
By Jeanne Madrid, LM

My first baby was born during the early years of The Farm. After spending a loving Saturday afternoon with each other, Mark and I topped it off with a long, warm bath together. After all that smooching and soaking, I started feeling a tingling sensation in my lower back. It wasn't long until it became stronger. I decided it was time to call my good friend, Mary Louise, one of our community midwives. She warned me the labor would probably pick up and continue to get stronger and reassured me I would be able to bear it. She was right.

She suggested that we all try to get some rest, since it was evening and we probably had the night ahead of us. It was quite comforting to curl up next to my man, listening to the sound of the woodstove crackling. We must have fallen sound asleep. Sometime around midnight, I awoke to the power of the contractions coming on stronger and stronger. Mary Louise checked me again internally. She was surprised and delighted to inform me that I was almost ready to push.

She called Ina May to check in with her, since the midwives worked in teams. While waiting for the midwives to arrive, I became nauseated, which is quite common in the transitional stage. Mary Louise and Mark continued comforting me. I tried focusing on all the other women around the world in labor with me. I just knew I wasn't the only one.

I don't remember having a strong urge to push. I do remember pushing and puking a lot. As horrible as it sounds, vomiting has its purpose. A good dry heave pulls the cervix open and pushes the baby down, but not enough to get the baby out.

Most of the night I was pushing in a semiseated position, pulling my knees back. Mark and Mary Louise took turns supporting me from the back. All night long: push, puke, push, puke. Anything the midwives suggested, I would attempt, but sometimes I was reluctant, just because I was plain tired. I wasn't exhausted, but I was tired. Everyone wanted me to squat. Oh, that hurt. They all cheered me on as I squatted. Ina May and Mary Louise continued to check for progress in the descent of the baby into my pelvic bones. Little by little, I made progress.

At one point, Ina May suggested that I not be so poised. She wanted me to be more athletic and to try speaking in a lower tone of voice. Okay, I thought. I used to be a competitive swimmer, and I was good at long-distance races. Now I remembered some of my training as a swimmer: to stay in control by getting my energy together, to set a pace, and to haul ass the last lap. I knew I could sing either soprano or alto in the church choir, so I chose to be an alto as the baby was being born. I shifted gears and kept on going throughout the night.

At dawn I thought, All right, the sun is up, and I've had enough. Is there an end to this? Just go ahead and cut me open and help get my baby out. Oops! I'm complaining. I know that will get me nowhere.

Someone gave me a striped peppermint candy, and it stayed down. Mark and the midwives continued to massage the tension out of my body. A little bit of sugar and love can go a long way.

Then I heard Ina May mention she would need to leave soon to pick up her husband. That was it. I decided to have the baby before she left. I

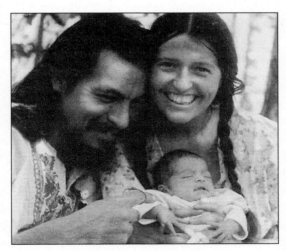

Mark, Jeanne, and Mulci

was determined. As I pushed with all my strength, she was inside me, pushing as hard as she could with both hands to help open my pelvis. Mark and I can both remember hearing my pelvic bones squeaking open with that push. The baby's head kept moving down, and the midwives cheered with every push: "We can see the baby's head. We love you. Look, you can see your baby's head in the mirror."

At last, I, too, could see her head, and I could feel its warmth with my hand. What a glorious feeling and sight. She was real. I burned, but I didn't care. I was so happy. Ina May helped the burning sensation by oiling her hands and supporting my stretching tissues with them.

With the next contraction, I took a big breath, grabbed my knees, threw my head back, and roared as loud as I could. Her head was coming out. Mark picked my head up just in time to see her body come barreling out. A girl, just as I thought. It was the greatest sensation in all my life. She was so beautiful and sweet. The midwives swaddled her with tender care and assured us that she was fine. In a short moment, she was cuddled in my arms. She was so perfect and so strong. All of that long labor was worth it.

The midwives watched over us until they were sure we were both stable and comfortable. Mark and I took a nap with our precious baby cuddled between us. We stroked her soft, fuzzy head as we fell asleep. When we awoke, we found that her head was miraculously quite round. It was Sunday, and we had been blessed. We named her Mulci, after Mark's great-grandmother.

◦❧ Robin's Birth—July 24, 1983
By Suzy Jenkins Viavant

We moved to The Farm two months before my son was born. I decided to have my baby there because, previous to my marriage, I had been a member of The Farm community and had spent my late teenage years surrounded by children who were born naturally. All of my friends had delivered their children naturally.

When labor began about 1:00 A.M., I woke up with serious contractions and told Chris to call the midwives. Ruth came immediately and started setting up the bed. Pamela, my good friend and midwife, was also there giving me coaching and her support. My water bag broke as I was dry-heaving, something I had done throughout the pregnancy.

At about eight centimeters, I was wishing I had never gotten into this. Then I realized I had to keep my attention on staying open, from my mind all the way through to my cervix, so that I would be like a hollow tunnel for the energy of life to pass through.

All I wanted to do was push and do something about my situation. I was determined to have the baby fast, because I did not want to push in the middle of a Tennessee heat wave. I wanted to have him before the day got hot. Chris helped by sitting behind me with his knuckles wedged in the small of my back as I leaned into him. He rubbed and kept the contractions coming on strong. I had invited all of my best friends to my "coming out" party, but my main attention was on Ina May while she kept checking me, breathing with me, and updating me on my progress. She was a great coach and told me to trust my body and that it wouldn't do anything it couldn't handle.

Pamela also gave me good advice by telling me to blow out from my diaphragm with each contraction to lessen the amount of pressure on my back. When I reached ten centimeters two hours later, I was ready to push. I worked incredibly hard for forty-five minutes. Finally when Robin's head came out, he was awake and looking around. The midwives wanted to give me a look at his head in the mirror. I was in such a hurry to get relief, I just wanted to push, and out he came with a big splash. They laid him on my belly, and Chris cut the cord. He lay there looking up at me, then holding his dad's finger. We all lay timeless in awe of the amazing journey we had just gone through, preparing for the amazing journey we were embarking upon for life.

❧ Vanessa's Birth—January 21, 1990
By Suzy Jenkins Viavant

After we had Robin on The Farm, we moved out west. I would have loved to return to The Farm to deliver Vanessa, but it was not practical for us at the time. After having my first baby in a cabin out in the woods of Tennessee, I was frightened about having my second baby in a hospital, especially because I had such a great experience with my first birth. I missed the trusting relationship I had had with my midwives. Although I would be delivering with a midwife at Kaiser, there would be no telling which midwife would be on call at the time of labor. This seemed to make it impossible to establish a relationship of trust.

Because we had just started on the medical program, my first visit with their midwife was only three weeks prior to my delivery. By the time I was dilated three centimeters, I had met only one midwife from the group. I had no feeling of security, not knowing who would attend my birth. I was afraid of having to fight tooth and nail against having an enema or an I.V. I especially did not want to be moved from a labor room to a delivery room while the baby's head was crowning. I knew from my first baby how impatient I would feel at that point.

While preparing to have our baby, we took a natural birthing class. During the class, we introduced ourselves and talked about how we had our first baby. When we said we'd had our baby out in a cabin in the woods of Tennessee after a labor of only three hours, we shocked everyone. The teacher announced that it was not "normal" to have a first baby that quickly and told the others not to expect that. She seemed to drill it into their heads that labor would be a very painful, long, and traumatic experience. I was glad that I had a previous experience so I knew it could be different. If I hadn't known better, I might have believed her. I think it would have made me uptight to be expecting the worst.

Labor began with the breaking of my water. There were no contractions. I called the hospital, feeling depressed, because my baby shower was scheduled for the following day. I asked if I had to come in, telling them I was having no labor pains. They said yes and that I should be prepared to stay.

An hour later, I started feeling light, periodlike cramps. We headed for the hospital. When they examined me, they said it was a good thing I had come in, because I was eight centimeters dilated. I still was having only light contractions. The baby's head was still high up the birth canal. I asked for the alternative birthing room, but they said they would have to qualify me first. My nurse, Alicia, came in the room and asked if I had delivered my first baby on The Farm. I said yes and asked how she knew. She had noticed on my chart that I had no previous hospitalization and that I had delivered in Summertown, Tennessee, so she put two and two together. I asked how she knew about The Farm, and she said she had been studying Ina May's book, *Spiritual Midwifery*. She said it had been her salvation throughout her years of studying nursing, preparatory to becoming a nurse–midwife. She now knew just what kind of care I was accustomed to, so she got me right into the alternative birthing room. She told the midwife about me, and they never tried to give me an enema or an I.V. I was immensely relieved not to have to fight about how I wanted to deliver my baby. I'm sure it made my delivery more relaxed, which, in turn, made it faster and more enjoyable.

At midnight, I had a moving sensation. Chris got Alicia, who said I was ten centimeters. I could hear the midwife in the next room yelling, "Push! Push!" to someone. I then told Alicia that I wasn't going to wait for the midwife and that I felt perfectly fine about her catching the baby. By this time I had developed a very trusting relationship with her. She said, "Well, that's just what is going to happen, so give us a little push." I started pushing, and then the midwife ran into the room, washed her hands, and caught the baby after only three pushes. A girl, born at four minutes after midnight! I had been hoping for a girl. Chris and I were so thrilled. Even though she weighed eight pounds five ounces and was born with her elbow and arm above her head, I didn't tear at all. She was beautiful, with jet black hair, and she looked like an Eskimo baby. They let her stay next to me for almost an hour before giving her a bath, so we had plenty of time for bonding. She remained in the room with us all night, and we checked out in the morning.

Alicia and the midwife both commented that they thought my attitude enabled me to have an easy birth and that they wished all their birthings went so smoothly. I attribute my attitude to living on The Farm, around children who were born naturally, among people who considered birth to be a normal, natural process.

✤ Lois's Story—May 7, 1977
By Lois Stephens

I credit daily visualization during my pregnancies for much of the reason why I was able to have fast, easy births. Every night as I was falling asleep, especially during the third trimester, I would picture the changes my body would need to go through for my cervix to open. (I was fairly well informed about the physical process of labor.) I would lie in bed, imagine being in labor, and imagine encouraging the sensations and welcoming the opening process. I would picture the baby's head pressing on the cervix and the cervix steadily opening. I had also learned from living on The Farm about the power of words, so I knew that when I was in labor, I could say "I just want to open up" or "I can integrate this" and that reality would sometimes follow the statement.

I was incredibly lucky to have lived on The Farm during those days when so many babies were being born, because I was friends with so many women who celebrated their birth experiences, and that was the only reality I knew. I did not have to sift through the confused and unrealistic subliminal messages women these days receive from the media, family, friends, and casual acquaintances. I never felt any fear of the home birthing process, although I did fear hospital birth.

I trusted the midwives implicitly. It is very important to trust your midwife or care provider. It is also important to have only people that you know and trust at the birth and not to be close when you're in labor with people whom you don't know or trust.

When my labor began, the rushes came on, one after another, like waves. They would get heavier and heavier and build up to a peak and then slip off a little and then build up again. I kept thinking things like, I want this to get heavier. This is for my baby. I want to open up. As soon as I learned to integrate one level, it would get heavier. Right then I'd have to stretch more to integrate the next rush. I couldn't space out at all.

As I was only three centimeters dilated, Mary left to spend a little time with her husband and said she would be back later. One of the midwife assistants stayed with me. Next time she checked me, I had gone from three to seven centimeters, so we called Mary right away. It took my complete attention to integrate the rushes by breathing as slowly and deeply as possible. When I did it right, the rushes didn't hurt but felt strong and pure.

Mary soon returned. She told me I should let Thomas touch my body more. She noticed I was a little irritable with him about that. I said "Yeah," and everyone laughed. I was grateful these beautiful women were helping me through this remarkable experience.

At one point Mary said, "This is the heaviest part," and I thought if this was the heaviest part, I could handle it. I started feeling like pushing before I was fully dilated. I leaned forward. Soon I could feel the baby's head enter the birth canal. My body just took over when I started pushing, and I loved it! Great, low grunts came from my throat while I pushed. I didn't even try to make the sounds. It wasn't long before they could see his head coming down.

His face eased out, and his mouth was wide open. I took a good look at him. After Mary checked for the cord, I just pushed, and he slid right out. I could hardly wait to hold him. Then he was on my belly. I put my hands on him, and waves of love flowed everywhere. I looked down at him, and he grinned. I felt lucky and happier than I had ever been.

✆ Climbing Out of Despair
*By Charmaine O'Leary**

My pregnancy tale started several years before my first daughter was born. I was spending my last free summer before leaving for graduate school vacationing in Vermont. The best part of the summer was spent living in a tree house with a wonderful man who was teaching me Italian. I had always been impeccable about my birth control before, but somehow I got sloppy and found myself knowing beyond a shadow of a doubt that I was newly yet definitely pregnant.

The thought of bringing a baby into the world at this point in my life was out of the question for me, yet I also felt the presence of the baby with me as I made my way south to see about my abortion. Somewhere in the back of my mind, I must have been having conversations with the baby. My hopes and dreams were that someday I would find a tribe of like-minded people who knew about babies, and I would try again to bring this baby down. I really hoped it worked this way, because the pain of having to arrange for the abortion was unbearable.

It worked out just exactly as I had wanted it to. Directly after graduate school I began teaching at the university. Some of my close friends in the graduate film department had heard about an intuitive community where people spoke the truth, ate vegetarian food, and birthed their own babies. I wasted no time in traveling to The Farm and joining the community.

I met my future husband on that first visit. He seemed intense and passionate, and we started dating soon after I moved to the community. I remember seeing many sides to him, including the angry young boy, yet I felt so very fancy and self-confident, because I had somehow conjured up this fabulous community of my dreams. Nothing

*A pseudonym.

could go wrong, I thought. I was on a roll, and besides, I thought, I could help him change.

We got pregnant right away, and I remember feeling so blessed to be carrying a baby. We were three months pregnant and visiting with my in-laws when it became apparent that my baby's father and I had very different lifestyle visions. Our relationship became a struggle from this time on.

The Farm midwives seemed to be very tuned in to the fact that the relationship was shaky. Yet this was only one of several things I was in denial about; the previous abortion was the other. The pregnancy went smoothly, but along with the baby's growth was a strange, haunting feeling of not being worthy or prepared for the task of child-rearing.

The birthing itself was a delightful break in what had become constant misunderstandings and hassling. The twelve hours of labor were for me a magical time of feeling connected. I had a strong sense of being linked to every other woman who had ever given birth before me. I wondered at each transition how elastic and powerful my bodily changes were as they revealed themselves.

The midwives slept in the back of our cozy school bus, and I felt their sweet presence. It was as if angels were afoot. All I had to do was trust the fact that I could handle what my body was presenting, and all would be well. I spent most of the night while everyone slept imagining I was meditating in a field of mosquitoes that were biting. It is interesting to me that we tend to pull on strengths that we have previously proved to ourselves. One never knows what will get you through.

Pushing the baby out became a huge party. The three midwives and my husband mooed loudly like cows with each push, and they got me mooing too, which was a lot of fun. The baby came out rather blue and limp. As my midwife jiggled and played with her, I felt that she might not be all right. I became completely detached from my body at this point, and what I saw next, I experienced from above, looking down. My beautiful midwife gracefully bent over my child and puffed two gentle breaths into her mouth. She filled with life in an instant, and her body turned from blue to pink from her heart first, then radiated the color change out to her extremities.

Much to everyone's surprise, the child who was not even breathing a few seconds before seemed intensely alert. She seemed to crane her head to look at everyone in the room. I remember telling everyone present not to rush to clean her up. I wanted to savor the moment, complete with birthing fluids, for as long as I could. We stayed for a long time in that state. I remember feeling an amazing amount of gratitude that I had been fortunate enough to find the very few people in this country who understood the sacrament of a home birth.

Postpartum depression was rare on The Farm. I think the midwives' attentive care in the weeks after birth helped prevent it. I experienced an acute case of postpartum depression that began about seven months after my child's birth. (I was not on The Farm at the time it began.) I tell our story to lend encouragement to anyone who may be going through this. It is a very frightening, yet completely curable disease.

I have always been a strongly intuitive person. I have great trust in my intuition, and it has always served me well. In fact, I like to put myself in adventurous situations that would stretch my intuition muscles, such as hitchhiking to far-off places, taking long trips to Europe and beyond by myself, and even riding an occasional freight train. Life is a great adventure, meant to be trusted and tasted deeply.

I would never have imagined not trusting that small voice inside. It had always seemed so right. Yet, at the time after my baby was born, certain circumstances led me to listen to a voice that was really misguiding me. This voice was angry, mean, and full of darkness. I think a lot of my inability to detect the fact that I was misguided had to do with the fact that, because I had killed my first baby through the abortion, I really did not feel worthy of being a mother. I felt that my own baby was going to be taken from me as punishment. All of this was subconscious at the time, because I literally never thought about the abortion until many years later.

I started becoming withdrawn. As this critical voice grew to huge proportions in my head, I started to believe that I was hearing the voice of God. Yet God was telling me to do awful things to my baby. I remember many a night holding my baby in complete terror while a loud, inner voice railed at me to trust God and bring harm to my dear little girl. I could tell no one about this desperate battle that was raging in my head for months and months. My own mother came to visit me and was horrified by the shape I was in. The outward appearances of the illness were mostly just a very terrifying look in the eye and a stiff way of moving and reacting, but my mother knew something was terribly wrong. She kept saying, "You are not yourself."

I kept my secret of inner torment and clung to my baby for dear life. After months and months of relentless guilt, I decided to take my own life. Then, at least, I would not bring harm to my baby. I ended up visiting a mental institution after this attempt—luckily—failed. It was here that an inmate pointed out that my marriage seemed to her like a complete failure and why didn't I strike out on my own and just be free of it? This comment broke one of my big denial issues, and when I faced just one of them, I was able to start climbing out of despair.

The journey back to health was long and difficult. I needed help for my baby; a kind couple watched her for me for a while, and she thrived in their care. I was brought to a household where people really believed that the personality can change, and I started changing myself just a little bit every day. I told myself that every day was my birthday, and I was a new being. I did a lot of sweeping floors and domestic tasks so I would be on the side that was helping, even if it was only in a small way. Finally, I learned again to discriminate and identify negative thoughts and cut them away from my mind. After months of slicing away this cruel critic from my mind, progress was made. I read up on nutrition and discovered I had a B vitamin deficiency. Correcting this helped a lot.

An interesting reward came from having lived through such a frightening illness: I could tell if a woman was experiencing postpartum depression. I have been able to work with women in this state quite well, because I feel I am living proof that it is curable. One phrase that seems to get a suffering woman's attention is to ask her if she is experiencing the "mythic plane." This is a place where the battle of good and evil takes place at all times. God and the devil are very real entities on this plane of reality. Directions to get out of this mythic plane have to do with willpower. The problem is that most people have no language to describe this experience. Another problem is that it can be seductively interesting, and some women I've met actually prefer it to reality, because it can be entertaining and a bit magical. These women need to be reasoned with and talked out of this idea, for their own sake and for the sake of their children.

The final healing of my illness came years later. My daughter was eight years old and watching me as I was bathing. She happened to ask me if I had had any other children before her. I told her honestly about the abortion. To my surprise, she very simply said, "Mom, that was me." I remember feeling the hair rise on my arms as I begged her forgiveness. She hugged me and told me very casually that it was all fine, I just hadn't found the right time to have her yet. I felt a strange relief that night as she left the bathroom.

✕ Travelers

Most of the people who traveled from another state to give birth at The Farm Midwifery Center originally made plans for care closer to home. The fact that well-informed, intelligent people will make such drastic changes in plan during pregnancy gives some indication that there is still not much choice available in how women give birth in many areas of the United States. The following stories were written by those who, for a variety of reasons, decided it was worthwhile to travel to a birthplace where they could feel secure.

Our rule of thumb in guiding women through labor is to let the mother choose her own way of giving birth. We midwives don't have a favorite position in which the mother should labor or give birth. Now and then a mother will choose a position that does not favor progress in labor, and only then do we advise her to find a position that will keep her progressing before she reaches the point of exhaustion.

✕ Sebastian's Birth—July 12, 1986
By Ellen Coss

I remember waking to the feeling of being adrift at sea. I glanced at the clock: 4:15 in the morning, and another wave crashed in. Five minutes later, the sensation reached a peak, and it dawned on me that my labor had finally begun.

I woke up Tom and called Deborah, hurriedly trying to collect myself. All I could think of was the baby I was soon to meet. Deborah arrived and prescribed activity. Tom and I walked to the swimming hole, played a little basketball, and tried not to look too excited about being in early labor.

By evening my labor was going ahead at full steam. I was still walking, but there was a stomp in my step now. I would storm about a bit and then lean heavily on Tom or throw myself down face-first on the couch.

Around midnight Deborah left to get some things, and Tom fell asleep. Left to my own devices, I prowled aimlessly, eventually heading for the bathtub, where I sat, hot water pouring over my body. When Deborah returned, I got on the bed, and she gave me a back rub, which soothed me into a semisleep state.

Soon enough I was back in the tub with Deborah guarding me. I was so punchy that she was worried that I might fall asleep in the tub. Eventually I felt calm enough to try once more to sleep. So, armed with a heating pad for my back, I went to bed and, indeed, to sleep.

Around three in the morning, my water bag broke. I was so astounded by the rushing fluid that I danced about. Even more astonishing was the intensity of my labor once the bag was broken. My first instinct was to crouch in bed on my hands and knees, my face buried in the pillows. Deborah, however, had other plans. She sent me walking the halls, pausing only for encouragement and thigh massages by her and Tom. Around this time, Joanne showed up to relieve Deborah. She and Tom tried to keep me sane while I howled, growled, and walked.

By the time I was eight and a half centimeters open, I wanted to push. Joanne said that my cervix was swollen and that I shouldn't push until she gave me the word. Deborah woke up at this point and took over monitoring me. Ina May also came in and gave me some strength. They all told me to keep my face relaxed, my eyes open, with my lips flapping while I exhaled during the most intense moments. I felt like a camel, but the technique really works. As I looked into their eyes, we would breathe calmly as one, and the discomfort would fade. They all brought me a great deal of courage.

Suddenly it was time to push. What a glorious feeling! I was so glad to be doing something. I ran around like a crazy person for a while and then squatted next to the bed. After two or three good pushes, I leapt up onto the bed. I felt as though I was going to split in two, but for some reason it didn't seem to matter. All that mattered was getting the baby out.

I watched in a mirror as a little purple bulge emerged and grew into an enormous head, all covered with dark hair. The baby's shoulders came out together, instead of one at a time, but because of my position (hands and knees), he did not get stuck. Suddenly the whole baby slipped out—a healthy boy, all parts intact.

Somehow they got me all arranged, baby in my arms. I searched for something momentous to say, but no words came, only a ceaseless joy, the sort that sets the soul ablaze with love for our boy: Sebastian.

☙ Moment of a Miracle—December 23, 1986
By Rebecca Salonsky

When I first discovered I was pregnant, I went to my gynecologist. I was excited and had lots of questions about giving birth. I wanted to know the percentages of episiotomies and cesarean sections that he had performed. He didn't know offhand, but I pressed him to venture a guess. With sixty-six percent C-sectioned and eighty percent episiotomied, I could relate to a scared chicken just before processing. Naturally, I began looking for an alternative.

After a couple of visits to The Farm, I had all the confidence I needed in my midwives and natural childbirth. They were genuinely interested in me, and I remembered how the obstetrician had seemed bored with my enthusiasm and offended when I questioned his routine.

Meanwhile, during my seventh month, I visited my sister, who works with a gynecologist. She asked me to come in for an ultrasound so she and my mother could know the gender of the baby. I clearly didn't want to know, but agreed to it if they wouldn't tell me. It turns out that they couldn't determine the gender anyway; the baby was breech and very large, they said. My family panicked.

When I returned to Tennessee, Joanne said calmly, "We'll give you some exercises to help turn the baby. If that doesn't work, we'll try to turn the baby manually." I was reassured, and the baby turned from my doing the tilt position.

The baby was due on December 23. I lost my mucus plug on the 20th and called Joanne. She told me to take my time but to come on down to settle in for the night. We did, and Deborah checked me out. The next day Pamela stayed with us. My rushes felt strong, but I wasn't opening up and my water hadn't broken. I needed to pee and couldn't. Finally, on the 23rd, they called the doctor to see if they should catheterize me. Just the mention of that did it! I peed.

Labor came on really strong, and they broke my water. What a relief! I felt like I'd had the baby already. They prepared me for transition so well, I never felt like I was going through it. The support I felt from my husband, Stephen, and the ladies was incredible. During a rush I felt like I was falling from a very high place at a rapid rate. When I'd ask Stephen to catch me, we would kiss, and it felt like he had put a big balloon underneath me to slow my fall.

At 7:32 at night, Taylor popped out with his eyes wide open. He was beautiful and alert. He wasn't upset until Joanne had to clear his air passages, but he quickly calmed down again. He just had to let everyone know he was numbered among the living. He even held his head up and smiled a little. They laid him on top of me and Stephen cut the cord—giving Taylor a life of his own. I felt so strong, primeval, and powerful. I experienced a trust in my own body that I'd never known before. While they took care of Taylor, I took a shower so I'd be clean to nurse him. No episiotomy, of course.

I'll never forget the song that was playing during my labor: "Morning with Roses." We had candlelight and champagne to welcome our little angel, who came out headfirst, at a very social hour, weighing only six pounds ten ounces on his due date, and rating a 9/10 on his Apgar score. Our pediatrician said babies are lucky to score a seven in hospitals.

But mostly, I'll never forget the sound of the gentle rain on the roof. It reminded me to be still and quiet in the moment of a miracle. I was, and it felt very holy.

Annah's Story—May 28, 1992
By Lais Sonkin

We are from Brazil. We came to the United States as tourists in 1990. We wanted to take a break from our jobs to see the world. We sold our house, bought a motor home in Miami, and began traveling. What we did not plan was my pregnancy.

Mauricio and I had been together for a long time already. He was forty-six, and I thirty-six. I was very happy, but it seemed that this would force us to go back home, and I didn't want to. I never thought I could combine having a baby with the lifestyle we were living in our motor home. After all, one of the biggest reasons we decided we could travel was that we didn't have kids!

We started my prenatal care every month, and everything seemed to be going fine. However, things weren't very relaxed. First, the attitudes and practices of U.S. obstetricians were not familiar to me. In my country you go to the doctor, who will see you when you have an appointment. He asks you questions, keeps his records on you, checks your blood pressure and the rest. He is the one who is there all the time, whether he is taking blood pressure or talking to you. In other words, he spends some time with you.

In the United States, whenever I went to an obstetrician when I was pregnant, I had to fill out a questionnaire and then see a nurse. Only then would I see a doctor for the few minutes when he would look at the questionnaire. Then I would go down a corridor with many doors. On each of the doors I would see charts with patients' files hanging there. When we got to an empty room, the nurse would show me the door. Then I would undress and lie there on the table until the nurse came back to take my blood pressure or whatever was necessary, while the doctor was consulting with another patient. I could hear all the doors opening and closing and the voices of the other people as I lay there. Finally the doctor would come back again, check me out, and leave again. Then the nurse would come back. I would then get dressed and wait again to see the doctor back in his office. I didn't like the arrangement at all; it was so impersonal, so unkind.

In Los Angeles when I was five months pregnant, I had a checkup and the doctor scared me. He recommended that I have some tests, because of my "advanced age," he said. He thought I should have amniocentesis and a screening for Tay-Sachs, since my husband and I are both Jewish. The doctor was cold, and so was the hospital where he sent us. He did the amniocentesis, and the baby was normal, as far as could be seen. But the episode alerted us, and I started to worry about all sorts of things, from the vibrations of traveling in our motor home and my age to the lack of continuous contact with someone during pregnancy.

At first I was planning to have my baby in a hospital somewhere. But I found myself homesick, missing my friends and wishing to find a better place than the emergency room of some hospital to have my baby. I was afraid of the injections and medications I would be given in a hospital. I had been in a hospital once before, and I had suffered both physically and emotionally.

Two months later, while we were in Louisiana, we remembered The Farm and got the idea to visit it, since we were within a few hundred miles of it. I had read *Spiritual Midwifery* a long time before and had been impressed by it. The Farm experience was famous, and many of my friends and I had dreamed of living in a community like The Farm. I remember that we in Brazil had looked at the pictures more than we read the stories.

I did telephone The Farm and got permission to come for a prenatal visit when I was seven months pregnant. Sometimes in life we forget our dreams, so it is really great when we have an opportunity to recapture them.

When Mauricio and I entered The Farm gate, we immediately felt comfortable. There was something in the air that felt new and friendly. Somebody immediately stopped their car and said hello, and that is something that does not happen very many times in the United States. At first we had come just to have a look, to visit the clinic, and to talk to the midwives. My husband had absolutely decided that we should have the baby in a hospital. I was not so determined as he was, but I did care about the safety of our child, and going to the hospital is what naturally came to my mind when I was thinking of giving birth.

We camped by the pond near the gate, went to the clinic twice, and met some people. As we relaxed, we started changing our minds. We met all of the midwives: Ina May, Pamela, Deborah, and Joanne, and we found out that we had been making a big deal out of bearing a child, while at The Farm, everybody—not just the midwives—is "professional" about this act. The people of The Farm showed us how simple things can be. In fact, that is the first gift the midwives gave us: They made it be simple.

We knew that in a U.S. hospital we could have all the technology we wanted. But I also knew that I would never have what I really needed in such a hospital: professional care combined with the friendship and compassion I found in the midwives. They made each prenatal visit enjoyable. The waiting room is a happy place, where people talk and laugh, everyone compares bellies, and you can feel the good vibrations. Even in the consultation room, you find the same climate of laughter. I don't mean to be sexist, but it was much easier for me to have something as intimate as prenatal checkups done by women who had had babies themselves. This fact also made it easy to expose my questions and fears to them in a way I could never have done with an obstetrician.

We decided to rent a little house on The Farm for two months, and we began preparing our nest for the birth. We made friends with the

Cramers and the Gavins, some Farm people who had had their babies at home. It was nice to see their healthy, beautiful kids. The kids themselves were very familiar with babies. They told us the stories about the children they had all taken care of—the adopted ones, the handicapped ones, and the thousands of births. I was enchanted when I realized that the whole community of The Farm is a birthing center.

My contractions—but I like the word the people here use: *rushes*—started at 3:15 in the morning. Mauricio was right beside me, helping me through the waves of differing intensity. When they became stronger, I had to go to the toilet every fifteen minutes. Sitting there during the rushes was more comfortable. When they started coming stronger and closer together, we called Pamela. It was 6:00 A.M. I wanted her to have a good night's sleep, and I wasn't feeling bad. She came and checked me out. Pamela is great, because it seems that she is always smiling.

"You are fully dilated," she said, after checking me for the first time. "Today you will have your baby."

I remember my surprise at hearing this, because I had had little rushes so often during my last month of pregnancy and thought they meant the baby was coming. I kept asking Pamela if she was sure. Soon Ina May and Deborah arrived.

The midwives work beautifully as a team. The three of them were around me, but they did not invade the tiny space of our bed. They were so good. They massaged me and cleaned me. I drank water, which was wonderful, because I am thirsty all the time, and I had been told at the hospital that they don't allow you to drink while you are in labor. The midwives talked to me in low, warm voices. While it wasn't dark in our room, we kept the lights turned to the minimum. I felt respected. I was incredibly sensitive to sounds, to lights, and everything else, and they understood all that. I didn't have to make any sacrifice while in labor and was able to take any position I wanted. When I began pushing hard, the midwives massaged me and helped me stay relaxed.

Suddenly, my baby was there, first in Ina May's hands and then in Mauricio's hands. He put her on my breast that sunny spring morning. This was the most wonderful emotion I had experienced in my life. Annah was born. I will be forever grateful to the midwives. Annah stayed in my arms. I couldn't let her go, and the midwives understood that. Nobody took her to wash her. Nobody carried her away. I didn't have to sleep. We stayed together, Mauricio, Annah, and I. Pamela, Deborah, and Ina May were there too, for a little while, but they were not there as staff members doing their duty, but as my friends, the midwives—just like the pictures in *Spiritual Midwifery*.

Sue and Chris Topf went through more adventures than most couples in traveling to The Farm to give birth to their first baby. They had no way of knowing that they would reach us in time for the birth, because they planned to cross the Atlantic on the Fri, *a small sailing ship. Before leaving Amsterdam, where I was visiting, I provided them with a small kit of essential supplies, in case their baby should be born at sea. We were all happy that Sue made it across the Atlantic and all the way to Tennessee still pregnant.*

Sue approached her first birth in a very flowing and instinctive way. Somehow it seemed that sailing across the Atlantic had been an excellent way of preparing for childbirth. Her slim body had presaged a short, intense labor, the kind that can be painful and frightening if the mother is apprehensive. (Thin women don't seem to have the muscle mass to resist what labor is trying to do that sturdier women have. Of course, there are always exceptions.) Sue never seemed afraid, though. Maybe her experience as a member of a sailing crew made her able to give her trust to us and the birthing process. Or maybe her having lived so close to the elements for the previous several months put her in tune with nature and her own instincts. Whatever it was, I remember being impressed with how well she "put her nose to the wind" and how little direction she needed to get through her labor. Chris's constant attention clearly helped Sue have a calm and beautiful labor. This birth had not been their first adventure together!

❧ Lisa's Birth—April 22, 1983
By Sue and Chris Topf

Sue: Our home, a community afloat in the form of a 115-foot sailing ship, was to act as a cargo courier for The Farm's international aid agency, Plenty (www.plenty.org), which was then delivering relief equipment to communities in the Caribbean. As we worked to prepare the ship for its journey from Europe to the United States, Chris and I discovered, to our delight, that I was pregnant.

We had met Ina May in Amsterdam, Holland, and had spoken to her about The Farm's birthing work. We contacted her in Tennessee, and it was soon arranged that we would have the baby there and become landlubbers for a few months while the ship did her Caribbean trip.

As a result of various delays and setbacks in the preparation of the ship for sea and spending many days becalmed in the gloriously hot mid-Atlantic, we arrived in the United States somewhat later than expected, only three weeks before Lisa's due date. It was another ten days before we were able to arrange transport to The Farm. When we arrived, it was with a big sigh of relief that we had come to the end of a long journey, ready to meet our baby.

We felt well prepared for the birth. At sea we had always faced the possibility of a crisis that we would have to deal with ourselves. Our copy of *Spiritual Midwifery* was well-worn from its use as a reference book by ourselves and some of our crewmates, who also wanted to be prepared, just in case! To be on The Farm and surrounded by midwives was a great luxury.

Two days before my due date I was experiencing a remarkable, heightened sense of awareness—colors seemed brighter, crisp and clear. I was feeling dreamy and soft. It was no great surprise when, shortly after we went to bed, I started rushing regularly.

My memory of the birth has no time sequence but is a jumble of great excitement, riding high on the rushes like a ship in full sail enjoying a fair-weather gale with a competent crew and a good suit of sails!

Chris: As Sue's labor intensified, time really lost all of its meaning. We cuddled up close, and I rubbed her back and the delicious belly, which erupted into quakes, making her navel point to high heaven. We welled into each other's arms and floated away on the waves of contractions. Ina May checked Sue's dilation and found her cervix thinning out and opening. She sent for Katsi, a Mohawk midwife who was visiting at the time, and Lidewij, a young Dutch midwifery graduate, both friends whom we had invited to attend the birth. Now the contractions were coming strong and regular, and Ina May advised me to get behind Sue, who was sitting on the bed. This way Sue could relax into my embrace, and I would rub her lower back, belly, or thighs as I felt each rush to be easing, or as Sue would let me know with a squeeze on my legs. It felt just too good to be true.

Gradually the contractions increased in force and some in duration, and, while exhaling, Sue started blowing bubbles through her quivering lips.

Ina May: I discovered that this type of lip-flapping exhalation works well to relax the cervix during an intense labor. Without any coaching from me, Sue began exhaling this way as she approached full dilation.

Chris: Katsi and Lidewij arrived, their eyes sparkling. They fit right in with the atmosphere in the room. The feeling was relaxed and holy. It all

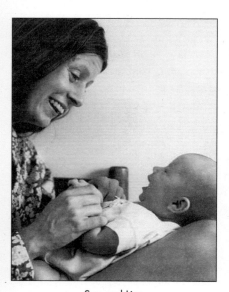

Sue and Lisa

felt just right, as if all of us were of one spirit, with the center being the one about to be born. Sue must have felt the same, as she was rushing stronger and stronger, and both the scale and volume of her sound effects increased proportionately with her dilation. During contractions she now squeezed my hands harder than a professional wrestler, and we both worked up a good sweat.

Time passed, and all the birthing paraphernalia was laid out in the nick of time. Sue opened wide, the rushes grew yet more intense, and so did the unearthly sounds that passed her lips. It felt so intense and yet so right and pure. In between these contractions, Sue would sigh and let her head fall back into my arms just long enough for a few breaths of relaxation and a sip of water before the next wave of contractions swept us away again. Charging ahead like this, full dilation was reached rather quickly, and the head started crowning with the next few pushes. Ina May asked Sue to pant for a spell, supporting the perineum so Sue could stretch around the head. This way the head emerged gradually, and it was born, slightly blue and very pointed, a few pushes later, facedown, then rotating toward Sue's right leg. From what I could see, she was all red in the face and crumpled up, pretty bald and covered with vernix. Out she slithered, surfing on the next push with a holler. A ripple of joy flooded my heart and body.

Sue: I remember reaching down and touching Lisa's head as she was crowning. With the next push, she slithered out. Within seconds she was in my arms and me in Chris's arms. Lisa was slippery and warm and absolutely beautiful. She didn't take long to find my nipple and begin nursing. We felt so strong, so full, so complete.

Chris: We were deliriously happy with this brand-new creature, whole and healthy, as she was handed up to Sue's belly. There she lay, tiny, blissful, perfect, and pink, announcing herself with a clear voice, and our hearts joined like three rivers mixing waters. Her lower lip was shaking, and her legs and arms were performing her first dance. Ina May clamped and cut the cord, and the little one tried for a first suck at her mother's breast. I just couldn't take my eyes off this perfect new being. No words can reflect these feelings flooding the gates of emotion on a first encounter like this. While we were acquainting ourselves with each other, Ina May gently tugged the cord and delivered the placenta. Everything went just fine, and Sue had neither torn nor bled. After a couple of hours and a few hugs, the midwives left us alone with the remaining night. Soon, first light was permeating the sky, tranquil and magic, and the first rain in a long while was beating on the tin roof.

Marbeth and Steve traveled from Haiti to The Farm Midwifery Center to give birth to Chelsea.

Chelsea's Birth—July 22, 1987

By Marbeth and Stephen Dunn

Marbeth: We came to The Farm a month early and moved into a rustic wooden house, which had housed many other birthing women in the past. We nested in and bonded with all the wonderful midwives here and gave the birthing up to God's hands.

On July 22, I felt something punch my cervix at six in the morning. I thought, There goes the mucus plug. Then the water broke, and my rushes started coming every seven minutes. Stephen called Deborah an hour later, and she was with us within two minutes. My cervix was dilated to two centimeters, so she called the other midwives to let them know my labor had started. As my rushes grew stronger, the other midwives arrived: Pamela, Joanne, and Ina May. There was also a medical student, Nan, who was sharing our house while she was learning what she could from the midwives. It was wonderful having all that feminine energy. Joanne had brought her daughter, Ida, to look after our five-year-old daughter, Shanna, while I was in labor.

As my rushes grew stronger yet, I kept affirming my gratefulness to God for my being here with all these wonderful midwives. I concentrated on opening up, on keeping my mouth loose, and on thanking God for giving me a perfect, easy birthing.

By three in the afternoon, I had dilated to ten centimeters and was ready for phase two—pushing out the baby. I had done quite a bit of reading about birthing babies. Shanna had been pulled out with forceps after an arduous seven hours of pushing, and I wanted this birthing to be different. I came across some literature that indicated that pushing was not desirable, because it made birthing like an athletic event. The author wrote that the uterus would push the baby out by itself. She had tried this at her second birthing and was thrilled at how easy this one had been, compared with her first birthing. Because of reading this, I decided that part of my problem with Shanna's birthing had been that I had exhausted myself by pushing before I was ready and that I wasn't going to push this time. I was going to let my uterus do the pushing for me.

The rushes grew in intensity, and the midwives told me that I would need to push to get the baby out. Deborah told me that she had had a

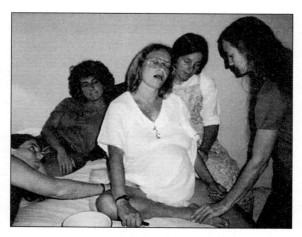

Marbeth in labor

similar situation once, and that in this case, pushing was essential. I agreed to push, and I did push on the stronger, more irresistible rushes, but something more was needed. Ina May decided to check and see how I was pushing during the rushes. By checking this way, she was able to direct my pushing energy to the right place, since I had been dispersing it before.

One of my problems was that I was afraid to make any noise for fear of frightening my daughter. However, when I expressed this to the midwives, they said to go ahead and make some noise. In fact, they encouraged me to really let go vocally. They explained to Shanna that I was okay and that I need to make noise to push out the baby. She handled it like a champion.

Something still wasn't quite right, and Ina May, looking at my breasts (I had pulled off my birthing gown by this time), suggested to Stephen that he stimulate my nipples to get some oxytocin flowing. He did, and the next rush was as powerful as a locomotive. All of the midwives cheered me on as I began to grasp what PUSHING was all about.

The baby still wasn't coming out, however, so Ina May reached in and pushed my pelvic bones apart with her hands, and slowly I began to make real progress. After a few pushes, she asked Pamela to take over for her, and I opened my eyes during one rush to see Pamela's arms shaking from the strain.

"Good! You moved the baby down half an inch!" she told me. It was getting harder to feel grateful, but I succeeded and blessed these wonderful ladies for their love and dedication.

Ina May thought that if two midwives could push on the top of my hips externally, it should help the bottom to open up (like squeezing the top of a clothespin).

Ina May: *I had learned this technique, called the "pelvic press," from Nan Koehler's book* Artemis Speaks *and first used it (successfully) at a birth made difficult by the baby's forehead-first position—the notorious "brow presentation," which is generally considered impossible for a vaginal birth.*

Marbeth: Deborah and Nan positioned themselves on either side and squeezed my hips on each rush. Stephen was still behind me, supporting me with his love and keeping the oxytocin flowing by manipulating my nipples.

Finally, Ina May added her strength to Pamela's on my pelvic bones, and the head was through! A few more minutes and my beautiful Chelsea Ray was born and snuggled up on my stomach. The total labor was twelve hours, and I pushed for three of those hours.

It turned out that Chelsea's hand was beside her head, impeding her progress down through my pelvic bones. After her head was delivered, Ina May reached in and pulled her hand and the rest of her came sliding out. Seven pounds eleven ounces of healthy baby.

I feel eternally grateful to have had this opportunity to push Chelsea out myself (with the midwives' help). I know what a hospital birthing would have been like (forceps, cesarean, or vacuum extractor). For me, there is no alternative to The Farm for birthing babies.

In 1976 a terrible earthquake devastated Guatemala. People who lived at The Farm's center in Mobile, Alabama, were some of the first who picked up the news of the disaster on ham radio, and they relayed this information to ham operators on The Farm. We had already begun an organization called Plenty to provide disaster aid in Tennessee and surrounding states, so Plenty sent a Farm couple to Guatemala to investigate how we could assist the recovery from the earthquake. Over the next few months and years Plenty established a relief and development team that included carpenters, farmers, soy-foods experts, emergency medical technicians, and paramedics. My husband, Stephen, and I traveled to Guatemala several times between 1976 and 1980 to oversee the project and to carry the Plenty crew from Tennessee to the areas where they would work.

During my first trip, I learned an important technique from a midwife named Etta Willis to free the shoulders of babies stuck during birth. Etta, who was originally from Belize, had received her formal midwifery training in that former British colony. By the time I met her, she had worked for several years as a midwife for the Guatemalan government. The indigenous midwives in her area whom she supervised taught her the technique she taught me for dealing with the complication of shoulder dystocia. Shoulder dystocia is the complication when the baby's shoulders become stuck after the birth of the head. These midwives attended the regular classes she held to make sure the care they provided was up to the standard set by Guatemala's public-health authorities. When I asked Etta what she did in case of shoulder dystocia, she told me,

"Turn the mother so she is on her hands and knees. That always works." She emphasized that the method she had learned from the indigenous midwives (who were all illiterate) was **superior** *to the maneuvers she had been taught during her own midwifery training.*

Back home in Tennessee, the next time I encountered this complication (which occurs in one or two percent of births), I followed her advice. See "Reuben's Birth" below. It worked each time my partners and I used it without injury to the mother. Usually, the baby was born quickly and easily. In severe cases, I found that in addition to changing the mother's position, I had to insert my first two fingers across the baby's armpit in order to pull the baby out or to locate one of the baby's hands and to grasp it and pull the baby's arm out so the body could be born. Once we adopted the use of the all-fours maneuver, there were no injuries to any of our shoulder dystocia babies. Shoulder dystocia is acknowledged to be one of those complications that sometimes results in injury to the baby and the mother when conventional techniques are used.

Our outcomes for thirty-five shoulder-dystocia births were published in the Journal of Family Practice, *June 1991, in an article cowritten by Dr. Anna Meenan and myself. Another article based on outcomes from a registry of eighty-two shoulder-dystocia cases dealt with by midwives and family-practice physicians was published in the* Journal of Reproductive Medicine, *1998; 3:439–443, with Dr. Joseph Bruner as my coauthor. With the publication of the latter article, I gained the distinction of becoming the only midwife in written history (that I have been able to find) with an obstetrical maneuver named after her—the "Gaskin Maneuver."*[1,2] *This method is now taught in Advanced Life Support in Obstetrics courses in the United States and the United Kingdom and in a major U.S. obstetrics textbook.*[3] *When I returned to Guatemala and asked the indigenous midwives where they learned it, the oldest of them pointed to the heavens and said, "Dios. We learned it from God."*

Reuben's Birth—April 15, 1977

By Barbara Bloomfield

We came to The Farm in the winter of 1977 to have our second child with the midwives. We tried to have our first child at home, without the help of experienced birth attendants, so after twenty hours of labor and pushing before I was fully dilated, we got discouraged. We drove forty-five minutes over winding roads to our backup, a doctor, who had his office set up for birthings. After he gave me some Pitocin and an episiotomy, my daughter popped right out.

We knew there was a gentler way to give birth. I never wanted to go to a hospital, which I consider an institution for treating serious illness. Even though my dad is a doctor, I don't feel comfortable in those surroundings and I never wanted to dwell on something going wrong, because I'm a healthy and active person and I see birthing as a natural process of our life cycle.

My labor with Reuben began as soon as I woke up in the morning after a good sleep. He was three weeks overdue, and I was anxious about having my baby, because my sister was getting married soon and I would miss her wedding if the baby and I weren't ready to travel. I began to feel the pressure of my muscles starting to open up at regular intervals. My husband, Neal, helped to get our twenty-two-month-old daughter off to a friend's house so we could concentrate on our task at hand. The midwives came and checked on me and let us be together throughout the morning as I gradually dilated. It was very reassuring to have them give me confidence and reassurance that all was proceeding smoothly. As the afternoon wore on and contractions were closer together and stronger, my little room slowly filled with midwives and trainees. I didn't know all of them, but my attention was so concentrated on getting the baby out that I was oblivious to many of those surrounding me. The exciting part of Reuben's birth was toward the end, when his head was born. I pushed and pushed but couldn't move him (because his shoulder was wedged behind my pubic bone). Ina May told me I would need to turn over, so somehow—with the help of Neal and the midwives—I got over onto my hands and knees. From my new position, I gave a few excruciating pushes and out came our ten-pound boy. I did tear a little, but Reuben was healthy and we were glad to have him in our arms at last.

✺ Mariahna Margaret's Birth—October 2, 1980
By Carol Nelson

Mariahna Margaret was my fourth child. On my due date I went for a walk, rode into town (which involved a bumpy ride on The Farm road), and then went for another walk later. I started having irregular rushes shortly after the second walk. After bathing the kids and tucking them in, I lay down myself and thought, I know I'm coming on to doing it, but it sure would be nice to get some sleep. I fell asleep quickly, slept very soundly for about forty-five minutes, and then woke up to my water breaking all over my bed. I felt very rested and ready at this point. Within about fifteen minutes, my rushes began coming very close together. Judith, our good friend and midwife assistant, came and checked me. I was open about four centimeters. GREAT! This is it! Everything I had been worried about during this pregnancy was gone at this point, and the contractions were coming on so strong that I had to keep all of my attention together to make it through each one. There was simply no time for worrying.

I could tell it was going to be a big baby—at least as big as our Sally Kate, who had weighed nine pounds nine ounces at birth. My labor was very fast and strong, taking about two and a half hours. I could tell I was having to open further than I ever had before. I think having the water bag broken makes the rushes feel stronger too, because you have just the baby's head pushing against the cervix instead of a cushion of water before the head.

I did everything I could to bring the labor on, even though it was so intense. Don and I sat crossed-legged facing each other, holding hands and looking into each other's eyes during rushes. We would melt into each other and laugh. He gave me a lot of strength, and laughing helped me relax. Eventually, it got to where I couldn't sit up any longer, so we lay down and cuddled and smooched. This made it feel very sensual and sexy. These feelings made labor easier to handle, and I could feel myself opening. Don and I were kissing, and this was helping me get through the strong transition contractions. Pretty soon I was making deep, throaty-sounding moans and felt the urge to push.

Mary, my midwife, checked me, always taking care to be gentle and unobtrusive. She found that I was almost fully dilated. I just had a little cervix left on the top, over the baby's head. I did a few more rushes and began finding it very hard to keep it together. I really wanted to push. Mary and the other midwives were doing deep massage on my thighs and calves, which felt heavenly and helped me relax. Mary checked again and found a little cervix still. However, she said I could go ahead and push slowly, and she would try to ease the cervix over the baby's head with her fingers. That worked. I was at full dilation and really ready to push.

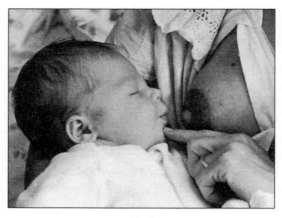

Mari

The baby moved down quickly with only a couple of pushes. I could feel her slip through the cervix, through the bones, and head down the birth canal. Such an intense but satisfying feeling. She started to crown. I was trying to take it slow, knowing this was the important part if I didn't want to tear. Mary gave me instructions on when and how much to push. When the baby's head was about halfway out, it felt so intense I started to wonder again if I was going to be able to keep it together. At that point, Mary gave me a progress report and said this was the fullest part and by the next push the baby's head would probably be out all the way. It was so good to get this kind of reassurance. I loved Mary so much for being so compassionate with me that she could know exactly what my sensations and feelings were. Okay, I thought. I can do this, no problem. With the next push, out came her very large, fat head—big relief! Mary checked and said there was no cord around her neck. At that point my rushes slowed down. I pushed a couple of times, but the rushes were not as powerful, and it started to become obvious that this baby wasn't going to come any further. Her shoulders were stuck.

Time was suspended at this point. Timelessness lets you see clearly what a very fine line there is between birth, life, and possibly death, if the right decisions are not made quickly. The seconds went by. I tried to push some more, and I pulled my legs back further. I moved one leg up and over, lying on my side a little, and tried pushing like that, but it didn't work. The baby's head was beginning to turn dark. Mary's hands were busy, and we were trying different things. I kept pushing but couldn't move the baby. The seconds kept ticking by. I could see the baby's head getting darker and darker. We all knew it was heavy and that we needed to figure something out soon.

Diane, another midwife, suggested that I turn over onto my hands and knees. Mary asked Don to help me do this. When I heard Diane's suggestion, my first thought was, She has to be joking. There is no way I can move! Remembering then the intensity of the situation, I immediately started to move, and Don began to assist me. Everyone moved quickly. Within a few seconds, I got over and pushed again. Right away I could feel some progress. The gravity helped, and I felt like I had a lot more strength and more leverage in pushing. I was also praying at this time. I knew we needed some help getting this fat girl out. I pushed again, and whoosh, out she came! I felt like turning over onto my hands and knees saved her life.

She had good muscle tone and started breathing right away, to let us know she was okay. She grabbed Mary's finger and held on to her. We gave her a little oxygen, and she cried and pinked up right away. It had taken about two minutes from the time her head was born to get her out, but she was obviously fine.

I turned back over and held her on my belly. She was so sweet, beautiful, alert, intelligent, and fat! It was very good to have her out, strong and healthy. The scale we had went only to ten pounds, and she was over that. The next morning she weighed ten pounds four ounces. She had already peed and pooped several times, so we know she weighed two or three ounces more than that. She looked a couple of months old but was so obviously newborn. How sweet. I loved her so much for being strong and wanting to be here as much as we wanted her.

I am grateful I was at home with trained midwives who knew what to do in this emergency situation. I didn't tear or need an episiotomy, which was great. Mary had used warm baby oil to massage my perineum as I was crowning. I really did try to stay relaxed delivering her head and with all the activity after. Keeping my face and neck muscles relaxed and making low-toned noises helped, along with lots of encouragement and reassurance from Don and the midwives.

We were all glad to have her out and healthy. It is very nice to get to have your babies at home with good friends who you know really love and care about you and your baby. I was quite grateful that the doctors we worked with were willing to let me have her at home even though this had been a complicated pregnancy.

Our video crew got a great tape of the birth. It shows clearly how to change positions and get into hands-and-knees position for a shoulder dystocia. It shows that it is easy and that it really works.

Liza was born during the late summer of 1990. At the time, I was traveling with Stephen. A couple of days earlier, I had lectured to doctors at the University of New Mexico at Albuquerque about breech births and shoulder dystocia. Little did I know that I would be called upon to attend such a birth while I was traveling. Shoulder dystocia is one of those complications that is hard to predict. While it happens most often with large babies, it can and does occur when the baby is less than eight pounds. The key to success lies in understanding the labor positions in which the mother's pelvic dimensions are greatest and that movement can often free a stuck baby.

✧ Liza's Birth—Esalen, Big Sur, California—September 19, 1990
By Karrie Dundas

Karrie: Liza's birth gave new meaning to the word *labor*. It felt like I was working hard, very hard, without exactly knowing what I was working toward!

Ina May: *Karrie's nurse–midwife stopped by the lodge where I was having dinner and said she would like me to assist Karrie. I said that would be all right with me, but I wasn't sure that Karrie would feel the same way, since we didn't already know each other. When I saw how deep into her labor she was, I said hello and then left. I was awakened around 1:30 A.M. by a man who said the midwife had sent for me to come to the birth.*

Karrie: By 2:00 A.M., I was five centimeters dilated. My bladder was completely full and blocking the energy of my contractions. Once the catheter was used to empty my bladder, I went full speed ahead with a lot of help from Ina May and her visualization technique. (Ina May: *I showed her with my hands how big she would open up to let her baby out.*) Within an hour I was fully dilated.

Ina May: *Karrie was laboring well when I reached her cabin on a cliff*

above the Pacific. I didn't actually check her inside because her water bag had been broken for some time, but her midwife said that her cervix was very thin and about six centimeters open. I told Karrie that opening up the rest of the way would not have to take as long as it had taken to get to where she was, which seemed to relieve her fears. Her next rush was even stronger than the one that had preceded it. When she began to toss her head from side to side, I suggested that she unwrinkle her forehead, hold still, and let her breath out slowly and easily—that this would help her cervix open the rest of the way. It seemed to do just that, and it wasn't long before she was ready to push.

Karrie's husband, Greg, was sitting on the end of the bed, as they had planned for him to catch the baby. I stayed there too, occasionally checking her progress and making suggestions about how to get more progress out of each push. She was looking pretty tired by now, and I didn't want her to reach the end of her strength. At first she was leaning back on pillows and pulling back on her legs. Then I suggested that she pull on the bar above the bed. That worked quite well. Later she went back to a sitting position, with me and one of the other midwives pushing on each of her hips to enlarge the outlet and shorten the time of pushing. Altogether Karrie pushed for about two hours, and the baby's head came to a nice, slow crown and came through without a tear or episiotomy.

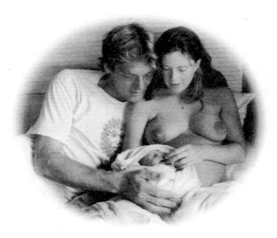

Greg, Karrie, and Liza

The first sign of trouble was that the baby's neck was not visible. Karrie's next push was ineffectual, so I asked Greg and the other midwives to help Karrie into the hands-and-knees position. One of the midwives took over for Greg at this point, but she was not able to bring out the baby's shoulders, even with me tweaking both of Karrie's nipples in order to stimulate a good push. The midwife then asked me to take over.

I had to reach way up to find the baby's posterior armpit. All I had in my mind was the thought, I have to get this baby out. My first attempt at traction was not successful, but the next time, I rotated the baby's body a little and brought her out to the waist. The rest was easy. The baby had made three attempts to breathe during this process of my pulling her body out, which took about three minutes. Her Apgar scores were good—eight at one minute and ten at five minutes. She weighed eight pounds twelve ounces.

Karrie: It really hurt when Ina May put her hand inside me to hook her finger under Liza's armpit. Now that I think of it, that was the only real pain I felt. The rest were just powerful movements that my body knew how to do.

Breathing really helped me. I was in a trance state most of the time, with my eyes closed. Even after Liza's shoulders were unhooked, I still had to push three or four times to get her body out. This surprised me, because I thought she would just slip out like a wet seal.

After I delivered, I turned over and saw her lying in her daddy's arms. I forgot everything that had happened in the last thirty-six hours and all kinds of energy flowed into me. When everyone had gone and my husband fell asleep, Liza and I gazed at each other in awe. We both knew this was just the beginning.

✂ How We Got Corbett—December 17, 1994
By Nancy Presley

I am forty-seven years old. I have eighteen- and fourteen-year-old sons. My husband, Van, came into our lives when the boys were ten and six and has been a wonderful father to them. Three years ago I had a miscarriage at four weeks, which was sad but reassuring that it was possible for us to put together a baby.

This pregnancy was a total surprise. We had become completely unattached to conceiving, and I had started lightly perusing the literature on menopause.

Once we got through the emotionally harrowing first weeks and could believe that we were going to make it this time with a healthy baby, I enjoyed the pregnancy. I started showing early and warned my coworkers that I always get really big when I'm pregnant. I'm small-framed, but I gained fifty pounds with each of my other two pregnancies, even though the boys were only six pounds twelve ounces and seven pounds fourteen ounces. I was confident of the delivery, because the others had been relatively uncomplicated, and the second so much easier than the first.

Fortunately, I had been on a fitness kick before I got pregnant and was at my goal weight and in fairly good shape. Fatigue was a factor in the early and late stages, though, and in the middle months I began to be troubled by hemorrhoids. These were the only things that seemed age-related in my pregnancy, but they did affect how much exercise I was able to get. By the middle of my seventh month, I had already gained fifty pounds and was dragging around the office so hard my coworkers were concerned about how big I was going to get.

By the time we set out for Tennessee to have the baby on The Farm (where I used to live and my other two had been born), I was rested and pretty well healed up. When we arrived, the midwives there confirmed that I was ready and told me that this baby was going to be bigger than my other ones. Two weeks went by. The moon was full, and it seemed to be a wonderful night to have a baby.

At 1:30 one morning, during a sound sleep, my water bag broke. I've never experienced a spontaneous rupture before, and Ina May had warned me that this was going to be a mess. And it was! It actually broke three times—once in the bed, once when I was standing next to the bed, and about an hour later, while I was sitting in the wooden rocker in our room. Van was really busy running around with towels.

Ina May and Pamela arrived around 7:00 A.M. I was really glad to see them. Ina May had been out of town for both my other birthings, and I appreciated that she wanted to be with me for this one. And Pamela had helped me have Asa, eighteen years ago. Another old friend, Cynthia, whose family was putting us up in their birthing room, was also with us for the birthing.

By 9:00 A.M. I was eight centimeters dilated and going strong. The rushes were getting very compelling by now, and I was integrating them by saying "Ohhhhhhhhh!" in a low register, so that as I got louder, I was sort of roaring. I was hanging out some of the time with Van alone, looking into his eyes, and as I approached transition I allowed my voice to express some dismay at the intensity of the feelings I was having. I saw all the color go out of his face and realized that this was his first birthing. I didn't want to diminish the experience for him or frighten him by complaining. This became very important to me and helped me keep it together. (Later, when I told him about this, Van reassured me that he just hadn't eaten in a while at that point and had not been frightened.)

Time has no meaning in a situation like this, so it wasn't until I read the birthing notes later that I realized that this stage of labor lasted for two hours. Carol Nelson, another of my midwives, kept massaging the little lip of cervix and reassuring me that it was getting smaller. She suggested I try different positions—hands and knees, for instance. At another point, she suggested I stand and that Van hold me up.

I wish I could say I was unwavering in my courage. I remembered Carol's video, how her eyes sparkled and she smiled as she blew gently through her rushes: "Whe-e-e-w..." My eyes were popping, and I had completely forgotten my delicacy at making noise in a house full of teenage boys. I was just roaring away. Between rushes I started saying things like "Is it gone yet?" (when she checked the cervical lip) and "I sure will be glad when this part's over." Carol is an old pro at keeping birthing mothers together, and she'd laugh and say, "You're still making progress," and "I'll bet you will."

I had no idea that she was going through a difficult decision-making process at the time. Someone suggested I try pushing against the cervical lip, that sometimes that would move it, but Carol told me later that I was turning red and putting out all this effort without pushing-type contractions working with me, and she couldn't feel anything happening at the baby's head. So she told me to stop. She and Ina May conferred with each other in another room about the possibility that I might be stalled at this point, making no progress and wearing out. Should they transfer me to the hospital for a cesarean section? "If you had been in a hospital," she said, "they would have wheeled you into surgery by then for sure."

They decided to check me one more time. This time Ina May massaged my cervix while I rushed, and then said, "It's gone, I don't feel it at all. You're ready to push!" What a joyful reprieve! The end was in sight!

My first and smallest son took an hour to push, my second about twelve minutes. We still didn't know what a big guy we had this time, but he took forty minutes. Van could see the head in five minutes, and I could feel it in my bones. For a time it moved down with every push but went back up between them. Van kept looking at me with his big blue eyes and saying, "You're doing great, you can do this." His faith in me meant everything.

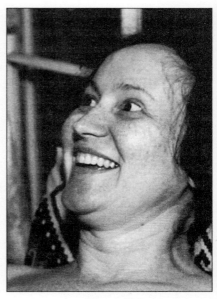

Nancy savors labor

Presently, Ina May asked me if I was pushing whether I felt like it or not. I honestly didn't know. I was locked into an endurance contest. She suggested I breathe and relax through the first part of a rush, then hold my breath and let the contractions lead me. It was wonderful advice. Now I knew what to do and so did my body. As soon as I held my breath, an overwhelming power came over me. Progress was still slow, but I felt that I was adding my strength to a natural force that made things happen.

My skin began to sting, and I knew the head was close. Van tried to gently hold it back so my skin could stretch around it. The big moment arrived and the head was out. Van said it looked like it was carved out of stone, an enormous warrior head. The neck wasn't out, and the shoulders were mightily stuck. Carol suggested to Van that he try to turn the head. He tried, but it wouldn't budge. He swept his fingers alongside the upper arm inside me to try to hook it out. He caught the armpit, but the arm wouldn't come. He tried the lower one, but there was no motion.

There was an inevitability about it that just felt like poetic justice of some kind. I don't remember thinking about it or having any trouble with it as hands appeared to help me roll over on my hands and knees. Van and Carol were a team now. Carol is not only an experienced midwife, she is an experienced instructor, having trained midwives in the hundreds. She knew how to let Van do all he could, and take over where necessary, and Van's instincts were very good. Ina May took a picture of all four of their hands inside me, manipulating this baby until the upper arm was out. With more work, they got the lower one out, and Van unwrapped the umbilical cord, which was looped around the back of the baby's neck and across the chest.

Even with all this help, my job wasn't done yet. I was instructed to push again to help get his barrel chest out, then again to get his hips out. This was the hardest work I've ever done; the baby felt like another being like myself coming out. I grabbed hold of the bed rails and gave it

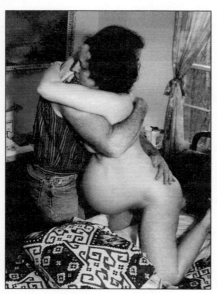

Van holds Nancy as she pushes

my all. There were sounds of exultation, exclamations that this was a big baby, a ten-pounder! When I could gather myself to turn around, I was astounded at what I saw. There were four pairs of hands on this young purple giant, who was moving and making little noises with his mouth, but not breathing. Ina May was listening to his heart and saying that his heart rate was good. Van and Pamela were massaging him. Carol gave him mouth-to-mouth. I was so grateful that he was in this peaceful, loving place with these wise people who cared so much about helping him to get started. Van said he looked calm and unafraid.

It had been four minutes from the time his head was born until he was fully born. He seemed to be satisfied just to be here, not really realizing the importance of breathing. When he finally did cry, it was sweet and polite, not the lusty gasping cry we wanted to hear. Carol waved the oxygen tube under his nose and he pinked up considerably. Van handed him to me. I cradled him in my arms and rested my lips on his sweet-smelling head, so grateful that he was here and all right. I knew I loved him from the start, but he really didn't quite feel like one of my children yet, because he was so big. I had to get used to skipping a whole stage of newborn.

I cannot put into words how it felt to see Van and his little boy. We had planned to name him Corbett Marks Presley.

So how was recovery for the geriatric mom from such a big baby? I'd have to say frustratingly slow, but absolutely complete. I was horrified at the hemorrhoids, which were beyond my wildest imaginings. But Pamela said, "Oh, that's nothing, they'll go away completely." I was astounded when they did, about three weeks later.

And I'm thoroughly enjoying the great cosmic joke of being a new mom again. It's just like riding a bicycle: You don't forget. And my pediatrician was right when he said that the late-in-life family additions in his practice seemed to be a great joy to their parents, who can appreciate every moment with the sure knowledge of how fleeting it all is and how fast it goes.

When Heidi and Rudy came to us for the birth of their first child, I quickly realized that their fears about birth were more pronounced than those of most of the expectant couples I had met. Their problem? Both were physicians in their last few months of training as obstetricians. They had dealt with plenty of frightening situations related to pregnancy and birth, and both knew that unnecessary surgery could be dangerous. During one of their prenatal visits, I learned that a couple of healthy women had died because of complications after their cesareans. (Neither death was caused by the cesareans the women underwent at the teaching hospital where Heidi and Rudy worked, but rather were related to their previous cesarean sections.) No wonder they wanted to give birth in a way that offered the maximum chance to avoid unnecessary surgery. Knowing that they must also have some fears about giving birth so far away from a hospital, at their first prenatal visit I gave them a spreadsheet of statistics from the nearly two thousand births we had attended by then, beginning with the first birth I ever saw.

ॐ M(idwife in) D(isguise)

By Heidi Rinehart, MD

After waiting seven years to conceive, my husband, Rudy, and I were expecting our first child. We waited through medical school, we waited through four years of residency training in obstetrics, and now it was our turn to do what all our patients were doing. Rudy and I were becoming parents.

I first was introduced to home birth in 1985 at a medical-student convention. The Humanistic Medicine Task Force of the American Medical Student Association (no relationship to the AMA) sponsored Dr. Stanley Sagov and Ina May Gaskin to speak about home birth. It made such intuitive sense that a new baby would arrive at home in the midst of his family! I cannot remember a single thing they said about home birth, but I remember thinking, This holistic approach to care is what drew me to medicine.

I didn't start medical school with a lot of fear about birth. My mother talked about birth being hard work—painful, yes, but an intensely physical experience with a tremendous reward when the work was done. I loved to hear her tell my birth story and those of my sister and brother. When she was pregnant with us, she refused to listen to the terrifying stories other women wanted to tell. My mother chose to be ignorant about birth over being in fear. She instilled faith in me that birth must be normal if there are this many people on the planet. It did not make sense to me that pregnancy and birth were taught in the same context as all those diseases that we learned in medical school.

Medicine concerns itself with the diagnosis and treatment of disease. As far as I could tell, it is not about health promotion, it is not about disease prevention, and it is not about empowering people to improve their overall well-being. Slowly it dawned on me that the detection of pathology and its treatment form is the dominant algorithm in medicine. By the time I realized that medicine was not the optimal career for health promotion, I had invested considerable time and money in my education, and it seemed that I could best effect change from the inside. So I continued with medical school, despite a nagging feeling that it wasn't the right place for me. My husband, however, knew exactly where my heart lay, and upon my graduation presented me with a desk plate that read, *Heidi Rinehart, MD—Midwife in Disguise.*

Rudy did not decide to go into obstetrics and gynecology until the third year of medical school, but I knew all along. We both found a fascination with reproduction, pleasure in working with women, an interest in how people value and make choices about their reproductive potential. We experience fulfillment at being present for birth.

Because medicine's focus is on pathology, I approached residency and training with trepidation. I knew that my residency would not train me to care for the majority of healthy women who do not require medicine's technology to give birth. I worried that I had four years of indoctrination into the culture of obstetric pathology ahead of me.

Medicine *is* a culture all its own; it has its own standards of acceptable behavior and mores. I knew I'd be immersed in this culture one hundred hours per week with little time to reflect on what we were doing. It is unbelievable to me how much beliefs and values of the medical culture influence the "scientific" search for knowledge and impact on its conclusions. Every scientific endeavor is influenced by the beliefs of those who do the work, but this is neither acknowledged nor challenged in medicine. When the prevailing belief is that childbearing is fraught with danger, how could I retain my belief in the normalcy of pregnancy and birth?

So I wrote to Ina May, saying, "Can I come to The Farm?" The Farm is a mecca for those reclaiming midwifery and normal births in the United States. By going there, I thought I could get some grounding in healthy, normal birth before I faced immersion in the culture of disease. The two weeks I spent there were a time of intensive study—attending births, reading, watching birth videos, observing midwifery care, and talking to the midwives. The experience profoundly changed my perspective. In the hospital, I hadn't perceived the anxiety and foreboding that permeated birth until I experienced the impact of its absence among the midwives. The peace, wonder, and intimacy were infinitely greater. What a compelling difference!

At one birth, the woman experienced heavy bleeding after the birth of her baby. Watching my reaction and that of the midwives made me realize that the skills of the caregivers (intellectual, manual, observational, and intuitive) define the quality of care, not the setting. Because of my training, I would have used medical tools without assessing if they were truly needed. The midwives intervened gently but did not overreact. And they used medical tools when needed, but their use was far more restrained than in the hospital.

I studied the safety of out-of-hospital birth. For healthy women with an experienced caregiver, home birth or birth-center birth is as safe as the hospital, in terms of the number of deaths. It is probably also safer in terms of numbers of procedures done to the mother or injuries to mother or baby. The small number of women who need to go to the hospital are, in fact, the minority, and the bad outcomes that occur out-of-hospital often could not be avoided in the hospital either (lethal birth defects, shoulder dystocia, and so on).

Residency training was as I expected it to be. It was grueling—the hours, the intensity, the stamina required, the tragedies witnessed. Normal birth was so infrequent. We did not learn how to facilitate or support it. The tools that we have applied have disrupted the process—I can look back on many instances where I used a medical tool (epidural, Pitocin, artificial rupture of membranes, even cesarean section), only to realize later that it had disturbed the normal process or precipitated a complication. Even as the least interventionist of my peers, I have felt compelled by the obstetric imperative to *do* something, when what was actually needed was support, careful reassessment, or patience.

I have tried to provide midwifery-like care to women I have taken care of in my clinic. It has been disappointing that even women who were motivated, well-informed, and had chosen me as a caregiver because of my natural-childbirth advocacy struggled with institutional routines that had their own momentum. Even small deviations from the hospital routine required forethought, negotiation, or "permission" for the woman to exercise her autonomy. The language everyone used reflected where control lay: "We *let* her eat, walk, not have an I.V. etc.," and "They *let* me keep the baby all night." It has been frustratingly difficult to change the atmosphere of hospital birth.

When we got pregnant, I knew that I wanted to be nurtured by midwives during the pregnancy, to give birth naturally, and to feel safe to be vulnerable during the pregnancy and the labor. The third one was the trickiest. Medical culture has indoctrinated me (and all my colleagues) that doctors aren't supposed to have doubts and questions or to be vulnerable. It was vital to me that my caregivers understand that I was sensitive and vulnerable like every other pregnant woman. They had to be able to meet Rudy and me where we were—knowing too damn much about obstetrics and all the bad things that can happen, but knowing too little about the physical and emotional experience. I needed not to feel performance anxiety or inhibition in labor. Rudy and I both needed reassurance and guidance as we waited for our baby and as we became parents.

We decided to drive to The Farm for our care (eighty miles each way), because Rudy and I felt most comfortable with the midwives there. Pamela Hunt and Ina May have three times more experience with vaginal birth than Rudy and me put together. That experience has given them confidence in themselves and their practice to the point that caring for two obstetricians was not intimidating in the least. It gave Rudy and me the confidence that they could guide us through a normal pregnancy and birth—territory that we sometimes *thought* we knew!

Rudy and I cherished how our long prenatal visits put the pathology we witnessed in its proper perspective and allowed us to verbalize the wonder of our pregnancy experience and to affirm the normalcy of pregnancy and birth. We felt tremendously nurtured, loved, and cared for by our midwives. They shared in our pleasure and helped us wrestle with our issues. I needed to talk about the fact that I have had a tremendous need to please authority figures, and what we were doing would *not* please the ones in our world! I also needed to talk about my many pregnancy dreams that were about problems I had recently seen. Rudy, on the other hand, was worried about baby care even though he had handled hundreds of newborns.

During the pregnancy, I also chose to get parallel care from an obstetrician. I did this for several reasons: One is that the physical and emotional stress of residency seems to cause doctors to have more than their share of preterm labor and preeclampsia. I decided that I wanted to have a relationship with an obstetric caregiver so that, if I needed hospital care, any negotiation about deviations from the routine wouldn't require establishing rapport too. Secondly, although we didn't keep what we were planning a secret, I didn't always want to talk about it. We had colleagues (nurses and doctors) who were supportive, those who were uninformed but curious, and those who did not ask what they did not want to know! When those who might not be supportive would ask, "Who's your doctor?" I could answer honestly. The doctor we worked with listened sensitively and perceptively to me, and, although he did not agree with our choice, he was very respectful.

Julianna's Birth—March 6, 1993

By Heidi Rinehart, MD

The day that Julianna was due, the contractions I had been having for weeks changed. They settled in my lower back and became a little more achy. My mucus had increased all week, and on her due date it was blood-tinged all day. Rudy and I realized that the baby could come any time. We went out for dinner that night, and I had contractions every five to ten minutes all through dinner. They were really mild. As we walked out to the car, Rudy said, "This may be the last dinner that is just the two of us."

At 2:00 A.M. I awoke with a strong contraction that was painful enough to startle me out of my sleep and make me jump out of bed to cope with it. I went back to sleep and had another like it at 2:30. At 3:00 A.M. the contractions started coming every five to ten minutes. They were mildly uncomfortable, aching in my lower back. Rudy dozed off and on and rubbed my back when it hurt. By 5:00 A.M. it seemed like labor had started, so we got up, showered, picked up some loose ends around the house, and had some cereal. I called Pamela to let her know we were on our way to The Farm.

The sun was up as we left the house; there was a little frost on the windshield, but it was sunny and bright. The drive down was calm. The contractions slowed to every ten minutes, but they were much more uncomfortable in the car. Pamela was waiting for us at the birth house on Tower Road when we got there about 7:30. We brought a few things in and settled down to chat for a bit. Pamela made some cereal for us. Carol, one of the other midwives, and Ina May stopped over. Ina May was supposed to give a talk at a health-care reform symposium in Nashville that morning, but she also really wanted to be at our birth. Three people had dreams that my labor was very fast, and since my mom had quick labors, it seemed reasonable to think mine might be too. I told Ina May she could go to the meeting, because the contractions were still mild and kind of irregular. When Pamela checked me, I was just three centimeters, so Ina May left for Nashville after leaving the number where she would be.

Since we had not slept a whole lot the night before and we knew we had some work in front of us, Rudy and I lay down for a nap, and Carol and Pamela left for a while. I kept having a few contractions, but they weren't really strong. Pamela and Carol peeked back in and saw that we were sleeping, so they were going to leave us a note. While they were outside writing the note, I had a really strong contraction that rolled me out of bed and had me leaning over the counter. At its height I had a moment of panic because I didn't know how to cope, and I suddenly wished Pamela and Carol would come back to help me. Just then they opened the door, and I said a bit pitifully, "That one really *hurt*." From then on they stayed. Carol suggested we go for a walk for a change of scenery about 10:15 A.M.

It was a beautiful day. It was early March, so there were a few daffodils, just a hint of green on the ground, and plump buds on the trees. The sun was shining, and the temperature was about sixty-five degrees. We walked along a dirt road among pine trees and between fields. We just walked along with Rudy rubbing my back. The contractions were mild, so we talked and teased. Rudy was concerned that he wouldn't be a good labor support, so he was already tallying his "debits and credits" as a husband. We were really enjoying being together, being outside, and were excited about being in labor. It was so beautiful, and we were so happy to be having our baby—that walk will always be a special memory. After we had been walking for about half an hour, I had a long, strong contraction that made me have to hang on Rudy. I could feel the baby move down. The sensation of her moving down triggered a bout of vomiting, which didn't bother me, but it left me a little trembly.

We went inside so I could wash my face and rinse my mouth. I put my contacts in, because it seemed like things were getting stronger and I might not be able to do it later. A good decision! When I went to the bathroom, there was a huge glob of bloody show. It was about 11:00 A.M. We thought about walking outside some more, but the labor had become a lot stronger. From here on, time was blurry, events didn't have a clear chronology, and my awareness of things changed. For example, much later in the labor, the other midwives, Deborah and Joanne, showed up and started to help. I was unaware of when they arrived or what they were doing, but at some point I noticed that they were there. I didn't greet them; I just kind of registered their presence.

Pamela checked me then, and I was three to four centimeters open. She decided to call Ina May and told her "not to dawdle," because she thought I could go fast. My back really ached with each contraction, way down low in my sacrum. It helped to have someone rub or press there during each contraction. Sometimes I sat on a chair with my forehead against Rudy's or Pamela's stomach and sometimes I stood hanging from Rudy's neck. By the time the labor was over, I had also been in the shower, knelt with my knees wide apart and my arms around Rudy's neck, sat on the toilet, and lay on my side. As each contraction started I'd call out, "Someone please get my back," if Pamela or Carol weren't already there rubbing. I guess Deborah and Joanne helped with that also, but I wasn't really aware of whose hands were there. Grunting and groaning helped a lot too. I never could have labored in bed on my side with a fetal monitor on; it was too intense and I couldn't have coped if I hadn't been able to move around a lot.

About 3:00 P.M. my dad called. He was piloting a flight that had an overnight in Nashville and was calling The Farm because we weren't at home as planned. Rudy had stepped out to get a snack, so I had to talk on the phone. I said, "Dad, I'm in labor and only have a minute. There are a couple of things I need to tell you."

Conversationally, he said, "How far apart are your pains?" I could feel a contraction getting ready to start, so I said, "Shut up! I only have a minute!" and told him what I needed to about getting into our house. The next contraction started before I could hang up, and since I hadn't started breathing deeply right as it was starting, it was significantly harder to cope with.

During labor I would sweat profusely, but then a few minutes later I would feel cold. I know the heat got turned up and down several times. Rudy and I both had thought that I might have a fever and an infection in my uterus making me feel this way, even though we should have known it was the intensity of the labor (or the exorcism of obstetrical demons!) that caused it. Each of us had many thoughts of pathologic reasons why different things were happening in the labor. For example, the baby's heartbeat was 140 most of the time, but one time that Carol checked, it was 160. That concerned me, because a rising heartbeat can be a sign of infection or stress on the baby. I asked Carol to check again a few minutes later, because it scared me. Of course, it was 140 again.

One thing that reassured Rudy and me throughout the labor was that the baby kept kicking and wiggling until she was born; I even felt her kick while I was pushing her out. And when I was hanging from Rudy's neck, both of us could feel her kicking between us.

Other things had us worried too. The baby stayed high in my pelvis until I was almost completely dilated. Rudy's and my teaching was that first babies who remained high in the pelvis late in labor would have trouble coming out and frequently required forceps or cesarean section. As the hours went by and it didn't feel like the baby had descended at all (based on the location of the sensations in my back), each of us wondered what was holding her up.

(Ina May: *We midwives all believed that Heidi's baby remained high because of the fear she and Rudy had.*)

Heidi: I continued to think that my pelvis was fine and the baby was not big, so the baby could come out. But I questioned if I could continue to cope with the back labor for as long as it would take. Rudy wondered if the baby could come out at all.

The next time Pamela examined me, Rudy asked to check me too. The midwives could feel Rudy's doubts about whether the baby could come out, so they thought it might help. They had absolute confidence that the baby would come, but Rudy didn't feel it and his help to me was no longer steadfast. A couple of times Rudy's touch during labor was uncomfortable; when we talked about it afterward, he told me that those were the times he was "examining" me out of fear rather than soothing me.

When Rudy checked me, I was about eight to nine centimeters and my cervix was soft and very thin. The baby's head was in a position that we obstetricians call "deep transverse arrest." He told me I had to push the baby down with the next contraction, and when I did, her head easily descended. At that moment Rudy's face lit up, he looked me in the eye, and said, "You can do it.... This baby will come out!" From then on, Rudy was unwavering in his cheerleading.

It helped me to have Rudy's confidence. Rudy is a terrible liar; he couldn't have feigned the look on his face and the tone in his voice when he said that I could do it. Even though I was even more vulnerable and sensitive as I dilated the last centimeter or two and began vocalizing my fears and feelings more freely ("You'd tell me if there was something wrong with me or the baby, wouldn't you?" and "Is the baby really coming?"), I was buoyed by Rudy's confidence.

When the labor was strong, it was overwhelming in its power. There was pain in my back that was hard to cope with, but I knew that the pain wasn't harming me in any way. The scary part was the power. It felt like I was running along a railroad track and a steam locomotive was bearing down on me, and I was about to be run over. I didn't realize at the time that unleashing that power made the labor progress and that I was in no

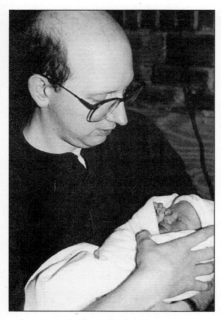
Rudy and Julianna

danger of "being run over." Afterward Carol and I talked about it. She described the sensation more accurately: It feels like you're riding on the front of a steam locomotive going 150 miles per hour. You're not going to fall off and get run over, but the ride requires that you have faith and surrender to the power of it.

When it got overwhelming for me, I would wish for a rest and the contractions would miraculously space out. I would lie down for a spell and close my eyes. This happened three or four times, and the midwives remarked that it seemed as though I could do it by will. The next time it got to be too much, I said, "I'd like to take a rest," and in fact, the labor slowed down. The trouble was that the breaks gave me a chance to think of new fears, which didn't make anything easier.

Ina May: *It was around this point that Heidi said she didn't think she could go on. I asked her to try saying something positive during her next rushes before she gave up. "I can too open another centimeter; I can too open another centimeter," she repeated during the rushes that took her through transition. This technique, called mantra in the Hindu tradition, is quite effective in dealing with deep fears, since the very act of making positive statements is empowering.*

Heidi: Finally I got to be nine centimeters and I asked Ina May to break my bag of waters, hoping that would speed the labor (and, by now I realized, the locomotive sensation) to a point where I could push the baby out. Soon I was pushing. The pushing was a welcome change, but the pain in my back didn't leave until the baby was quite low.

The sensations I felt as she started to crown were wild. I could feel the muscles in my lower vagina spread apart as her head passed. The sensations were distinct enough that I could appreciate different muscle groups. That was weird! As her head emerged, I held my hand over my vulva, because it seemed to help me slow down to ease her out. I expected it to hurt more as she was born; instead, it was just intense, because every sensitive nerve was firing. After about an hour of pushing with fifteen minutes of crowning, Julianna was born at 7:48 P.M.

What relief...physical relief and release, relief of our fears, because she was healthy and started breathing right away, and relief that the struggle was over. At first I was stunned; I don't remember much except a floating sensation of well-being. I asked the midwives to cut her cord, because it was short and pulling on me when they laid her on my belly. Rudy and Joanne were busy checking her out while I got cleaned up. Then we got to hold her and haven't stopped since.

I am so grateful for everyone's help; Rudy and the midwives were wonderful. I couldn't have labored without medication in the hospital, because I would have been too inhibited to do the things that really helped (being nude, groaning, holding myself as Julianna crowned), and I would have felt constrained by the hospital's routines. The intimacy and emotional intensity of our birth added to the wonder. Talking about it afterward, Rudy and I were glad that the labor was not very short. We needed the time to learn how to work with the labor, and we both needed time to distance ourselves from what we thought we knew about birth. Rudy and I are very grateful for the experience.

I treasure the experience of Julianna's birth and especially what that meant for her first hours on earth. She was completely alert, since I had had no medication, and we were never separated. Joanne handled her lovingly as she examined her and dealt with her eye ointment. She has never had anyone handle her roughly or impersonally. We got to shower her with love the whole night after she was born. What a blessing!

The following is one of our second-generation birth stories, for Mariahna's mother gave birth to her on The Farm, too, as is recounted on p.100.

✤ Ajahna's Birth—May 14, 2000
By Mariahna Nelson-Schaefer

It was Thursday night, May 11, 2000. I really hoped to have my baby this weekend even though she wasn't due for another week. I couldn't sleep, and around midnight mild contractions started. They were irregular, coming every half an hour. I tried to get some rest in between the contractions. My husband, Eric, was away and wouldn't be back until the next night, so I was trying to hold back. I knew I had to hold tight until Eric got here.

The next morning I was having regular contractions. My mom (who is also a midwife) checked me, and I was about two centimeters. I had contractions all day, which got stronger and closer as the day went on.

Before Eric got home that night, I went for a walk up to the area where some of my friends were having a big bonfire. The fire was so bright that I could see the dancing flames from quite a distance as I was walking up the road. It was a beautiful night. The moon was full and luminous, lighting up the trail as far as you could see. It felt so magical. I could feel the energy of the baby all around me.

When Eric arrived, we hung out for a while. Then we made love. We knew it would be the last time for a few weeks. That really made the contractions stronger. Eric slept through the night, but I didn't get much sleep. The contractions were close enough and strong enough that they kept me awake.

I was six centimeters open at five the next morning. Well, that was encouraging—over halfway there! But then, at the same time, only six! It seemed to me that I should be more open than that. I had been having regular contractions—even though they weren't real close—for a day and a half already. I had been eating and drinking to keep my energy up, but I was still getting tired.

I changed positions a lot. I was all over the place. I walked, squatted, lay on one side and then on the other side. I got on my hands and knees. I went up and down the stairs. I took a few hot baths and showers. I would stand and bend and move my hips around, sometimes dancing, while I listened to some of my favorite music. I was on and off the toilet frequently. It felt good just to sit there. I walked outside, sat in a tree for a while, and even hung from one of the branches. I also had some contractions straddling the limb of the tree and leaning on the tree. This all felt so natural. I didn't want to stay still. I had to keep moving, trying to figure out what felt good and would help me get more comfortable but also what was going to help me make progress. I had a lot of emotions going through me. I was so happy and loved everyone, but at the same time the sensations were so strong and intense. I laughed, I cried and felt frustrated, sometimes all in the same contraction. Sometimes I cried because it hurt so badly.

My nephew, Lance, who was three at the time, would come up to me and look sad and hold my hand. At one point he said, "Aunt Mari, do you think you'll ever stop hurting and get better?" I assured him that I probably would, after the baby came out.

I kept trying to stay focused and relaxed, but it was hard to do. The contractions were strong—like nothing I had ever felt before. Sometimes they felt like strong cramps. Sometimes a tightening came that was so strong that I thought my uterus was going to rip apart and break from the force. Sometimes I rubbed my stomach, squeezing it hard during the contractions, and that felt real good. It made the contraction stronger but felt like it was helping me make progress. I walked a lot. I breathed slow and deep through each contraction. I breathed so deep I could feel my breaths going to every cell in my body. I tried to take each contraction one at a time and not think about what was coming next. This seemed to help a lot. I had a lot of lower-back pain and pressure. It felt good for someone to rub my back with oil. It also felt good if someone rubbed and pressed on my whole spine and tailbone. I used a hot-water bottle often. The warmth felt good. It helped me relax and helped relieve some of the pain.

When they checked the baby's heartbeat they used a Doppler, and you could hear it in the room. It was so nice to hear. It gave me confidence and let me know everything was all right. I knew I wouldn't be hearing her heartbeat inside of me for very much longer. Soon she would be out.

My mom checked me again around 10:00 P.M. She said I was about fully dilated but had a lip of cervix. I had been this far along for several hours already. At that point she said that if I didn't make more progress soon, we would need to think about going to the hospital. She felt like something wasn't right, like something was holding the baby up. She knew that I was getting very tired, and this would be my third night in labor.

I decided right then I was going to have to just let it hurt more. I was determined to have the baby at home. I had a small lip of cervix that wouldn't go back. My mom tried to get it back a few times, but I just couldn't handle it. She applied some evening primrose oil to my cervix about 11:15 P.M. At 11:40 P.M. my other midwife, our friend Sharon, helped push it over the baby's head. Once I got fully dilated and started pushing, it helped. It was 11:45 P.M.

We had a mirror so I could see my progress. Once I saw her head and hair, I was determined she was going to come out, no matter how much it hurt. There was no turning back. It was so intense, it felt like my cookie was going to crumble. There was a lot of pressure. Her head was making me stretch. It felt very sharp and stung intensely. I really wanted her to come, but I also wanted to wait until Mother's Day, which was rapidly approaching.

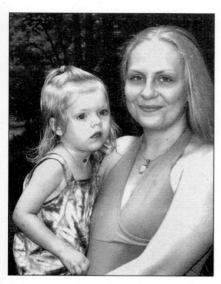

Ajahna

When she came out one minute after midnight, it was such a relief. I'll never forget how warm and soft and silky she was. She smelled so good, so sweet and newborn. She was such a little cuddle bug! She weighed eight pounds four ounces and was 21½ inches long. She latched right on and started nursing within minutes.

It turned out that she had both of her hands up by her face. They call that a "nuchal arm." With her, it was both arms! That's what was taking so long. That's why I had such strong back labor. Her little elbows were pushing on my spine and then on my tailbone.

It was all so intense, I was so glad it was over. She is now twenty months old and still puts her hands up by her face and ears when she is nursing or sleepy. She was such a sweet-smelling squishy little snookums. She was a lot of hard work but so worth it. I love her very much!

I am grateful that I didn't have to go to the hospital and that Eric, my midwives, my friend Lily, and my family were there for me. My sister Sally videotaped the whole thing. I couldn't have done it without all of them. I am so thankful for having such a loving, supportive family.

Ajahna Kaya Sky Nelson-Schaefer was born 12:01 A.M. on May 14, 2000. I'd gotten my wish. It was the weekend, Mother's Day, and she was a beautiful, healthy, sweet, little smiling girl.

Notes

1. Meenan, A., and Gaskin, I., et al. A new (old) maneuver for the management of shoulder dystocia, *The Journal of Family Practice*, 1991; 32:625–29.
2. Bruner, J., and Gaskin, I., et al. All-fours maneuver for reducing shoulder dystocia, *The Journal of Reproductive Medicine*, 1998; 43:439–43.
3. Gabbe, S. G., Niebyl, J. R., and Simpson, J. L. *Obstetrics: Normal & Problem Pregnancies*, 4th ed. New York: Churchill Livingstone, 2002.

II

THE ESSENTIALS OF BIRTH

INTRODUCTION

It almost goes without saying that the birth stories told in Part I differ from those of most American women. Overall, the stories are too positive; there is too much talk of joy, ecstasy, and fulfillment. These stories do not describe the usual proportions of forceps, vacuum extractor, or cesarean deliveries that are representative of these interventions. (For the women who gave birth at The Farm Midwifery Center, the approximate rate of such interventions combined was less than two percent. This compares with a rate of at least thirty to forty percent in the general U.S. population of birthing women.)

These births, for the most part, took place in a small birth center or in homes, and the number of midwives present at many of the births is far larger than would be typical of the U.S. mainstream. Given these differences, you may wonder whether these stories, and the overall experience of the women whose births were attended by my partners and me, can have any significance for you.

If the women who shared their birth stories were special beings, the answer would be no. But if it is true that the women who gave birth at The Farm are much like other U.S. women in their intrinsic physical capabilities—and I am certain that this is the case—then our experiences *do* have something to teach. Enfolded within the stories are lessons that can empower you, too, to give birth to your own child without technological intervention, wherever you decide to give birth. But birth in our social context has become somewhat complicated to fathom, given a collection of widely accepted cultural myths about this physiological act. Contrary to myth, for instance, intrinsic physical characteristics only rarely interfere with the capacity to give birth. In other words, your pelvis is probably big enough for vaginal birth. Nearly every woman's is. Mental attitudes and emotions, on the other hand, interfere with the ability to give birth far more than is generally understood.

Part II explains why we at The Farm Midwifery Center were able (with good and timely help from various doctors, hospitals, and community members) to achieve excellent results, even from the beginning when my partners and I had practically no experience. *Before the first cesarean became necessary, 186 babies were born* (the 187th baby was lying sideways in the womb and couldn't be turned). The second cesarean was the 324th birth. We achieved this remarkably low intervention rate without endangering women or their babies.

The reason that the statistics for The Farm Midwifery Center (See Appendix A) are so good is that we as a community managed to do right a great many of the things that could be done right or wrong. We got a lot right before we read any research. And the more things you do that are right, the more synergic they become. Each might seem small to someone looking for a magic bullet. What?—Turn birth over to women? Feed them? Just let them sleep? Wait for them to go into labor? Don't scare them? Yet the combination of these simple protocols produces a gestalt that leads to relaxed, happy, enthusiastic mothers and healthy babies. Yes, we still need hospitals and obstetricians, but the statistics from The Farm illustrate how infrequently this is necessary among healthy women who are well-prepared for birth. Part II also explains what routines you are likely to encounter in hospital maternity wards that may influence the course of labor and how these might affect the normal physiological process.

I make the point about our having done many things right from the beginning because it illustrates an important truth about birth: Birth is a normal physiological process. In no field other than midwifery could my partners and I have entered as amateurs, arranged for our own education, and still have managed to safely produce results that far outstripped those of medical professionals in hospitals with the most up-to-date technology. We could not have become dentists or surgeons this way.

I share my midwife's experience to encourage and to inform you.

It is important to keep in mind that our bodies *must* work pretty well, or there wouldn't be so many humans on the planet.

The information in this book is special because it was discovered and *realized* by a group of women who collectively learned that developing a women-centered style of maternity care made it possible to know things about their innate physiology that they had never before heard of.

1

The Powerful Mind/Body Connection

Do you ordinarily think of your mind and your body as separate from each other? If so, you are like most women brought up in Western cultures. From early in life, most of us are bombarded with messages that teach you to think that your thoughts and feelings don't matter when it comes to the functioning of your body. In the same way, Western medicine assumes a total separation between mind and body. Thoughts and feelings are considered irrelevant to physical welfare. When something goes wrong with the body, our culture teaches that pharmaceutical medicines or surgery will be necessary.

The well-documented placebo effect is a notable exception to the medical philosophy that assumes the irrelevance of mind to body. This phenomenon occurs when a person, given a "medication" that is in fact a sugar pill, believes that there is actually some curative agent in the pill. Some people given such pills experience a complete cure of whatever ailed them. In cases like these, the person's mind is fooled into believing that the body will recover. This belief then precipitates or hastens the actual recovery. A placebo is a way of tricking people into positive thinking. Despite medical culture's recognition of the placebo effect, orthodox medical theories about labor and birth generally take little notice of the intimate connection between mind and body.

Two of the first ten births I attended taught me how powerful the mind/body connection can be during labor and birth. The first eight women had labors like the ideal described in midwifery or medical textbooks. Contractions began, and the woman's cervix (the circular opening at the lower end of the uterus) dilated at a steady rate. However, in these two cases, after opening to about seven centimeters (ten centimeters is full dilation), the woman's cervix remained tightly locked for many hours, no matter how slowly and deeply she breathed, no matter how calmly she accepted each rush (contraction). In neither case did the woman's cervix appear to be any different from those of the other women, but clearly each was behaving differently. I wondered why, but my obstetrics text offered no hints as to the possible cause.

In the first case, a visit from a close friend of the laboring woman made a dramatic difference in the course of labor. On being invited into the birth room, she asked, "Has Sheila [the laboring woman] told you about her mother yet?" My body tingled all over on hearing those words. I then learned that the woman in labor had been adopted and had confided to her friend that she had grown up afraid that her biological mother had died in childbirth. She was apparently too embarrassed or too far beyond speech to admit that she was afraid of dying if she surrendered to the power of her labor. Once this profound fear was mentioned aloud, her cervix relaxed and displayed abilities it didn't seem to possess earlier. It wasn't long before it was completely open. A healthy baby was born within two hours of the mention of the secret fear. I was quite impressed to know that an unspoken terrible thought could so powerfully alter a woman's body's ability to perform a normal physiological function. At the same time, I was delighted to realize that a verbal solution to such a situation could remove any need for medication, mechanical intervention, or surgery.

In the second case, the laboring woman's cervix had also dilated to seven centimeters and stayed there for more than a day, despite strong rushes. Like the woman mentioned just above, she was having her first baby and was happy about her pregnancy. I was certain that Pamela wasn't afraid of dying in childbirth, so I was puzzled at her lack of progress for so long. After many hours of unproductive labor, I asked her if anything was worrying her. To my surprise, she answered yes. Her mind kept going back to the wedding vows she and her husband had written for their ceremony several months earlier. She had wanted to include promises about lifetime commitment, whereas he had been reluctant to go that far. As she told me this, I experienced a tingling over my body identical to what I felt upon hearing the other woman's friend explain about her situation.

Not knowing what else to do, I decided to consult Stephen, my husband, who happened to be a close friend of Pamela. He offered to give the couple a chance to repeat marriage vows that included the "as long as we both shall live" promise. When I asked them if they were willing to do this, they agreed. Between rushes they repeated these more comprehensive vows, and within two hours their healthy son was born.

I have never forgotten these births. My memories of the first several hundred births I attended are especially vivid, and these were among the first I witnessed. One reason they carved so deep a niche in my memory is that these two taught me something extremely precious that I hadn't realized before. I learned that true words spoken can sometimes relax pelvic muscles by *discharging emotions* that effectively block further progress in labor.

Another birth I attended a couple of years later is especially memorable because it taught me how closely coordinated a woman's mind/body can be during labor. I was traveling with family and friends and happened to be staying briefly in the city where a friend would be giving birth. Dawn's first baby had been born at home, attended by my midwife partners. She would have had this second baby at home as well, if her baby had not threatened to be born several weeks prematurely. She found that the hospital for high-risk pregnancies in her city was conducting a trial of a new medication to halt premature labor. By enrolling in this trial, a nurse–midwife could attend her birth, but the birth would have to take place in the hospital, even if the pregnancy went to full-term, as it did.

To my surprise, I was summoned to the hospital when Dawn went into labor. I wasn't sure what was expected of me as I walked through the wide halls of this brand-new hospital with its glistening floors and state-of-the-art birthing beds. As I entered the maternity ward, I saw a large green board on the wall, which listed the name of each woman in labor, her room number, and the amount her cervix was open. Suddenly, a loud alarm bell rang, and people began scurrying around in all directions. A nurse ran to the board and wrote the word *Complete* in the dilation column after one woman's name, as farther down the hall a doctor and several nurses dashed into the room of the woman about to have her baby.

When I arrived at Dawn's room, her nurse–midwife introduced herself and quietly invited me inside. She informed me that she saw the impending birth as a chance to give her client what she most wanted—to have me serve as her midwife—at the same time that she herself could witness her first "home birth." She quickly explained that her training as a midwife had not given her the opportunity to observe birth in any setting besides a hospital, adding that she had been present when her dog had puppies. As she spoke, she walked over to the door and showed me a feature of the room that I hadn't noticed: a lock, which had been installed to ensure that there would be no unwanted interruptions to women in labor. She turned it. There we were, secure in the knowledge that the calm atmosphere we were about to establish in the midst of the frantic pace of a large regional high-risk hospital would not be shattered by intruders or curious staff members.*

Dawn was so relieved that the plan she had devised with her nurse–midwife was coming to pass that she smiled with gratitude throughout labor. After a while I checked her internally to see how open her cervix was. She said, "I just want to open up and let this baby out." As she spoke these words, her cervix yawned open another two centimeters beneath my fingers. Now I was experiencing behavior that *I* didn't normally see, since I had never heard a woman express the wish for her cervix to open while I had my fingers on it to confirm that it was happening. Pretty fancy, I thought, to be able to tell your body exactly what you want to happen and have it comply. I wondered if I could have done that. Not long afterward, Dawn pushed her baby girl out into my wait-

*Incidentally, this birth happened in the mid-1970s during the height of the home-birth movement. Hospitals sometimes bowed to the wishes of laboring women and midwives then, which was probably the reason why inside door locks were installed. It has been a long time since I have heard of inside door locks in U.S. hospitals.

ing hands. Except for a couple of pairs of gloves, a cord clamp, scissors to cut the cord, and receiving blankets, we had no need for the many items that had been assembled for the birth. Dawn had her "home birth" in a hospital, and one hospital-based midwife had a new sense of what birth can be when it occurs in a setting where calm and confidence reign instead of anxiety and fear.

Years later I was in Edinburgh, Scotland, addressing an audience of midwives and mothers. I had just related the story about my friend whose cervix had opened when she wished aloud that it would. A woman in back of the meeting hall caught my attention with her animated facial expression as she listened to this story. She wanted to talk about her experience during her labor with her first baby. She had been sitting on her bed in the first stage of labor (during which the cervix is opening), encircled in her husband's arms. He whispered in her ear, "You're marvelous!" and she was sure that she felt her cervix open when she heard his words.

"Please say that again!" she told him.

He repeated the words, and she again felt her cervix open.

"I *know* you're going to think I'm crazy," she said, addressing both him and her midwife, "but would you just keep saying that?"

Her husband, joined by her midwife, kept up the chant. Soon, her cervix was completely dilated, and she pushed her baby out.

I think that everyone in that room felt blessed to have heard this wonderful story of the possibilities when female and male energy combine in a powerful and graceful way. What I love about stories the most is the power they have to teach us of possibilities that might not occur to us without them. What can be more liberating to an expectant father than to know that his loving words to his partner may give her strength and energy to make her birth crossing easier—even to the point where sometimes it ventures into ecstasy?

Another way in which the mind/body connection is made obvious in birth may occur just after the birth and the separation of the placenta from the uterine wall. Sometimes a woman's uterus does not contract sufficiently to shut off bleeding from where the placenta was attached. In cases like these, medications or herbs are most often used to stimulate harder contractions to stop the bleeding. At times, though, words are enough. Several times, I have told a mother to stop bleeding, and she has done so.

If any bodily process ever required a maximum degree of relaxation, it is birth. Babies are the biggest things that pass through any of our orifices. Ever.

My midwife partners and I at The Farm learned by observation and experience that the presence of even one person who is not exquisitely attuned to the mother's feelings can stop some women's labors. All women are sensitive. Some women are extraordinarily so. We learned this truth by observing many labors stop or slow down when someone entered the birth room who was not intimate with the laboring mother's feelings. If that person then left the room, labor usually returned to its former pace or intensity.

In my third year of attending births, I observed something I had never seen nor heard of before. I noticed that it is possible for a woman's cervix to "go into reverse" after dilating more than halfway. Judith, a friend of mine, was in labor with her first baby. She had been laboring along for three or four hours in what seemed an easy and relaxed manner. She and her man cuddled and smooched during the rushes, occasionally joking with each other and us midwives. Judith asked me to check her, and I found her cervix to be almost fully open (eight centimeters). Around this point, her labor took another course from what we had observed before. She got that inward look that women take on when they feel another rush approaching and they know it's bigger than anything they have experienced before. Throughout it, she held herself as if she were sitting on the most fragile of eggshells. Afterward she was quiet, alert, and very serious. The next few rushes were considerably easier—in fact, they were so mild that she asked me to check her dilation again, knowing that I was scheduled to leave on a trip within a couple of hours. That was when I made my thrilling discovery—that her cervix had cinched down from eight centimeters to about half that amount. Having been with her continuously throughout her labor, I knew that she had done it with her mind, because she had been sitting rather still as it happened.

Intuitively, I felt that Judith could probably help her cervix to open again if she allowed herself to surrender to laughter. "Try to lighten up if you can," I said to her in the gentlest, most encouraging way I could.

She did just that. It wasn't long before she delivered her baby daughter, well in time for me to stay with her. Excited about my new knowledge, I began researching what others had written about the phenomenon of a woman shutting down or actually reversing labor, whether voluntarily or involuntarily. After going through innumerable obstetrics, midwifery, and nursing texts and asking many audiences of nurses and nurse–midwives if they knew of such references, I realized that I wasn't going to find anything. Too many hospital-based midwives and nurses told me that if there was a difference between their measurement of cervical dilation and that done by a doctor (as there often is), the doctor is always believed (never the midwife or nurse). They also said that doctors in these cases rarely, if ever, believe that the cervix truly had been more open before. For them, it is easier to believe that the nurse or nurse–midwife is wrong than that women have unknown abilities that aren't always noted in medical textbooks. This kind of miscommunication is rampant in the medical model of birth care. Only rarely do doctors in training have the opportunity to sit continuously with laboring women for hours. Most are taught to intervene in the normal process so often and so early that they have never witnessed a normal labor and birth. Obviously, continuous observation is the best way to learn about the mind/body connection, because it alone affords the observer the chance to witness the subtle nuances of emotions as they ebb and flow throughout labor. It is the only sure way to correlate emotional changes with physical changes.

I later learned that the doctors who wrote textbooks never had the chance to observe the behavior I watched. I began to wonder whether medical textbooks had always been so blind to this particular instance of the mind/body connection in labor. Digging into texts written before birth moved into hospitals, I found that earlier generations of doctors still retained some of the common-sense knowledge that was transmitted by medical textbooks throughout the nineteenth century. In this category were many references to the reversal of labor I had observed. Some women, it seems, can just suck their babies back in if they really don't like the way things are going. It was as true then as it is now, but more people knew about it then. Nineteenth-century doctors had much to say about the importance of staying out of the laboring woman's bedroom until birth was imminent or medical attention was deemed necessary by the women helpers at the birth. They taught their medical students (always male in those days) to respect the consensus of the female birth helpers.

- Betschler (1880) mentioned a case "in which the pains were suddenly suspended by a violent tempest, so that the neck [cervix], though widely dilated, closed again, nor did the labor recommence until nineteen days had elapsed."[1]
- Cazeaux (1884): "Every day, indeed, we witness a suspension of the pains for half an hour, and sometimes even for several hours, upon visiting women whose modesty is shocked by our presence."[2] Male birth attendants were still comparatively rare in those days.
- Dewees (1847): "In 1792, I was called to attend a Mrs. C, in consequence of her midwife being engaged. As I approached the house, I was most earnestly solicited to hasten in, as not a moment was to be lost. I was suddenly shown into Mrs. C's chamber, and my appearance there was explained by stating that her midwife was engaged. As I entered the room, Mrs. C was just recovering from a pain—and it was the last she had at that time. After waiting an hour in the expectation of a return of labour, I took my leave, and was not again summoned to her for precisely two weeks. And Dr. Lyall says, 'We have been informed by a respectable practitioner, of a labour that had nearly arrived at its apparent termination, suspended for more than two days, in consequence of a gentleman having been sent to the patient, against whom she had taken a prejudice.' Every accoucheur [birth attendant] has experienced a temporary suspension of pain upon his first appearance in the sick chamber; but so long a period as two weeks is very rare."[3]
- A. Curtis (1846): "As soon as you arrive, let the husband, or some familiar friend, inform the lady, and then you should remain in the ante-chamber till she requests your presence. A sudden surprise, especially if attended with the fear of severe treatment, will greatly retard the process, and, in many cases, cause the foetus to retract. When you enter the room, let your mind be calm and collected, and your feelings kindly sympathize with those of the patient."[4]

- Francis H. Ramsbotham (1861): "On arriving at the patient's residence it is better not abruptly to obtrude one's-self into her presence, unless there be some immediate necessity for our attendance. Information should be sought from the nurse, on such points as will enable us to judge whether labour has actually commenced. On being ushered into her chamber, we may engage her in some general conversation, which will give us an opportunity of observing the frequency, duration, strength, and character of the pains; and our conduct must be framed accordingly."[5]
- W. A. Newman Dorland (1901): "On The 'Pains,' or Uterine Contractions: Mental emotion of any kind will temporarily diminish their intensity or even absolutely suppress them; the entrance of the physician into the lying-in room may have the same effect."[6]

I was fascinated to learn that most doctors once knew that an unwelcome or upsetting presence could stall labor. They knew it the same way that farmers knew about the birthing behavior of their animals—it was common knowledge, accumulated through observation, that was passed down from one generation to another. But when the pool of home-birth knowledge dried up, knowledge that once was common became rare or even extinct. The fact is that doctors are no longer in a good position to note that their own presence in the birth room or their hurried manner often can retard labor. We must remember that the mind/body phenomenon described in the nineteenth-century textbooks is no less true now than it was then.

The problem is that doctors today often assume that something mysterious and unidentified has gone wrong with labor or that the woman's body is somehow "inadequate"—what I call the "woman's body as a lemon" assumption. For a variety of reasons, a lot of women have also come to believe that nature made a serious mistake with their bodies. This belief has become so strong in many that they give in to pharmaceutical or surgical treatments when patience and recognition of the normality and harmlessness of the situation would make for better health for them and their babies and less surgery and technological intervention in birth. Most women need encouragement and companionship more than they need drugs.

Remember this, for it is as true as true gets: *Your body is not a lemon.* You are not a machine. The Creator is not a careless mechanic. Human female bodies have the same potential to give birth well as aardvarks, lions, rhinoceri, elephants, moose, and water buffalo. Even if it has not been your habit throughout your life so far, I recommend that you learn to think positively about your body.

Notes

1. Betschler 1880, quoted in Engelmann, G. *Labor among Primitive Peoples*. St. Louis: J. H. Chambers, 1882. Reprinted New York: AMS Press.
2. Cazeaux, P. *Obstetrics: The Theory and Practice*, 7th ed. Philadelphia: P. Blakiston, Son & Co., 1884.
3. Dewees, William P. *Compendious System of Midwifery*, 4th ed. Philadelphia: Carey & Lea, 1830.
4. Curtis, A. *Lectures on Midwifery*. Philadelphia, 1846.
5. Ramsbotham, Francis H. *The Principles and Practice of Obstetric Medicine and Surgery*. New York, 1861.
6. Dorland, W. A. Newman. *Modern Obstetrics*. New York, 1901.

Said the plumber to the maiden as they lay there by the sea, "Shh! Someone's coming!" Said the maiden, "Hush! it's me!"

—Author unknown

2

WHAT HAPPENS IN LABOR

The physical changes that take place in a woman's body during labor are perhaps the most dramatic that occur in humans. They involve more movement, more shape-changing of various organs, more prolonged physical sensation, and considerably more effort than do other physiological functions of the body such as yawning, swallowing, burping, sneezing, coughing, laughing, crying, digesting, breathing, peeing, vomiting, pooping, farting, and coming—the functions we experience on a more regular basis. Birth—as experienced by the mother—is the Mount Everest of physical functions in any mammal. Unless we have seen it before, we can barely imagine that something so relatively huge can come out of a place that usually looks so small. And yet, it happens every day.

Since it is not immediately obvious how this can happen, let's take a look at the basics, beginning with what happens to the uterus in pregnancy and labor.

There is no other organ quite like the uterus. If men had such an organ, they would brag about it. So should we.

The membranous, nearly transparent bag of salty fluid—a miniature ocean—contains the baby and its umbilical cord. The cord leads to the placenta, a short-lived but wondrous organ that, maintaining its attachment to the baby at the navel, is planted in the rich uterine lining of blood vessels and serves a multitude of purposes in pregnancy. The placenta does the work that will later be taken up by the baby's lungs, digestive system, liver, excretory organs, and the two chambers of the baby's heart that mostly don't function during intrauterine life. In some languages, the word for placenta translates as *mother cake*, perhaps in recognition of the vital role it plays in the baby's intrauterine growth. The placenta literally feeds the baby.

The cervix (the word means *neck* in Latin), the circular opening like a bottleneck at the lower end of the uterus, is a powerful band of muscles that holds the uterus tightly closed until labor begins. Picture a knit purse with a gathered opening held tight by a string. This thick cervical muscle has to be strong enough to hold the uterus shut despite the pressure of approximately fifteen pounds of baby, placenta, and fluid against it—and considerably more in the case of twins and other multiple pregnancies. The cervical muscle is the kind that is able to remain closed without exertion in its prelabor state. (Once labor begins, its task is to thin and get out of the way.) The cervix is sealed during pregnancy with a plug of thick mucus, which is expelled during the hours before labor begins. Usually this mucus is slightly tinged with blood, giving it a pinkish, reddish, or brownish color. When this mucus, called *show*, is expelled from the cervix, it signals that labor will soon begin.

The top part of the uterus is also muscle tissue, but of a different type from the cervix. The three layers of muscle fibers of the main body of the uterus are amazingly powerful yet stretchable and flexible. They must expand to contain even a multiple pregnancy and still be able to expel everything inside when labor time comes, no matter how large or small the baby or bits of tissue may be.

Before pregnancy occurs, the uterus is a hollow muscular organ the shape and size of an inverted pear. It is located in the lower half of a woman's belly, held in place by strong ligaments. After conception, the fertilized egg is swept from the fallopian tube to the interior of the uterus. There it burrows into the uterine lining and develops a placenta and a water bag containing a future human. As the baby and placenta grow, the uterus expands with them. During pregnancy, the uterus grows to approximately the size of a large watermelon if there is just one baby inside—even larger if there is more than one baby. By the time a baby is ready to be born, the top of the uterus has risen above the lower rib cage and has pushed the stomach above its usual position. (This is why pregnant women often find it necessary to eat smaller, more-frequent meals during the last weeks of pregnancy to avoid heartburn. Some don't avoid it.)

At the time of labor, the walls of the uterus are relatively thin. Even so, their power to squeeze during a labor contraction is sufficient to push a big baby through the open cervix and out the vagina, which must also expand and open.

During the last few days of pregnancy, hormones called prostaglandins cause the thick cervical muscle to begin to soften and thin in readiness for labor. This process is called *ripening*. The cervix, which feels something like a nose during pregnancy, becomes extremely soft to the touch when ripe, losing its distinctive necklike shape. No longer a bottleneck, it becomes part of the bottle.

The part of labor when the cervix is opening is called the *first stage*. Given the choice, most mammals are restless during this part of labor, for this is the time when the baby is pushed, jostled, wriggled, and turned into the most advantageous position to pass through the maternal passageway if she is not already well-positioned. Hoofed mammals tend to be born feetfirst. Primates, such as humans and the other apes, are usually born headfirst, although bottom- or feet-first babies can be vaginally born as well.

Once the cervix is pulled completely open, a combination of uterine contractions and some pressure from the abdominal muscles pushes the baby outside of the mother's body. This is called the *second stage of labor*. It lasts until the birth of the baby. Gravity can greatly affect progress during this part of labor. So can a lot of other things, but we'll get to that later.

As for the water bag, sometimes this breaks before labor, sometimes during labor, and sometimes it is intact at birth and has to be broken and peeled away so the baby can take her first breath. Sometimes the bag is intentionally broken in an effort to speed labor. Breaking the bag intentionally can be dangerous when the baby's presenting part is still high enough to leave room for a loop of umbilical cord to be swept out of the uterus by the downward-rushing fluid. In cases such as this, the circulation of oxygen-rich blood to the baby can be pinched off when the cord is caught between the baby's head and the opening cervix.

Rhythmic contractions of the upper part of the uterus thin and pull back the cervix during the first stage of labor. During the second or pushing stage of labor, these contractions also push the leading part of the baby down through the lower part of the pelvis. Only rarely do the dimensions of a woman's pelvis significantly interfere with the birth of her baby. (Civilized nineteenth-century women, though, often suffered from pelvic deformities caused by vitamin D deficiency, and such deformities did obstruct vaginal birth.) Meanwhile, the baby's skull (which, like the pelvis, is made up of separate bones held together with flexible ligaments) is able to temporarily mold itself for easier passage through the maternal pelvic bones.

One of the best features of labor is the rest periods that occur between these rushes. Hardly anyone seems to talk about these in birth preparation books, but they are one of the most brilliant features of labor. Savor every second of them. Appreciate them. They are your chance to relax and enjoy feeling "normal" and alive. These rest periods may be ten—even fifteen—minutes apart in early labor. In the second stage of labor, they may be only a minute or two apart until the birth of the baby.

The *third stage of labor* lasts from the birth of the baby until the expulsion of the placenta. The uterus continues to contract after the birth of the baby, quickly diminishing its size to that of the placenta. Further contractions shear the placenta from the uterine lining. This event is usually signaled by the expulsion of dark red blood within fifteen or twenty minutes after birth. More contractions then expel the placenta. Gravity and gentle traction on the umbilical cord by an attendant may aid this process.

The *fourth stage of labor* is the postpartum or newborn period, roughly the six weeks that follow childbirth. This is the time during which the mother's body adjusts to new motherhood and returns to the nonpregnant state.

Labor for a first-time mother lasts from less than an hour (this is relatively rare in our culture) to twenty hours or significantly more, as we have seen from some of the stories in Part I. Much of this time in the latter case, however, is not "hard" labor. Subsequent labors are usually somewhat quicker, but there are exceptions.

> Over thirty years of experience as a midwife have not lessened my awe and respect for the efficiency and beautiful design of the female body as expressed in labor and birth. In fact, the years only increase my sense of wonder about how well our bodies can work—given the right circumstances. The outcomes of our births at The Farm Midwifery Center demonstrate how rare it is for complications and difficulties to occur when women are properly prepared for birth and when technological interventions are kept to a minimum—that is, used only when necessary. Ninety-four percent of women gave birth at home or at our birth center. Fewer than two percent had cesareans. Fewer than one percent had their babies delivered by forceps or vacuum extractors.

The Hormones That Regulate Labor and Birth

An intricate and exquisitely balanced combination of hormones is necessary to trigger all of the functions of labor and birth described above. The subtle, complex interplay of changing hormone levels during the birth process is one of the most fascinating and little understood aspects of pregnancy and birth in the modern world. Prostaglandins, oxytocin, adrenaline, and endorphins are some of the most important natural chemical combinations produced within the woman's body during labor and birth. They play key roles in regulating and timing uterine contractions during labor and birth. They stimulate the maternal and infant responses (emotions and actions) that are vital to the survival of the newborn.

I mentioned earlier that natural prostaglandins act on the cervix to soften and thin it in readiness for labor. Oxytocin causes the uterus to contract. Later on, when the bulk of the baby passes through the vagina, a sudden rise in oxytocin levels in mother and baby stimulates the chain of instinctual dance between them that is most often called falling in love. They gaze into each other's eyes with gratitude and wonder.

Now we come to adrenaline. If oxytocin is the accelerator of birth (since it stimulates the contraction of the uterus and makes it work harder to open), adrenaline is the brakes. Adrenaline "pumps us up." High adrenaline levels increase the heart rate and make us stronger and faster so that we can either fight or flee. They can sometimes—as I discussed in the previous chapter—make labor stop. The effects of adrenaline should not be underestimated, especially in births that take place in busy hospitals. I believe that high adrenaline levels are the reason that so many women in labor find themselves no longer in labor when they check in to a hospital.

I'll never forget the woman who told me that her first birth was attended by a young resident (doctor in training) who was not good at hiding his horrified expression when her baby's head parted the lips of her vulva. It seems that the baby was coming face-first, and it was the first time the resident had seen this (usually the top of the baby's head comes first). He imagined that he was seeing some horrible defect. His facial expression terrified the mother, who instantly felt her baby retract inside her body with such force that one of her ribs cracked. A cool-headed obstetric nurse took charge at that point and managed to restart the second stage by pushing down on the woman's uterus. The baby was born in good condition.

My sister's first birth was an example of adrenaline having the opposite effect—of speeding up labor instead of slowing it down. When an impatient doctor warned her that a cesarean would be necessary if she wasn't fully dilated in twenty minutes, she managed to dilate the five centimeters necessary to escape surgery. "I really didn't want to get cut!" she told me later. French physician Michel Odent calls my sister's experience an example of the *fetal ejection reflex*—a sudden rise in adrenaline gives us the surge of power necessary to complete the job of birth.

The third major hormone category involved in labor is the endorphins. Endorphins are nature's opiates. When we expend a lot of physical effort, endorphin levels rise correspondingly, especially when we are warm enough, feeling loved and supported, and, above all, when we are not frightened. Endorphins are a blessing, because they actually block the reception of pain. Endorphins give us that feeling of pleasure that comes with a job well done or a work-in-progress.

That, in a nutshell, is what happens in birth. When Jessica Mitford, author of *The American Way of Birth*, sought to describe the essence of birth, she reverted to her mother's description (as women often do): "It's like trying to push an orange out through your nostril." I liked everything in her book but this statement. Birth is nothing at all like pushing an orange out of a nostril. Nostrils weren't created to do anything of the kind. Nothing larger than a little mucus comes out of them. A vagina is able to accommodate the size and shape of what it contains, whether we are talking about a penis or a baby. The big "secret" is that it is better able to accomplish this task when we can imagine or "picture" this happening.

We need to always remember that mothers who are afraid tend to secrete the hormones that delay or inhibit birth. This is true of all mammals and is part of nature's design. Those who are not terrified are more likely to secrete in abundance the hormones that make labor and birth easier and less painful—sometimes even pleasurable. In the next chapter we'll examine the mind/body connection more deeply to gain some understanding of how it relates to the normal progress of labor.

The more cultured the races of the earth have become, so much the more positive have they been in pronouncing childbirth to be a painful and dangerous ordeal.

—Grantly Dick-Read, *Childbirth Without Fear*

3

THE PAIN/PLEASURE RIDDLE

The message that childbirth is extraordinarily painful has traveled far and wide. No one questions that labor and birth can be physically painful experiences for many women. Less well known is the fact that some women in all cultures have labors that are essentially painless. This raises two questions: First, how is it possible that the same physical act can be experienced in ways so completely different? Second, what can we learn from this about preparing for labor?

To answer these questions, it may help to try thinking of labor and birth from a different angle than the usual one. Let's consider another act that involves the same female reproductive organs as labor does—the sex act. Sexual intercourse may be extremely painful or ecstatically pleasurable, depending upon the skill and sensitivity of the sexual partner and the willingness of the female involved. The size of the object inside her vagina actually has less to do with the physical sensations she experiences during the act than do the factors just mentioned. The same can be said of the sensations experienced upon the insertion of a tampon. To begin with, tampons are smaller than the penises of adult men. Yet the same size tampon may be inserted in a painful or painless fashion, depending on whether the woman had too much coffee that morning, how cold it is, or the speed with which she tries to insert it. A lot depends upon how ready she is for the experience. Looked at from this perspective, it should be somewhat less surprising that there is such a wide variation in the way different women describe the sensations of labor and birth.

Another interesting aspect of the pain question is that women's perceptions of labor pain vary a great deal depending upon their country or culture of origin. In some countries, including the United States, probably a majority of women consider it a hardship to labor without some form of anesthesia. There are exceptions, of course, including the women of The Farm and Old Order Amish communities, among others. In other countries of similar wealth (the Netherlands and Japan are prime examples), most women do not expect to be given anesthesia for a normal physiological process such as labor and birth. If there is pain, it is not something to focus on. It is part of nature and therefore not to be feared. In both the Netherlands and Japan, midwives attend most of the births—in contrast to the United States, where midwives, although growing in numbers, still attend only about ten percent of all births.

A study comparing a group of Dutch women's expectations of labor pain with those of a group of U.S. women found striking differences.[1] Both groups of women were having hospital births and were asked the following questions within two days after they gave birth: What were their expectations of pain, did they take pain medication, and how they would prefer pain to be managed in a future labor? Both the Dutch group and the U.S. group were informed of the potential negative effects of pain-relieving medications for labor. Nearly two-thirds of the Dutch group received no pain medication, in contrast with only one-sixth of the U.S. women. Two-thirds of the U.S. group were given narcotics during labor, along with some type of nerve block for birth. The U.S. women *expected* labor to be more painful than the Dutch women did, and they expected to be given medication for pain. In both groups, the proportions of women expecting pain to those who actually received medication were nearly identical.

Anthropologist Brigitte Jordan commented on the difference in attitudes about labor pain between Dutch and American women in her important book, *Birth in Four Cultures.* She wrote: "There is in Dutch birth participants a deep-seated conviction that the woman's body knows best and that, given enough time, nature knows best and that, given enough time, nature will take its course."[2] When I visited Japan, I found similar attitudes among the women and midwives with whom I spoke. "Birth is natural," several said. "I would be afraid of an earth-quake, but not of having a baby without anesthesia. That's just the work that women do. Besides, if you take anesthesia, you miss the ecstasy. You miss the euphoria."

Another study compared perceptions of labor pain between two different groups of U.S. women: those who gave birth in the hospital and those who gave birth at home. The hospital group rated childbirth pain *significantly higher* than did the home-birth group.[3] There are some good reasons why birth pain seems to be less for women who have home births. First, they are far less likely than women having hospital births to be confined to lying in bed during labor, to be denied food and drink, or to have strangers around them as they labor. The normal creature comforts of everyday life—moving around freely, eating and drinking at will—are just as compelling during labor, if not more so than they usually are. Women who have out-of-hospital births are also more likely than are women in U.S. hospitals to have the continuous help of someone they trust, another factor that has been shown to reduce the perception of labor pain.

Pain is a strange category of human experience in certain ways. We women seem to think about it in different ways, according to what we think causes it. Probably all of us have had stabbing or wrenching pains from trapped intestinal gas—what a friend of mine calls an impacted fart. Understanding that the small displacement of the intestines from a tiny amount of captured gas can cause severe, knifelike pain makes it easier to comprehend why pain is often part of the experience of labor and birth.

Labor pain is a far more subtle, changeable set of sensations than our cultural mythology admits. When I say "subtle," I am not talking about the *feeling* of labor pain so much as the change in attitude that can alter our perception of it. I have seen many laboring women go from hell to heaven within seconds as they moved from stark terror to a realization of how to work with the energy of birth.

Of course, it is much more possible to pay attention to such subtle mind changes when you are being given continuous encouragement by someone who is not herself (or himself) frightened of labor. You may feel during a rush as if you are being horribly injured inside, but your midwife's calm, steady manner or soothing words tell you that no injury is actually taking place. This knowledge at such moments is so reassuring that it becomes possible to feel either the pain diminish or your own ability to bear whatever you are feeling increase. I can't count how many times I have seen a woman's eyes widen with fright at the sheer power of the rushes that accompany the full dilation of the cervix. When I see those eyes, I know the words that will relieve the kind of unreasoning fear that has seized her.

"Don't worry," I'll say. "I've never seen anyone explode or tear in half." Relief is usually instant and complete.

"Only the baby will come out," I'll go on, if I notice my words are having a calming effect. "Your body is very wise. It only pushes out what needs to come out."

What happens in cases like these is that with relief and gratitude comes a rush of endorphins, nature's opiates. Pain diminishes. This causes still more relief and gratitude and a stronger endorphin effect. The woman gains a new appreciation of the wisdom of nature as expressed through her body. When she starts to understand that being amused and grateful actually moves the process of labor along more efficiently, she starts to work toward these feelings herself. Hard work may continue, but she now has the heart for it. Instead of fearing her body, she experiments with trusting it.

> *We are, indeed, fully prepared to believe that the bearing of children may and ought to become as free from danger and long debility to the civilized woman as it is to the savage.*
>
> **—Thomas Huxley**

Painless Birth

As I mentioned earlier, there are women who have painless birth experiences. Some don't even realize they are in labor until the baby is actually emerging from their bodies. My friend Mary thought that the cramps she was feeling at nine months' gestation with her first baby were caused by an intestinal flu that was going around. She went to sit on the toilet. A couple of minutes after she sat down, her son was born, caught by his father a second before he dropped into the water. I should mention here that my own birth experiences were nothing like this. I always knew when I was having a baby. Still, some women have experiences like this, even with their first baby. Occasionally, the father of the baby experiences more pain than the laboring woman herself.

I watched three women tell their stories of surprise, relatively painless births on Maury Povich's talk show in 1996. Each had been unaware that she was pregnant. One had never given birth before (she had previously been told by a doctor that she couldn't conceive), and she did not have pain severe enough that it occurred to her to go to a hospital. Having had sensations as strong from a stomach flu, she just submerged her body in her bathtub and never realized that she was having a baby—until her baby's head emerged.

Stories as remarkable as these are sometimes written down. A childbirth preparation book written by Alice B. Stockham a century ago included these:[4]

- Dr. Douglas's experience of being called by a family in London in 1828, only to learn that the baby had been born *before* he was called. The woman had actually given birth in her sleep and became aware of this only when she was awakened by her frightened five-year-old daughter, who'd heard the cries and felt the movements of the newly born baby.
- In another case reported by Dr. Douglas, "A lady of great respectability, the wife of a peer of the realm, was actually delivered once in her sleep; she immediately awakened her husband, being alarmed to find one more in bed than there was before."
- Alice Stockham's neighbor had each of her four babies before Dr. Stockham could reach her, despite the fact that she lived across the street. After the quick arrival of the first baby, she made Dr. S. sleep with her shoes already laced when her time was near.

One of my sisters taught me that some women come to their first birth with life experience that has prepared them well for putting labor pain into perspective. I had just helped her and her husband with the birth of their first child at home and happened to mention that she had seemed to have an especially easy time for a first birth.

"I kept waiting for the rushes to get as painful as my period cramps," she told me. "I used to get cramps so bad that I had to go to bed with them on the first two days." A woman who has had a miscarriage or who is used to severe menstrual cramps already has some life training that should help her to give birth without becoming terribly frightened of pain itself.

In his classic book *Childbirth Without Fear*, Dr. Grantly Dick-Read told the story of one of the first births he ever witnessed as a young medical student in London in 1913. Believing, as he did at the time, that childbirth was always painful, he was surprised when the laboring woman refused his offer of a whiff of chloroform. This was the first time in his admittedly short experience that any woman had declined to take chloroform. When he was about to leave after the birth, he asked her why she had refused the mask.

"She did not answer at once," he wrote, "but looked from the old woman who had been assisting to the window through which was bursting the first light of dawn; then shyly she turned to me and said: 'It didn't hurt. It wasn't meant to, was it, doctor?' "

During World War I, when Dick-Read was a battlefield doctor, he witnessed two unforgettable births. The first asked for a doctor, and Dick-Read made a private space, examined her, and found her to be in advanced labor. Soon the baby was born and all was well. Seemingly with no consciousness of the war around her, the young woman "sat up on the stretcher, laughed, and took the child in her hands at once."

The second was a Flemish woman who was leaning against a bank in a field where she had evidently been working. Something about the way she was standing told him that something was happening to her. They didn't understand each other's languages, but she managed to communicate that she was having a baby, that she wasn't frightened, and that she didn't really need his help. He decided to stay nearby, smoke his pipe, and be available if he should be needed later on. Meanwhile, the woman was all laughter and smiles and happiness. When her contractions returned, her face became "set, not with pain or fear, but with a sense of stern expectancy." The baby was soon born. The mother smiled almost immediately but left the baby lying on the ground for a few minutes.

After what seemed a long time, the baby began yelling, and the mother picked it up and somehow tore the cord free. She wrapped the baby in a piece of cloth that had been around her shoulders, turned to the amazed Dick-Read, and "gaily laughed." Five minutes later, she had some contractions and the afterbirth was expelled with no apparent bleeding. Dick-Read never forgot the experience, which was so unlike the hospital births he witnessed of women who were more frightened. He wrote:

"One thing that appealed to me was the spirit of joy, the spirit of happiness and pride at the arrival and sound of the child.... My visions of postpartum hemorrhage, blue babies that would not breathe, uteri that would not contract and placentas that would not separate, all seemed entirely foreign to this exhibition of labour, conducted more efficiently than I have ever visualized in my most ambitious moments."[5]

I read *Childbirth Without Fear* at sixteen. Reading it prepared me well for labor—if not how to escape the routines of U.S. hospitals in the mid-1960s that prevented women from having unmedicated labor and birth without episiotomy, forceps or vacuum extractor.

The question of whether childbirth was meant to be painful has been discussed for at least a century and a half—the approximate time during which various anesthetic drugs have been used to quell the pain of labor. John Dye, a nineteenth-century U.S. doctor, posed an interesting question to those who believed that childbirth pain was attributable to divine wrath over a female ancestor's disobedience (sometimes called the "Eve goofed" theory of childbirth pain). His question was this: If this is indeed the design and pain is truly necessary for birth, why do some women suffer so much more than others? Besides, Dye wondered, why were those doctors who were most ready to assign responsibility to the Creator for women's suffering in birth so quick to turn to man-made drugs to interrupt this divinely ordained pain?[6]

Grantly Dick-Read's fascination with the riddle of why some women feel pain while others do not guided his entire life and career. As a medical student watching experienced midwives work in a London hospital, he noticed that sometimes women who entered the hospital in the agony of a difficult labor could be eased and soothed by the attention of a sympathetic midwife. A midwife could go to a woman who had been the "picture of agony and torture," stroke her hair, and talk to her in such a way that the pain, if not the effort, would seem to disappear. Time after time, he watched the way attentive midwives, nurturing each laboring woman in a motherly way, could bring peace and comfort to those who had been sent in as "terrified abnormal cases."

Orgasmic Birth

In some cultures—including ours—a lot of women accept or demand pain medication before they have tested what the unmedicated experience might be like. I once asked an audience if anyone had ever heard that some women experience orgasm during labor or birth.

Scanning the faces of the audience, I saw mostly expressions of surprise and curiosity. Then I spotted a petite blond woman, whose face was especially animated. "Yes! I'm so glad to hear you say that! *I* had the most amazing, prolonged orgasm when I gave birth seventeen years ago," she declared. "I thought I was the only person in the world this ever happened to and that maybe I was just weird."

She went on to explain that her determination to go through labor without pain medication had been met with pressure from her doctor.

"You're not going to get a medal for refusing medication," he told her. As the intensity of labor increased and birth became imminent, she said that she began to feel tingly all over. Then she did something she later regretted: She told her doctor that she felt like she was having an orgasm.

"Do you know what he told me?" she asked. "He said, 'You are a lunatic! You are the strangest patient I have ever had!' That's what he told me. Now I realize that all the embarrassment I have felt when I remember the birth was because of his ignorance and rudeness."

She paused for a moment and then added, "But the orgasm was great!"

I have met a number of women whose experience was much the same: Whatever their expectations had been about how labor would feel, they discovered that parts of it at least felt extremely good. A few were taken aback to find themselves experiencing such exquisite pleasure while surrounded by strangers who were oblivious to what they were feeling—especially since they had never before heard that it was possible to feel pleasure while giving birth. Caroline, a childbirth educator from South Carolina, told me that she decided it would be a good idea not to mention her feelings to the doctor and nurse who were attending her. "I just went ahead and enjoyed myself," she said. "And I've never told anyone else about it until just now. I have always wondered why no one ever seems to talk about this."

Curious about how many women I could find who had orgasmic experiences in labor or birth, I decided to conduct a small survey among some close friends. Of 151 women, I found thirty-two who reported experiencing at least one orgasmic birth. That is twenty-one percent—considerably higher than I had expected. Most of the women had their babies on The Farm, but interestingly, some said the orgasm occurred during a hospital birth. I have included some of the women's comments below, as they perhaps shed some light on what factors are present when women have birth experiences such as these. (I have changed the women's names out of respect for their privacy.)

Julia: *I had an orgasm when I had my fourth child. It happened while I was pushing. We went to the hospital after I had been "stalled" at nine centimeters for a while, attempting a home birth with some midwives who made me nervous. I no sooner got inside the door than I began having overwhelming urges to push that baby OUT!!! I orgasmed as she was being born. They just barely got me onto the delivery table in time for her birth, but I was oblivious to all that because it was feeling so good to get her out.*

Margaret: *I had a cosmic union orgasm, a bliss-enhanced state. In a way, this has had a permanent effect. I can still go to that place.*

Vivian: *Being in labor felt like work; but giving birth, the actual process of passing the baby's entire body out of my womb (which did happen quite quickly), was indescribably incredible, particularly the first time.*

Marilyn: *My last birth was very orgasmic in a sustained sort of way, like I was riding on waves of orgasmic bliss. I knew more what to expect, was less afraid, and tried to meet and flow with the energy rather than avoid or resist as I had the first time. The effect was probably mostly psychological in that it gave me tremendous satisfaction just to have accomplished such a difficult passage safely. I felt great for months afterward, which helped me feel positive about myself in general. This, in turn, affected how I felt about myself sexually. I also think that, for me, learning to let go and let my body take over in labor (as opposed to thinking about it with my mind all the way through!) helped me tap into a part of me I never knew before and helped me feel more willing to let go while making love.*

Janelle: *Giving birth was like pre- and postorgasm by the second or third birth but did not contain the pulsation felt at climax. Being in tune with rushes, pushing, deeply relaxing in between was a very sexual and powerful experience but higher than orgasm, because orgasm can seem more self-gratifying and is short-lived. Giving birth is such a spiritual experience, so miraculous, you are very in tune with God and seeing the divinity in everyone that the sexual part is not that important. You are totally immersed in selfless love and so the blissful and sexual feelings are a by-product, a gift of allowing your body to do what it knows how to do while your consciousness is very expanded.*

Paula: *I have been pondering this question for some time. I have always felt that labor and birth were like one big orgasm. The contractions were like waves of pleasure rippling through the body. I only found the final few centimeters of dilation as extremely strong and slightly less pleasurable. But I felt like labor and birth were/are a continuous orgasm. I can't say that it is like the orgasm experienced during sexual intercourse, where I find myself being engulfed and lost in the wave of orgasm. The type I experienced during labor and birth was a more all-consuming feeling that required more of my attention than that experienced during sex. However, I do feel that it is an orgasm. The birth itself is very orgasmic as the baby comes through the birth canal—extremely pleasurable and rewarding.*

Maria: *I had to think about this one for a few days. At first I thought "no," but there certainly were sensations in the first stage during dilation that were incredibly intense when Ted would kiss me or I would bury my face in his neck during a rush. I did not have a particularly hard time during the first stage of any of my births and remember enjoying the birthing process for the most part. The general excitement, rushes of energy, and all the touching were very pleasurable. The sensations weren't the same as an orgasm exactly, but when the rushes would end, the total splash-out [relaxation] was very similar to how I feel after*

orgasm now (which I call the wet-noodle effect). For me, however, the second stage was another story. I remember not liking that part because of the intense stinging of the tissue stretching. I always thought I was weird since I liked the first stage and couldn't really get into the second stage. Anyway, it goes without saying that good energy rushes are enjoyable and, even though I don't know if my inner muscles were twitching rhythmically or not, having a baby was the greatest energy sweep ever. I think it is very probable that it is much larger than an orgasm rush, or certainly different.

One other thing I think might be true—I think it is possible that I hadn't perfected the art of having superorgasms back then when I was so young and having the babies. Since then, over the years, I have become quite good at it, so I'm not sure if that lack of experience could have kept me from experiencing some of those sensations during labor and birth.

Some of the women described, instead of orgasm, a euphoria that had some similarities to the bliss they associate with sexual pleasure.

Elayne: I didn't have an orgasm, but I felt a little bit like it when I had my first baby. And that was only at the transition shortly before pushing. For a moment I felt like being shortly before orgasm—being high, having pain, and being afraid what's coming next. And I felt all this at the same time.

Alicia: No, I can't say I would describe the experience as "orgasmic." Rather, it was "euphoric." To say it was orgasmic would describe the experience in almost a base way. Rather, it was spiritual.

Nanette: I wouldn't say I experienced orgasm either in labor or giving birth. However, I would say the sensation of out-of-controlledness (!) was comparable. My sister says that giving birth was "like" the biggest orgasm ever—but only "like" it—so it sounds like a qualitative difference. I remember you telling me that my brain had migrated to my pelvic area, which was where it was needed, and I think you were right—the births of all three children are a delightful blur that was so much just being there and experiencing it with my body and not my head.

Before I move on from the subject of orgasmic birth, I want to note how infrequently this possibility is mentioned to women who are preparing to give birth. There is more than one possible explanation for this silence. One is that most childbirth professionals simply don't know that it can and does happen. Another is that when it does happen, no one mentions it, since orgasm is generally considered to be too private a matter to talk about in polite company. Still another reason is that those who know it can happen don't want to raise the expectations of women, who might then come to expect it and feel cheated if their experience doesn't "compare" with the description of someone else's. Finally, from what I can tell, orgasm during labor and birth doesn't seem to happen very often in women whose labors are medicated with narcotics, epidurals, or barbiturates. Since so many women in our society do have medication of one kind or another during labor, this may be a significant reason why this phenomenon is so unrecognized by birth professionals and most of the general public.

Birth Pain Is Different from Other Pain

The women from The Farm know that birth usually hurts—at least the first time you do it—but they know it as a different kind of pain from the pain of injury. When you are injured and feel pain, its message is "Run away!" or "Fight! You are being damaged." This is survival information. The pain of labor and birth has an entirely different message. It says: "Relax your pelvic muscles. Let go. Surrender. Go with

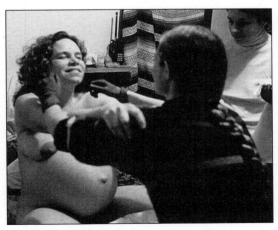

Kathryn finds a comfortable, effective position
for pushing

the flow. Don't fight this. It's bigger than you." This is far different from the message of "Protect yourself!" or "Run away!" that accompanies injury.

Yet many women react to labor pain in the same way they react to the kind of pain they experience when wounded. They think of med-

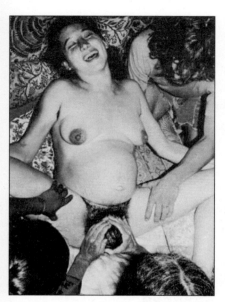

Unmedicated, first-time mother (Terese) experiencing birth ecstasy

icating it and see no gain from experiencing labor without medication. They don't know that a change of position, of attitude, of atmosphere in the birth room, and a host of other factors can utterly change the inner sensations of labor. They usually aren't aware of the extent to which you can ease your own tense reaction by declining to think in terms of "uterine contractions" and thinking instead of "interesting sensations that require all of your attention."

Probably the last thing you want to hear about labor pain (if you have already felt it) is that there is anything subtle about it. Of course, it is much more possible to pay attention to subtleties when you are surrounded by your close friends,

who happen to have a lot of experience helping other women with birth. You may even feel like you are being horribly injured inside during a contraction, but your midwife's calm, understanding manner or words tell you that no injury is actually taking place. This knowledge at such moments is so reassuring that often it is possible to feel either the pain diminish or your own ability to bear it increase.

I have heard many discuss their reasons for having an epidural as early as possible in labor, saying they can't stand pain at all. Naturally, I take a statement like this more seriously when the woman speaking doesn't have pierced ears, tattoos, or breast implants, hasn't had cosmetic surgery, and doesn't wear uncomfortable shoes. In all these instances, the woman has *chosen* pain that is traumatic to some degree because she perceives a kind of gain that comes along with it.

Some have characterized giving birth without painkilling drugs as some sort of "extreme sport." Women who choose natural birth have been derided as martyrs or superwomen exhibiting some demented female version of machismo. This is caricature, not reality. In fact, many women who choose to labor without medication do so because they fear the consequences of unnecessary intervention, including the trauma and postbirth pain of cesarean section. The women at The Farm have a healthy respect for surgery and generally seek to avoid it if there is any way around it.

Please realize that I'm not promising you an orgasm or a completely painless labor if you refuse pain medication in labor. No one can make such promises. I just know that when I was facing my childbearing years, I wanted to be aware of all of the possibilities of women's responses to labor.

Why is the woman on these pages smiling? Certainly not because of drugs, because she didn't take any painkilling medication or sedative during labor. She's smiling because she is in a state of ecstasy. This baby, an eight-pounder, is her first. Her labor lasted for twenty-four hours. None of these factors ruled out orgasm. My guess is that it doesn't happen as readily in women who are discouraged, frightened, or angry—at least, I haven't seen it in women in these emotional states. It's the women who do their best to understand the rushes and work

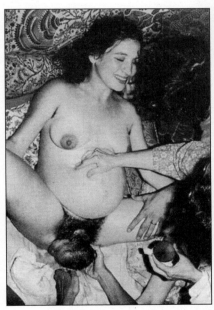

Happy as can be

with them who seem to me most apt to have an orgasmic birth. At the same time, as we have seen above, some women have orgasmic births who never knew it was a possibility.

Scary Birth Gets High Ratings

Most women in North America now gain their first ideas of birth from television portrayals of birth in hospital dramas or sitcoms. Commercial television feeds on the sensational and the danger-charged moment. If birth is written into a show's script, dramatic tension in the plot usually requires a mishap, death, or prosecution. Typically, there will be either a courtroom scene or an operating-room scene. Women who have little real knowledge of what birth can be are especially vulnerable to the negative messages embedded in these dramas.

The demands of commercial television and film have led to the propagation of many myths and misconceptions about labor and birth. Here's an example of how our cultural mythology of birth is affected by them: In real life, labor usually starts rather gradually. In dramas, it usually strikes like lightning. One minute a character is brushing her hair or enjoying dinner in a restaurant, and within seconds her labor overwhelms her with such force that she is immediately carried away to the hospital to be saved from it. Women and girls raised on this sort of thing without a source of more accurate knowledge learn to equate labor pain with danger. Pain is portrayed as if it could be fatal. My mother-in-law used to call this being "too well bred to breed well."

Television *could* be an effective way of decreasing women's fear of birth. If we were allowed to witness what really happens when the sexuality of birth is honored, I believe that our extreme fear of birth would begin to subside. I have included a list of excellent birth videos in the Resources section.

I believe that the pain of normal labor does have meaning. The interesting thing about pain is that it is clean. When you are finished experiencing pain, it is over. You cannot reexperience its sensation by remembering it. Labor pain is a special type of pain: It almost always happens without causing any damage to the body.

When avoidance of pain becomes the major emphasis of childbirth care, the paradoxical effect is that more women have to deal with pain *after* their babies are born. Frequent use of epidural anesthesia drives up the rates of cesarean section and vacuum-extractor and forceps births. Epidurals cause long-term backache in approximately one woman in every five. Sometimes the use of forceps and vacuum extractors results in injury to the baby or the mother. Intravenous lines are painful as long as they are in place and for a couple of days after they are removed. The more you move and disturb that plastic in your vein, the more it hurts. Women who have cesarean operations must have a catheter inserted in their urethra before the surgery is performed. This hollow tube will be kept in place for at least twenty-four hours. While the catheter is in place, many women experience a constant urge to urinate. Of course, since they are constantly "peeing," there is no way to satisfy this urge. Cesareans usually involve the placement of a surgical drain sewed in the part of the wound most likely to efficiently drain away blood and lymph from the abdominal cavity. Women find the removal of this drain on the third day painful, particularly when they haven't been given pain medication an hour or so before the procedure. Finally, the formation of intestinal gas after any abdominal surgery (including cesarean operation) is acutely painful for women. Postsurgery soreness can interfere with a woman's ease in handling her newborn baby. Each of the procedures and conditions I have mentioned above involves pain *after* birth.

The woman who gives birth without interventions, on the other hand, is more apt to be *through* with pain when her baby is born. Often, she is euphoric, buoyed on the hormones released after the birth of the baby. Oxytocin, the love hormone, is released with the final stretch of the perineum around the baby's head and body, a pleasant sensation for most women. Pain, if present seconds earlier, is often erased or pushed into the background. Not only that, the woman has developed powerful relaxation techniques, practiced during the most intense and memorable experience of her life. She has learned how breathing slowly and deeply can change her bodily sensations, as well as the tenor of her thoughts. She has probably developed a new respect and appreciation for her body. She has experienced the extraordinary mixture of vulnerability, power, and contact with the female principle that characterizes labor and birth.

Notes

1. Senden, I. P. M., et al. Labor pain: A comparison of parturients in a Dutch and an American teaching hospital. *Obstetrics & Gynecology,* 1988; 71 (4).
2. Jordan, Brigitte. *Birth in Four Cultures: A Cross-Cultural Investigation of Childbirth in Yucatan, Holland, Sweden and the United States.* Montreal: Eden Press, 1983.
3. Morse, J. M., and Park, C. Home birth and hospital deliveries: A comparison of the perceived painfulness of parturition. *Research in Nursing Health,* 1988; 11:175–81.
4. Stockham, Alice, MD. *Tokology.* 1882.
5. Thomas, A. N. *Doctor Courageous.* London: William Heinemann Ltd., 1957.
6. Dye, J. N. *Painless Childbirth.* Buffalo, NY: Baker, Jones & Co., 1888.

I will praise Thee; for I am fearfully and wonderfully made.

—Psalms, cxxix, 14.

4

SPHINCTER LAW

Sphincter Law is what I call the set of basic assumptions about birth that my partners and I follow. We obey Sphincter Law. We're sure it rules.

Instead of proceeding from an understanding of Sphincter Law, most U.S. women and virtually all obstetricians believe in a set of assumptions that obstetricians call the Law of the Three Ps. The Three Ps are the Passenger (the baby), the Passage (the pelvis and vagina), and the Powers (the strength of uterine contractions). I think this so-called law creates misunderstandings of the true capacities of women's bodies for both women and doctors, causing in the process lots of unnecessary cesareans, births involving forceps and vacuum extractors, and other complications. Probably the major philosophical difference between Sphincter Law and the Law of the Three Ps is that the latter blames the woman for what medicine calls "dysfunctional labors."

(That's the kind that Pamela and Sheila had—see pages 134–135—except we didn't call them dysfunctional; we just thought they were longer than usual.) According to the Law of the Three Ps, if a woman's labor doesn't produce a baby in the time allotted, it is her fault: She grew too big a baby, has too small a vagina or too weak a uterus. According to Sphincter Law, labors that don't result in a normal birth after a "reasonable" amount of time are often slowed or stalled because of lack of privacy, fear, and stimulation of the wrong part of the laboring woman's brain. I'll elaborate on how this works in this chapter.

Obstetricians generally don't understand Sphincter Law as it is related to obstetrics, because they haven't been taught it during medical education and rarely—if ever—have a chance to see what would happen if it were observed. Instead, they are presented with the Law of the Three Ps, almost as if having a baby were a problem of physics rather than a millions-of-years-old *physiological* process. What is interesting about the Law of the Three Ps is how little it explains in practical terms. One of the most meaningless diagnoses in obstetrics is cephalo–pelvic disproportion (CPD), a term based upon the Three Ps theory—the baby being too big to fit through the maternal pelvis. The rate of CPD varies widely from hospital to hospital, as well as from country to country. My partners and I have attended successful vaginal births for many women who were previously diagnosed with CPD (see Diana's story, p. 53, for instance).

In a few extreme cases, too great a mismatch in size *does* prevent a normal vaginal birth. Problems of this kind were far more frequent in the nineteenth century, when many women had misshapen pelvises from rickets. (Few women have rickets anymore in developed countries.) In the labors of most women, a problem with one or more of the Three Ps is *not* the reason so many end up having obstetrical interventions such as oxytocin augmentation, episiotomy, cesarean section, forceps, or vacuum extraction when birth does not follow several hours of labor. Failure to respect Sphincter Law is one of the more likely causes.

To qualify as a law of obstetrics, a description of a biological truth ought to be true all of the time, not just occasionally. Take these examples of the law of gravity:

- Every time we hold something in the air and then let it go, it falls.
- Water always flows downhill.

If the Law of the Three Ps were truly descriptive of the intrinsic abilities of women, there would be little variation in the number of women requiring obstetrical interventions in birth. The Law of the Three Ps does not begin to explain how The Farm's consistently low cesarean rate (always less than two percent) exists in the same country that has an overall rate of more than twenty-four percent. The problem with the Law of the Three Ps is that it ignores the considerable evidence demonstrating the importance of emotional, psychological, and spiritual aspects of birth. This leaves many physicians thinking that a large percentage of U.S. women are born with some deficiency that prevents them from giving birth without enormous technological intervention, when in fact almost all would be able to give birth given the right care and circumstances. Some midwives have proposed that the Law of the Three Ps should be expanded to include other Ps—such as Psyche, Position, Professional Provider, Place of birth, People, Politics, Procedures, and Pressure—since all of these may influence how difficult or easy giving birth may be.

When I came up with the concept of Sphincter Law to describe the basic assumptions that guide my work, I was, of course, thinking of the sphincters involved in excretion, labor, and birth. Knowledge based upon Sphincter Logic has been embedded in the birthing practices of traditional cultures all over the world since time immemorial. Cultures such as these, which sustained themselves for thousands of years, may indeed have something to teach our technological society about childbirth wisdom. Intellectually curious physicians have long wondered why women from traditional cultures generally have an easier time giving birth than women whose connection with the natural world is more tenuous.

To explain what I mean by Sphincter Law, I will first describe the general function and properties of the various excretory sphincters of the body—the bladder and the rectum, along with those involved in the process of labor and birth, the cervix and the vagina.

THE BASICS OF SPHINCTER LAW

- Excretory, cervical, and vaginal sphincters function best in an atmosphere of intimacy and privacy—for example, a bathroom with a locking door or a bedroom, where interruption is unlikely or impossible.
- These sphincters cannot be opened at will and do not respond well to commands (such as "Push!" or "Relax!").
- When a person's sphincter is in the process of opening, it may suddenly close down if that person becomes upset, frightened, humiliated, or self-conscious. Why? High levels of adrenaline in the bloodstream do not favor (sometimes, they actually prevent) the opening of the sphincters. This inhibition factor is one important reason why women in traditional societies have mostly chosen other women—except in extraordinary circumstances—to attend them in labor and birth.
- The state of relaxation of the mouth and jaw is directly correlated to the ability of the cervix, the vagina, and the anus to open to full capacity. (I recommend that you remember this if you ever suffer from hemorrhoids and are afraid to poop, as this aspect of Sphincter Law is helpful in this situation as well.)

The Excretory and Reproductive Sphincters

Sphincters are circular muscle groups that ordinarily remain contracted so the openings of certain organs are held closed until something needs to pass through. Each sphincter's job is to relax and expand so that it can open comfortably and wide enough to allow the passage of whatever must move through. Elimination and birthing both involve the opening of sphincters.

Michel Odent, the well-known French physician, has contributed greatly to our understanding of the physiology of birth by explaining the function of the human brain in labor and birth. He distinguishes between the neocortex—the newer, rational part of the brain, which plays a role in abstract thought—and the primitive brain, which governs instincts. The primitive brain, or brain stem, is also considered to be a gland that releases hormones. All female mammals, including humans, release a certain number of hormones such as oxytocin, endorphins, and prolactin in the process of giving birth. Stimulation of the neocortex, on the other hand, can actually interfere with the birth process by *inhibiting* the action of the primitive brain in hormone release.

How is the neocortex stimulated? It can be done in a number of ways: by asking the laboring mother to answer questions that require thought, by being near her in a way that makes her feel self-conscious, by subjecting her to bright light, and by failing to protect her privacy.[1] Many statements made by nineteenth-century doctors (when most women still gave birth in their bedrooms), including those I quoted on pages 140–41, illustrate that the medical profession then had a better working knowledge of Sphincter Law than physicians of the present time. Of course, they didn't call it Sphincter Law then; instead, they talked about "modesty."

A recent study of the brain[2] was designed to examine the ways the primitive brain center coordinates the smooth muscles of the bladder with the relaxation of the sphincter muscles. Brain-imaging technology was used. The researchers' first task was to identify people to participate in the study. In order for the imaging technology to be used, the subjects of the study had to be able to urinate in the presence of an observer. Understanding that not everyone can accomplish this task, the researchers began by choosing people who could pee in their own homes while being observed. This group was then to undergo the same process in the hospital while their brains were being imaged. However, the researchers had to deal with a snag they had not fully anticipated: A high proportion of the people who could pee at home in the presence of an observer could not perform the same function while in the hospital.[3] Women who labor in hospitals have to contend with these inhibiting factors.

The urinary and anal sphincters enable the bladder and rectum to function as reservoirs capable of holding their contents so that elimination takes place at convenient intervals rather than continuously. In infants, these sphincters have not yet fully developed their ability to remain contracted until it is socially acceptable for them to relax. Learning to maintain this measure of sphincter control is the goal of potty training, which usually takes place during the second or third year of life for infants in the industrialized world.

For most people who have grown up in industrialized societies, some measure of privacy or familiarity is required for the grip of the sphincter muscle to be relaxed enough to allow elimination, even in the presence of a strong urge. (There is some difference in this respect between the bladder and the rectum, obviously, since the bladder has smaller absolute limits compared to the rectum.)

Sphincters, like the involuntary muscles, are affected by the emotions. They function most comfortably and smoothly in an atmosphere that is relaxed and free from discordant emotions. Probably because our organs of elimination are in close proximity to or, in the case of men, double as organs of reproduction, public toilets are usually segregated on the basis of gender. Our societal norms demand the privacy afforded by walls between stalls and doors that lock.

Understanding the true process of labor and birth becomes easier when we learn that the opening of the womb (the cervix) and the vagina are also sphincters. In many ways they function like other sphincters of the human body. They perform normal bodily functions. Labor is obviously hard and intense work (hence, its English name). It demands all of the mother's attention and may require hours of work, sweat, and heavy breathing. Still, it remains a normal physiological process that human and all other mammalian females have experienced for as long as we have existed. To understand this physical process, it is necessary to understand how sphincters work.

The Properties of Sphincters

Sphincters Do Not Obey Orders

It is a fairly common practice in hospitals in most of the industrialized world for laboring women to be strenuously commanded to push once they reach full dilation. Such commands are often given without the awareness that, in most cases, the urge to push will arise spontaneously in the mother. Pushing will take place without the mother requiring someone to shout at her when and how to do it. Many women may be able to push their babies into the world while being yelled at, but it is likely they accomplish this in spite of, not because of, such a distraction. There is no more compelling bodily urge than the uterine contractions that move the baby down the birth canal once the cervix is fully dilated. I am reminded of Dr. Christiane Northrup's observation when, in labor, she first experienced the urge to push. She had just completed her obstetrics residency training. She vowed that never again would she tell a laboring woman to *stop* pushing when she felt the urge, as she had been taught to do by some professors.[4] Those who have never felt what it is like to give birth while being shouted at can better understand how this can interfere when they try to imagine what it might be like to poop while a stranger stationed a few feet away yells at them how to do it.

Sphincters Function Best in an Atmosphere of Familiarity and Privacy

A close friend of mine gave me a practical lesson about this axiom during a seven-day road trip from Iowa to California. This was during our student days in the early 1960s. We camped in national parks to keep our costs to a minimum. In those days, the standard toilet facilities in national parks were usually outhouses or other nonflush toilets. This was my friend's first cross-country trip. She found all the toilets between Iowa and California so unsatisfactory that she became more constipated as each day passed. She could pee, but that was all. Each morning she gave me her daily constipation report. No matter how clean the gas-station rest rooms along the way, she was not able to relieve herself while we were traveling. When we finally reached her relatives' home in southern California, she headed straight for the bathroom. A few minutes later, she emerged, smiling with great relief. What made the difference, she said, was that she felt at home in the bathroom of a relative. That difference made it possible for her body to function in the normal way. When we remembered this trip together recently, she told me that she had just returned home from a half-month trip to Czechoslovakia. Having no Czech relatives was apparently a problem, because she didn't have a bowel movement for the entire two weeks. Some things just don't change over time.

North Carolina midwife Lisa Goldstein's childbirth-education classes for couples in her area of rural North Carolina include a humorous and effective way of teaching fathers a lesson about how inhibition can affect the opening of sphincters. First she shows them a fifty-dollar bill. Then she places a medium-size stainless-steel bowl on the floor with ten or fifteen couples circled around her. She then offers that bill to the first man who comes forward and pees in the bowl in front of everyone. In all the years she has repeated this routine, she has never handed over that fifty dollars to anyone.

Sphincters May Suddenly Close When Their Owner Is Startled or Frightened

Sphincters may "slam shut" without the volitional act of their owner. The sudden contraction of previously relaxed sphincter muscles is a fear-based reaction. This is part of the natural fight-or-flight response to perceived danger. Adrenaline/catecholamines rise in the bloodstream when the organism is frightened or angered. Female animals in labor in the wild, such as gazelles and wildebeest, can be on the point of giving birth and yet suddenly reverse the process if surprised by a predator. This is just one of the ways all mammals have programmed-in protection during the vulnerable process of labor and birth. These same evolutionary behaviors take over in us humans when we go into labor, without our necessarily understanding the evolutionary wisdom of our own behavior.

Numerous practical jokes are based upon people's knowledge of this particular physical reaction. My husband assures me that in the case of men standing at a urinal in a public toilet, if someone suddenly and noisily bursts in, a number of those men will find their "water cut off." It may take a few moments of relaxation before they are once again able to resume urination.

I remember a birth that taught me that a rough and uncompassionate pelvic examination can reverse a mother's cervical dilation. I was attending the labor of a first-time mother, who developed a fever. It soon became evident that it was caused by a bladder infection. Although she had reached seven centimeters of dilation, she was not moving past that point. I decided that I should transport her to a hospital. When we arrived at a hospital in Nashville (with her dilation still at seven centimeters—I checked just before we got there), her care was assigned to an obstetrician who was rather sullen and unfriendly in his manner. With no pleasantries or permission, he examined her internally so roughly that she cried out in pain—a reaction she had not had during my previous examinations. He muttered that her cervix was only four centimeters dilated and left the room for a few minutes. While he was out, I confirmed that her cervix was four centimeters dilated with my own examination. I was sure it was his painful, rough examination that closed her cervix that much. Her labor never reestablished itself after the obstetrician's rude internal examination, so this mother's baby was born by cesarean. To the woman's neocortex, this man may have been an obstetrician. To her cervix and her primitive brain, he was a predator.

Given the inherent mystery of women's bodies, it is only the observations based upon continuous presence that can convey an appropriate depth of experience. What could be more mysterious than a bodily process that changes according to who is nearby?

Some skeptics may wonder if there ever was a good reason to exclude males (other than family members) from the birth room. Can their presence, or that of females who are strange to the laboring mother, truly inhibit labor?

I am certain that the answer to both questions is yes. The presence of a strange person in the birth room, especially if that person is male and not an intimate companion of the laboring woman, frequently (although not always) slows or stops labor. Nowadays, of course, it is possible to restart or to intensify labor with synthetic oxytocic drugs delivered intravenously. This may be convenient when truly necessary, but intravenous drugs used to keep women in labor also prevent them from moving around freely and cause more painful contractions. Changing positions, walking, being nourished, and being upright during labor are important to women's ability to give birth under their own power. (See pages 226–31 for a fuller discussion of these important activities during labor.) And no drug given in labor or birth is without undesirable side effects.

Laughter Helps Open the Sphincters

Pain-numbing endorphins, nature's opiates, are instantly effective and have no negative side effects. A smile is good. A chuckle is better. A good belly laugh is one of the most effective forms of anesthesia. A young woman who recently attended one of our midwifery-assistant workshops told me that she had spontaneously discovered how much laughter could help her reach her goal of an unmedicated, wide awake, beautiful birth.

"I giggled almost constantly during labor," she said. "I always do that in stressful situations. Like on airplanes during takeoff and landing."

I remember the slumber parties of my early teenage years. My friends and I used to get a big laugh going and keep it happening until someone began to pee her pants. Of course, I know it's hard for anyone who has had a painful labor to believe that laughing could have helped to cut the pain. However, only those who have tried it really know.

Forget puns and witticisms. They won't work. Weird jokes, bawdy jokes, toilet jokes—these are all possibilities, depending on your mood. As an example of the last category, I like to tell about my father-in-law in the hospital. He was a stern man with a deadpan expression most of the time. One morning, a nurse stopped by his bed and brightly asked, "Have we had our B.M. today?"

"I've had mine. Have you had yours?" he asked her.

Most of my bodily function jokes use the one-syllable, Anglo-Saxon words for body parts, fluids, and performance. They provoke more laughter than their Latin equivalents. Jokes such as these have a double function. Not only might they stimulate a few laughs, but they also reassure the mother that I will not be revolted if she poops a little during the pushing stage. This kind of reassurance keeps her from fearing humiliation and embarrassment, which could slow or stop her labor.

Slow, Deep Breathing Aids the Opening of Sphincters

Other factors and practices affect the ease with which the sphincters can open. Deep abdominal breathing causes a general relaxation of the muscles of the body, especially muscles of the pelvic floor. This kind of breathing is taught by teachers of yoga. Yoga instructor Ruth Bender teaches the following method in her book *Yoga Exercises for More Flexible Bodies.*[5]

> *Lie on your back and bend your knees with your feet on the mat or floor. Put your hands on your belly just below your belly button so you can feel better what is happening. Now let your belly go out gently (without pushing it out) and then draw it in slowly. Only your belly should be moving during this process. Don't think about breathing. Just let your belly move out and draw it in*

again. Do this in a slow, relaxed way, about ten times, without making any jerky movements.

Repeat this exercise with your eyes closed, so you can really notice what is going on in your body. You will feel that when your belly goes out, you are inhaling. When you draw in your belly, you are exhaling.

Many women have been conditioned to feel bad about relaxing their abdominal muscles, as if they are afraid that this might cause them to develop a large belly. However, relaxing and contracting the abdominal muscles in turn is actually a good way to strengthen and firm these muscles.

This deep abdominal breathing is not only relaxing to the heart, the nervous system, and the mind, it also allows for the greatest lung expansion. This increases the amount of oxygen that can fill your lungs. It can help you relax enough to go to sleep. Besides that, it gives your abdominal organs a gentle massage, increases the wavelike squeezing movements of your intestines, and strengthens the blood circulation in your abdominal organs to help them function properly.

More Factors That Help the Sphincters Open in Labor

Immersion in a warm water bath can also be very calming to a laboring mother. Holding your muscles stiff and rigid is very difficult while you are immersed in water.

If it becomes necessary to gain entrance to a vaginal, cervical, or anal sphincter, it is a much less unpleasant experience when certain principles are kept in mind:

- First, permission must be asked. This is basic politeness, but it is also practical. When permission is given, there is less resistance of the sphincter muscles, and therefore less discomfort or pain will occur.
- Second, it helps if a finger is gently placed on the rim of the sphincter and held still for four or five seconds.
- Third, once you have felt the sphincter relax, slowly and gently move inside. The same gentle principles hold true for examination of cervix and vagina. When they are followed, reversal of cervical dilation is much less likely.

Early in my midwifery career, I observed another fascinating relationship pertaining to the Law of the Sphincter. I noticed a strong connection between the sphincters of the mouth/throat and those of the cervix and yoni. A relaxed mouth means a more elastic cervix. Women whose mouths and throats are open and relaxed during labor and birth rarely need stitches after childbirth. As long as they don't push the baby out too fast, they tend to give birth without tearing or being cut. On the other hand, women who grimace and clench their jaws while pushing have a greater tendency to tear, because their perineal tissues are more rigid. Many times I have observed the release of tension in the perineal tissues when a woman pursing her lips or clenching her throat and jaw relaxes all the muscles. This relaxing tactic has avoided and lessened tears and episiotomies over the years. Most women can figure out how to relax their jaw more easily than their bottom.

Understanding the connection between top and bottom can ease pain and discomfort of constipation, premenstrual tension, period cramps, labor and birth, and afterpains. If you feel like grinding your teeth or clenching your jaw, catch yourself! Take a deep breath and exhale, relaxing your mouth and throat muscles. This effect is enhanced with an audible sigh when you exhale. Make a sound pitched low enough to vibrate your chest.

In spring 1972, one of my friends was giving birth to her first child. She became quite distressed and panicked as her baby's head began to move down her birth canal. She wanted to get up and run away from the pain. I needed to find something she could do to calm herself so that her baby's head could emerge without tearing her perineal tissues. It was just as important that she not kick me off the bed. Then an idea occurred to me. She was a singer, so I knew she had already disciplined her mouth and throat. This was a strength we could use, so I suggested that she sing during her next push. She readily agreed, appreciating *anything* that might help her keep some composure. As soon as she began her song, hitting and holding all the notes perfectly (she wouldn't have been able to scream while singing), her baby moved down to crowning. Within minutes her baby was born.

Not every woman is a professional singer, but everyone can find something to sing while having a baby. Singing will maximize the ability of the body's sphincters to open. The sounds that accomplish this best are the notes that come from as deep down in the body as possible, the ones that vibrate the entire chest. Even the woman who makes *no* sound as she gives birth can deliberately hold her mouth and throat in a loose, relaxed position as she pushes. If she holds her mouth and throat open rather than clenching her jaw or biting down, her perineum responds accordingly. Its muscle tissues instantaneously become more flexible and stretchy and thus more able to slip around the baby's head and body without tearing or being cut.

I cannot count how many times I have observed women experiencing similar relaxation of the cervical sphincter that correlated with positive and loving words spoken during the most intense phase of labor (usually around the time when the cervix is almost completely open). After Dawn's birth (see pages 135–36), I sometimes told her story to mothers in labor—how the words she spoke affected her labor. I especially wanted to illustrate the beneficial effect that positive words can have on the body/mind of a laboring woman. Quite often, a mother would realize she had nothing to lose by speaking positively. Then she would tell her husband, her baby, her midwives, her friends who were helping her, how much she loved them. I can say this categorically—I have never noticed *anyone's* cervix remain tight and unyielding while speaking loving and positive words.

Other times a woman's cervix has opened a couple of centimeters as my fingers were testing it. Early in my career, I observed many women laboring with open mouths and throats, relaxed, making the sounds associated with pleasurable lovemaking. Knowing how this works, I have often demonstrated the sounds that help dilation: low-pitched moaning and orgasmic sighs. A mother needing help with this phase of labor can repeat the sounds. My partners and I have also found that many women find it helpful to be told that mooing like a cow is a good way to keep the throat open and relaxed. If they think it's funny to hear these sounds, so much the better, since being amused also aids relaxation.

During the early years of my career, I developed another relaxation technique to help women keep their mouths and throats relaxed during labor. This is called "horse lips" or "raspberries." When a person totally relaxes the lips and blows a good amount of air through them at considerable pressure, softly flapping them together in the process, it is reminiscent of the soft, lip-flapping sound that horses make. I find that when women in labor attempt to make this sound (even if they don't quite succeed), it significantly relaxes their mouth, throat, and, at the same time, their bottom (cervix and perineum). Women who have tried this during menstrual cramps have found it surprisingly helpful in alleviating pain. I also recommend it to the extremely constipated person—including the one who has hemorrhoids—who has reason to be afraid of the pain that may be involved in opening the anal sphincter during the next bowel movement. Incidentally, I don't recommend this to *replace* hemorrhoid treatments, such as stool softeners and change in diet, but to complement them.

This horse-lips technique is helpful in another way too. I recently attended the home birth of a large baby—the mother's second child. The mother's cervix was open almost to its full extent, but the last little bit of stretching that was necessary was taxing to her. She did not feel sure she "could keep doing this." At that point, her two-year-old son toddled into the bedroom, wanting to see his mother. His father helped the little boy climb up to sit between him and the mother. I continued to encourage her by telling her that she was almost ready to push, that she could continue, and that I understood what a challenge it was to do what she was doing. Then I demonstrated horse lips to the mother, telling her that trying it could help her cervix dilate the rest of the way. Just then her son did it. He looked so cute that she forgot how discouraged she had been and smiled at him. Of course, he was happy to see her smile again, so he kept doing horse lips, and she joined in too. The combination of her amusement, her smile, and the horse-lips technique enabled her to dilate the rest of the way within a few minutes. Soon, her ten-pound seven-ounce daughter was born.

Developing an understanding of Sphincter Law is an important part of learning about the mind/body connection. Because trust is such a valuable and powerful feeling, it is important for pregnant women to be cared for by people whom they trust. Love is another very powerful healing and easing emotion. Trust and love make relaxation possible. I believe the best midwives are those who feel a special kindliness and love for the women they care for. This means that they do not view the women in a critical way, noticing faults or shortcomings. Instead, they appreciate the women just as they are. When the mother loves and trusts her midwife or physician, she is going to find it far easier to relax her bottom in the presence of this person. This feeling of safety will not only make labor and birth more efficient, it can also make it significantly less painful.

I once made a joke that had a good result. A young woman having her first baby was resisting the sensation of what the Amish call her "push-pains." From experience, I knew that she was having trouble believing she had room for something as big as that baby's head to pass through, so she was trying to protect her bottom. I had a hunch that she was in the kind of mood I remember when I was a miserable, sick eight-year-old who wanted to redesign the universe for her own comfort (in my case, I wished that my mother could pee for me so I wouldn't have to get out of bed).

"It's times like these when it's easy to start thinking Nature could have had a better design," I said. "Like, for instance, that babies' bones would form *after* birth, instead of before. That would mean you could just ooze them out."

When I told her that, she brightened a little. But logic forced another thought, and I added, "But then you'd have to carry them around in a mixing bowl for a while so their bones could develop."

She laughed about what an unsatisfactory situation that would be. With her next push-pain, she got down and pushed and soon had her baby.

One of the births we attended at The Farm Midwifery Center during the 1980s promised to be a challenge. Six years earlier, this mother (I'll call her Sara) had her first baby with us, a six-pound four-ounce girl. That birth was one of our few forceps deliveries. I had not attended the labor myself, but my partners told me that it had been long. After trying for several hours, Sara became too exhausted to push her baby out. Sara came back to The Farm a month before her second baby was due. Feeling the baby in her belly, I could tell this baby was already bigger than six pounds four ounces. If she had her baby at the normal forty weeks, there was a good chance this baby would weigh close to eight pounds. I needed to know if any dimensions of Sara's pelvis were narrow. Three of us examined her and agreed that her pelvis was big enough for the vaginal birth of a baby around eight pounds. We could not be sure of what the problem had been with Sara's first labor. Sara remembered that she had never felt an urge to push and believed that pushing without a good urge had tired her out.

This time when she went into labor, Sara's attitude could not have been better than it was. She was grateful to be in labor. She accepted each rush, willing to surrender to it. Between rushes she conversed with her husband, Mark (who sat behind her on their bed), and us midwives. Mark is a big bear of a man. Sara clearly enjoyed leaning on him. One of us mentioned how well that seemed to be working for them.

"Oh, he does feel good to lean against," said Sara. "I leaned on him just like this when I was in labor with Candace. As a matter of fact, I wouldn't let him move for the entire fourteen hours."

"That's right," said Mark. "And I had to pee for the last twelve of them!"

All four of the midwives looked at one another. We were thinking the same thing: Leaning against a big vital man who was not able to fully relax himself might be what prevented Sara's own optimum relaxation. This would certainly slow down cervical dilation. One thing was clear: No one was going to be sitting around at *this* labor trying not to pee. We shared a lot of jokes about that.

Sara and Mark's second baby weighed almost eight pounds. She was pushed into the world by her mother's power alone and never had to feel the steel grip of forceps.

Optimum functioning of our various sphincters is easier to obtain when we understand how to better accommodate our thoughts to the needs of our bottoms. I often say that our bottom parts function best when our top part—our minds—are either grateful or amused at the antics or activities of our bottoms. It is amazing how much better our bottoms work when we think of them with humor and affection rather than with terror, revulsion, or, worst of all, look away from them in shame. Lord knows, we can't turn our backs on our bottoms.

Notes

1. Johnson, Jessica, and Odent, Michel. *We Are All Water Babies*. Berkeley, CA: Celestial Arts Publishing, 1995, pp. 56–60.
2. *Brain*. November 1998.
3. Ibid.
4. Northrup, Christiane. *Women's Bodies, Women's Wisdom*. New York: Bantam Books, 1994.
5. Bender, Ruth. *Yoga Exercises for More Flexible Bodies*. Avon, CT: Ruben Publishing, 1978.

5

WHAT YOU NEED TO KNOW ABOUT YOUR
PREGNANCY AND PRENATAL CARE

The Two Models of Maternity Care

The birthing stories and the previous chapters have provided you with some basic information about the wondrous capacities of the human female body, the kinds of atmosphere in which labor proceeds best, and the factors that can shut down or even reverse labor. This section is intended to give you an idea of the range in maternity care available in the United States, as well as some criteria for deciding on the right caregiver for you.

It is important to know that there are two distinct ways of thinking about pregnancy and birth in the United States, as well as in many other countries. Out of these very different conceptions of women's bodies and the meaning of birth have come two separate models of maternity care: the midwifery or humanistic model of care and the techno-medical model of care.

Sociologist Barbara Katz Rothman was the first to name and describe the differences between the models.[1] She pointed out that the midwifery model of care is female-centered. Within it, birth is something that women do—not something that happens to them. The birth-giving woman is the central agent in the ancient drama of life bringing forth new life. The midwifery model of care recognizes the essential oneness of mind and body and the power of women in the creation of new life. The midwifery model of care conceives of pregnancy and birth as inherently healthy processes and of each mother and baby as an inseparable unit. According to this model, the emotions of the woman have a very real impact upon the well-being of the baby. When the woman's emotional needs are filled, there is less risk for the baby. The reality is that the baby has no choice but to feel what the mother feels. Prenatal visits within the midwifery model tend to be much longer, allowing for more questions to be answered than in prenatal visits in the medical model. The midwifery model of care recognizes the importance of good nutrition as the best way to prevent the most common complications of pregnancy. It emphasizes the importance of companionship and encouragement during labor as a way to minimize technological intervention in the birth process. It does not impose arbitrary time limits in physiological processes.

Good research shows that when the midwifery model of care is applied, between eighty-five and ninety-five percent of healthy women will safely give birth without surgery or instruments such as forceps and vacuum extractors. Within the midwifery model, medical intervention is inappropriate unless it is truly necessary. Labor has its own rhythms, so it is not expected to conclude within any rigid time limit. It can start and then stop, speed up or slow down and still be normal. A laboring woman may move around freely, drink, eat, and be sexually playful with her partner within this model (if that is what best stimulates her labor). All of these activities help labor to progress. The midwifery model of maternity care, of course, recognizes that medical intervention is sometimes necessary and that it should be applied in these particular cases. At the same time, it maintains that medical intervention may be harmful when it is used purely for convenience or for profit.

The techno-medical model of maternity care, unlike the midwifery model, is comparatively new on the world scene, having existed for barely two centuries. This male-derived framework for care is a product of the industrial revolution. As anthropologist Robbie Davis-Floyd[2-3] has described in detail, underlying the technocratic mode of care of our own time is an assumption that the human body is a machine and that the female body in particular is a machine full of shortcomings and defects. Pregnancy and labor are seen as illnesses, which, in order not to be harmful to mother or baby, must be treated with drugs and medical equipment. Within the techno-medical model of birth, some medical intervention is considered necessary for every birth, and birth is safe only in retrospect. According to this model, once labor starts, birth must take place within twenty-four hours.

Mind and body are considered to be separate within the techno-medical model of birth. Because of this, emotional ambience is of importance only when it comes to marketing the service. Where the techno-medical model of birth reigns, women who give birth vaginally generally labor in bed hooked up to electronic fetal monitors, intravenous tubes, and pressure-reading devices. Eating and drinking in labor are usually not permitted. Labor pain within this model is seen as unacceptable, so analgesia and anesthesia are encouraged. Episiotomies (the surgical cut to enlarge the vaginal opening) are routinely performed, out of a belief that birth over an intact perineum would be impossible or that, if possible, it might be harmful to mother or baby. Instead of being the central actor of the birth drama, the woman becomes a passive, almost inert object—representing a barrier to the baby's eventual passage to the outside world. Women are treated as a homogenous group within the medical model, with individual variations receding in importance.

The techno-medical model of care has been dominant for a century in North America. By the 1920s the United States and Canada had become the first societies in human history to do away with midwifery, only to find out some decades later that women still wanted midwives and that some (like my partners and me) would reinvent midwifery if they had to. Many people share the goal of reclaiming midwifery and ensuring that in the not-too-distant future there will be enough midwives in Canada and the United States that every women who wants one can have one. Even though midwifery is legal in the United States and Canada, midwives still attend fewer than ten percent of all births in each country. These percentages are far below those of the nations of western Europe and the rest of the world, where midwives attend the vast majority of all births. More than seventy percent of babies born in the countries with the lowest rates of maternal and newborn deaths are born with only midwives—no physicians—in the birth room. In Germany, a federal law ensures that a midwife must be in attendance at every birth—even in cases when an obstetrician must perform a cesarean section or an instrumental delivery.

Distinguishing between the midwifery and the techno-medical models of care is not always as simple as you might think. In the first place, there is a whole spectrum of practice styles between the two models. For instance, although most physicians practice the techno-medical model of care, some doctors practice according to the midwifery model of care and may employ (or be employed by) midwives. Practices like these are distinguished by their low rates of medical interventions such as cesarean section and instrumental deliveries and by the amount of freedom women have to labor according to their individual needs. In the same way, although you might expect that all midwives practice according to the midwifery model of care, the reality is sometimes different. Many midwives work as employees in large hospital practices, where the techno-medical model of care is still the rule. In practices like these, midwives are used to attract women who desire midwifery care, but they may in fact be under constant pressure to practice within the techno-medical mode. You will likely need to look at more than surface answers to your questions to find out whether a maternity service is closer to the midwifery or to the techno-medical model of care. Try to talk to other women who have given birth with any of the practitioners you are considering. See Appendix C for the Ten Steps of the Mother-Friendly Childbirth Initiative.

The Underestimated Importance of Good Nutrition

There is perhaps no greater area of disparity between the midwifery or humanistic model and the techno-medical model of care than the perspective of each toward the role of nutrition during pregnancy. According to the midwifery model, one of the most important things that you can do during pregnancy to be healthy and to prevent complications is to eat a nutritious diet. Through eating and drinking well, you will give yourself and your baby some of the best pregnancy insurance possible. One of the most common and deadly complications of pregnancy, metabolic toxemia of late pregnancy (MTLP, usually called preeclampsia, eclampsia, or HELLP syndrome), can largely be prevented through good nutrition and the lowering of stress. A good diet can also prevent various anemias and infections in mothers and babies. Toxemia is characterized by elevated blood pressure, protein in the urine, and generalized swelling beyond the normal that most women experience during pregnancy because of expanded blood volume. In its most severe form, the disease causes abruption of the placenta (the placenta detaches itself prematurely from the uterine wall, endangering the baby), convulsions, and death to the woman and her baby. Between fourteen and twenty percent of first-time mothers in the United States develop toxemia, as well as about six or seven percent of women who have already had babies.

The Farm Midwifery Center experience supports the view that most cases of toxemia *can* be prevented with good diet. In a published study of the prenatal records and dietary histories of 775 women from The Farm community, only one woman developed a case of preeclampsia (0.1%). Her case was mild, and her babies were all born vaginally.[4] Women from our community eat high-protein vegetarian diets (with protein sources such as soybean products, various varieties of dried beans and nuts) that also include plenty of vegetables, whole grains, and water as the main beverage. We midwives do not restrict women's use of salt during pregnancy. Women in our care salt their food as much as tastes good to them. Several studies carried out in a variety of locations have lent support to the benefits of assuring good nutrition during pregnancy and the role nutrition plays in lowering the incidence of toxemia. [5-9]

In telling you that toxemia can be prevented, I have given you the good news. The not-so-good news is that the techno-medical model of birth does not recognize any connection between toxemia and poor nutrition. The assumption about toxemia underlying this model of birth is that it doesn't matter what a pregnant woman eats or drinks, because her baby is somehow able to extract what it needs from her, regardless of how poorly she eats. One of the most important reasons for this missed connection between good nutrition and good health is that obstetricians receive virtually no training in nutrition during their medical and clinical education. Instead, they continue to be taught that the cause of toxemia is unknown and that it cannot be prevented.

Obstetricians have responded to toxemia in a variety of ways over the past two centuries. During the nineteenth century, doctors treated it by bloodletting.[10] During the 1930s and 1940s, they began recommending no-salt starvation diets during pregnancy as a way to prevent toxemia. During the 1960s and 1970s, they added the prescription of powerful diuretic drugs (water pills) to keep women from gaining more than twenty-four pounds during pregnancy. My obstetrician for my first pregnancy was particularly severe, in that he allowed only twelve to fifteen pounds of weight gain and required that I take diuretics. These drugs are no longer routinely prescribed as they were in the 1960s and 1970s, but many obstetricians still restrict salt intake when high blood pressure readings are found, whether or not these readings are associated with toxemia or one of several other possible causes. Within the techno-medical model of care, the favorite ways of dealing with toxemia today include "treatment" by early delivery, whether by induction of labor or planned cesarean section, and the prescription of magnesium sulfate, Valium (diazepam), or calcium.

Tom Brewer, author of *Metabolic Toxemia of Late Pregnancy*, is a U.S. family practice physician who has devoted his life and career to understanding the cause of toxemia and to educating women and caregivers about how to prevent it. Between 1963 and 1976, he ran a prenatal-care project in Contra Costa County, California, for a population of over seven thousand mothers from the lowest income group in the San Francisco Bay Area. By all odds, most of the women in this population would have been considered likely candidates for developing toxemia and having low-birth-weight babies. In similar populations during the same period, the incidence of toxemia ranged between twenty and thirty-five percent.[11] That is not what happened in the Contra Costa County project, where because of Brewer's intensive work, the women received extensive nutritive counseling during pregnancy. There, the incidence of toxemia was only 0.5 percent, with no cases of convulsive toxemia.[12] The published results of this study convinced many midwives but few physicians or researchers, ostensibly because Brewer's work was not based upon randomized controlled trials. This research method (in which women are assigned by chance to groups receiving different treatments, whose outcomes are then compared by researchers unaware of the group to which each woman belongs) is often called the "gold standard" of research because it is designed to eliminate bias. However, the problem with applying it to the thesis that good nutrition can prevent most cases of toxemia is that it requires the deliberate malnutrition or starvation of a group of women to be compared with a group of well-nourished women. Unfortunately, in the modern world of techno-medicine, cures and treatments involving drugs and surgery are often more researched and quickly accepted by most obstetricians than are preventive measures.

Gardeners know that you must nourish the soil if you want healthy plants. You must water plants adequately, especially when seeds are germinating and sprouting, and they should be planted in a nutrient-rich soil. Why should nutrition matter less in the creation of young humans than it does in young plants? I'm sure that it doesn't. Farmers, ranchers, and veterinarians know that pregnant animals must be well-fed and given enough water and salt to give the best chance of survival to their young. It doesn't make sense that the human species could be the only one whose newborns have the power to extract from their mothers nutrients that their mothers aren't eating themselves.

I know of no zookeeper who would feed pregnant animals in zoos junk food and expect optimally healthy young to be born. Common sense says that eating well is a good idea. Even if it made no difference in the incidence of toxemia (which I doubt), what is there to lose by eating a good diet?

So eat well. This means eat food. Avoid eating anything that isn't food, such as preservatives, chemical additives, and anything that nature didn't produce. Read labels. The same goes for what you drink. If you are addicted to carbonated, sweet beverages, swear off them during pregnancy and breastfeeding and drink water. Make sure that you get enough protein by eating about fifty to seventy-five grams per day of food such as dairy products, dried peas or beans (legumes), nuts, or meat. Drink as much as you like, and salt your food to taste. Eat dark, leafy greens such as spinach, kale, or collards and yellow vegetables such as carrots, yams, and sweet potatoes, as these are high in the kinds of vitamins you most need during pregnancy. See Resources for more information on nutrition and pregnancy, including Tom Brewer's published writings and his Toxemia Hotline.

Whether you choose a practitioner from the techno-medical model or the midwifery model, there are certain tests that are performed at each prenatal visit. Your urine and your blood pressure will be checked. The height of your uterus will be measured. Your ankles will be felt. These signs and measures of health are recognized as essential in both models of care.

A battery of several optional prenatal tests has been developed over the last quarter century. These technologies include ultrasound, chorionic villus sampling, amniocentesis, and maternal serum alpha-fetoprotein screening. Each was at first envisioned for use only in a relatively small number of women who had some kind of high-risk condition, but their use has since expanded in many practices. Within the medical model of birth care, most North American women are now given some form of prenatal diagnostic screening as a routine part of their prenatal care. Most insurance plans pay for diagnostic screening, leading many women to decide to go forward with such tests. But there is some reason to be cautious about allowing yourself and your baby to be tested, especially if you would be opposed to terminating your pregnancy regardless of the genetic or chromosomal status of your baby. Virtually none of the women who gave birth at The Farm Midwifery Center decided to undergo prenatal diagnostic screening, with no expressed regrets.

Ultrasound

Ultrasound scanning came on the scene a few years after a large study demonstrated an increase in cancer among children x-rayed in utero.[13] During the 1970s ultrasound rapidly gained popularity among physicians and birthing women. It was introduced by a Scots obstetrician who borrowed an industrial ultrasound machine for detecting flaws in metal and used it on pregnant women, despite the lack of scientific evaluation of possible hazardous effects. By 1980, obstetric ultrasound had become routine in many countries, including many in which the scans were funded by taxpayers.

The use of ultrasound is especially unregulated and popular in the United States. The Food and Drug Administration (FDA) bowed to pressure from industry and organized medicine to relinquish control over the amount of sonic energy that can be emitted by the new ultrasound devices used in obstetrics. Currently, there are no federal or state regulations requiring periodic calibration of obstetric ultrasound machines, written consent of the pregnant woman, indications for the procedure, the type of equipment used, the amount of exposure, or the identification and qualification of the sonographer.[14] Anyone can buy an ultrasound device and use it on pregnant women, whether to determine the sex of the child or to make ultrasonographic photos for family albums.

Research about the safety of ultrasound has been limited, considering the extent of its casual use. No problems have been detected in the short-term for children exposed during pregnancy and labor, but ultrasound has not been used long enough to identify any long-term hazards. We truly have no idea what long-term effects there may be from exposing fetuses to ultrasound.

The notion that ultrasound makes pregnancy or birth safer for all women is a misconception. Several major studies have been carried out to evaluate the effectiveness of routine diagnostic ultrasound, but so far none has shown routine use to improve maternal and infant outcome over ultrasound used only when medically indicated. Ultrasound can be useful to diagnose if a fetus is alive, the age of a fetus (only in early pregnancy), how many babies there are, the location of the placenta, the position of the baby, and, when two scans are done two weeks apart, how the baby is growing. Ultrasound can show the sex of the baby, but you should know that it is quite possible for sonographers to make a mistake in determining the sex. I know lots of cases where this happened, despite repeated ultrasounds, and of cases of twins mistakenly diagnosed when there was only one baby. I have also known of weight estimates by ultrasound to be off by as much as five pounds.

Within the medical model of care, the routine use of ultrasound is often assumed. It makes sense to consider how having an ultrasound will enhance your pregnancy before choosing to have one. Having that early look inside is not always reassuring, nor does it always prepare you for what is to come. I remember my cousin who told me that she felt like she grieved through the second half of her pregnancy because she had learned her baby's gender (which was the same as her older child's). She later fell in love with her second child, but she spent several months burdened by information that did her and her baby no good.

If you would prefer not to have an ultrasound that your doctor or midwife has asked for, I suggest that you ask what specific information they want. If the effort is to try to confirm your due date, you may be able to use other information (such as accurate records of your last period or temperature charts) to determine when your baby was conceived. In any case, state your preference that the ultrasound not be used. Competent practitioners can learn a lot by using their hands, as midwives and doctors did before the invention of ultrasound.

Some obstetricians use ultrasound to measure women's pelvic dimensions. In my experience, this is a poor use of a technology whose long-term effects are still unknown. The midwives at The Farm Midwifery Center understand pelvimetry as more of an art than a science—an educated guess rather than an exact system of measurement. In our view, such a judgment is better made by hand than by the use of imaging technology such as ultrasound or X ray. I say this because my partners and I have taken care of more than twenty-five women who were told by their doctors that their pelvises were "inadequate" on the basis of X-ray or ultrasound measurements—too small for the normal birth process to take place successfully. With just two exceptions, these women were able to give birth vaginally. At The Farm Midwifery Center, we have always measured pelvises and babies' sizes by hand rather than with any mechanical or radiological means. None of us has found X ray or ultrasound to be necessary or even particularly helpful in predicting women's ability to give birth to a baby of any given size. Our hands know how big a pelvis is in relation to the baby who must come through it, the same way all people who do the same task repetitively learn to measure things by feel.

Another reason to refuse an ultrasound ordered to obtain your pelvic measurements is that these dimensions actually change according to the position you assume. (Most physicians don't know this, by the way.) One of the greatest weaknesses of measuring the pelvis based upon ultrasound is the idea that the female pelvis is fixed in its size and shape. This would be true if the pelvis were a solid ring of bone. In fact, it is composed of four separate bones connected with ligaments at the joints. The hormone relaxin loosens these ligaments in late pregnancy, in preparation for birth, making it even easier for them to shift in relation to one another. The pelvis that might be a little small while you are lying on your back becomes significantly larger when you are on your hands and knees.

Janet Balaskas, well known yoga teacher and childbirth educator, describes a wonderfully empowering exercise for creating awareness of this ability. Here's a quick take on how it's done. Stand or kneel with one hand on your pubic bone in front and the other on your tailbone. Notice how far apart your hands are. Now lean backward as far as possible (taking care not to hurt yourself) and continue to notice how far apart your hands are. Next, lean forward until your torso is parallel to the ground.[15] Most people find it surprising how much their hands move with this exercise. Most feel a noticeable increase in the distance between their pubic bone and tailbone after leaning forward. No wonder monkeys (who are built much like we are) tend to lean forward during birth!

Chorionic Villus Sampling

Chorionic villus sampling (CVS) is an invasive technique for testing for chromosomal abnormalities (such as Down syndrome). It is done before twelve weeks. Its main advantage is that it can be done earlier in pregnancy than amniocentesis. Women who have already had a child with chromosomal abnormalities, as well as women over thirty-five, are likely to be offered the test. CVS, like other invasive procedures, can cause miscarriage. The rate of pregnancy loss after CVS was about four percent in a large register organized by the World Health Organization. Rarely, CVS can cause damage to arms, legs, fingers, and toes of the embryo.

If you know that you would not have an abortion if screening tests indicated that you might have a baby with Down syndrome, you should decline the test. In a case like this, having the test would likely make the pregnancy more stressful.

Amniocentesis
Amniocentesis is another invasive procedure that can reveal certain conditions and disorders in the fetus. It involves removing a sample of amniotic fluid through a long needle while the doctor uses ultrasound images to lessen the chance of accidentally sticking the fetus. Like ultrasound and CVS, this test can reveal the gender of the baby. In addition, it checks for chromosomal abnormalities and neural-tube defects such as spina bifida and anencephaly. Within the medical model, amniocentesis has become standard for women over thirty-five. The age thirty-five was chosen as the cutoff because at this age the likelihood of having a baby with a chromosome condition is about the same or greater than the risk that the test will injure the fetus or cause a miscarriage. There is about a 1.5 percent chance of miscarriage or fetal damage following amniocentesis. Amniocentesis began to be offered to younger women after a spate of "wrongful life" lawsuits, in which parents who had a child with Down syndrome sued doctors who hadn't told them about the availability of amniocentesis. Amniocentesis is done between fifteen and eighteen weeks of pregnancy, and analysis takes another two or three weeks. Occasionally, the test has to be performed more than once.

Some women find amniocentesis reassuring, but others wish they had been warned about the feelings that often follow while waiting for the analysis. By this time, the baby's movements are usually clearly felt. Sociologist Barbara Katz Rothman has written eloquently about the conflict this causes for many families. Amniocentesis, in her words, "asks women to accept their pregnancies and their babies, to take care of the babies within them, and yet be willing to abort them."[16] For any woman who has an amnio, there are two remote possibilities that go with the procedure: one is the possibility of having a child with Down syndrome, the other is having a miscarriage caused by the amnio. Remember: an amnio never cured anything.

Maternal Serum Alpha-fetoprotein Screening
Maternal serum alpha-fetoprotein screening is not a diagnostic test but rather a screening procedure, as its name states. At sixteen weeks, this

test is now routinely offered to almost all women during pregnancy (within the medical model of care). What you should know is that AFP screening does not tell you that your baby is okay. This simple blood test tells you the chance of your baby having certain abnormalities, but it cannot tell you whether or not your baby has these conditions. When AFP screening indicates there may be a problem, your physician will usually order an amniocentesis or an ultrasound. About five percent of these initial AFP screenings will produce an abnormal result, even when the fetus is absolutely healthy. This high percentage of mistakes is partly due to miscalculation of the gestational age or the presence of twins.

When the AFP-screening test kit was first introduced, the FDA regulated it and allowed its use only in research settings. However, pressure from physicians and laboratories prompted the FDA to withdraw from regulating AFP screening. The American College of Obstetricians and Gynecologists (ACOG) advised its members to offer the test to all pregnant women, as part of a *liability alert*.[17] This alert was for the benefit of doctors, not women. It was meant to prevent lawsuit. Although the test is promoted as reassuring, those women for whom the test shows high AFP levels (including those for whom the test shows a "false positive" result) find it anything but reassuring. The results of the AFP may be quickly analyzed, but the follow-up amniocentesis that is usually indicated involves weeks of waiting. The routine use of this procedure has been questioned because it subjects so many women to tests and unnecessary anxiety when so few actually will have any problems. One thing is certain: If you are already having an amniocentesis, you do not need AFP screening.

Screening for Gestational Diabetes

If your caregiver works within the medical model of care and large babies run in your family, you will likely be offered screening for "gestational diabetes." Gestational diabetes (GD) is not really a disease. Rather, it is a higher level of blood sugar than average during pregnancy, as determined by a glucose tolerance test (GTT). GD differs from diabetes mellitus in that GD goes away after the baby is born. Diabetes mellitus does not. Many doctors recommend this test for all pregnant women, to be performed between twenty-four and twenty-eight weeks of gestation. The test, unfortunately, is not very reliable. Between fifty and seventy percent of women, if retested, will have a different result than they got from the first test. The best evidence we have says there is no treatment for GD, either with diet or with insulin, that improves the outcome for mothers or their babies. In short, the anxiety that is often produced by this test simply isn't worth the information gained from it. Sometimes, when the test is positive, you may be urged to undergo further expensive tests and treatments with no proven benefit.

Beyond the routine testing with urine dipsticks at prenatal visits, my partners and I use a little device called a glucometer to help us identify the women who can benefit from dietary changes if we find that their blood-sugar levels are varying too widely. The glucometer is a finger-poker that measures the sugar level in a drop of blood. We use it when we notice several of the following symptoms at twenty-eight weeks or thereafter:

- fast weight gain
- feeling "funny" or "dizzy" after meals
- constant thirst
- craving for sugar
- family history of diabetes
- previous large baby

We get a glucometer reading fifteen to thirty minutes after breakfast and again one hour later. We have encountered a few cases in which a woman's glucose was high (250) within that time range and back to normal (120 or less) within an hour. These are the women who feel funny after a meal and whose high sugar reading wouldn't be detected by a GTT. We usually find that they have been eating something that they don't tolerate well during pregnancy—sugar and white flour, for instance. In the short term, the best way for the woman to bring down the sugar level in her blood is to get up and exercise if possible. For the rest of her pregnancy, her best bet is to completely eliminate white flour, pasta, other starchy foods, and sugar from her diet.

Screening for Beta Strep (Group B Streptococcus)
Although we tend to think of bacteria as disease-causing organisms, there are varieties that live in our bodies—in our throats, vaginas, and bowels, for instance—and cause us no harm at all. One common variety,

group B streptococcus—also called beta strep—does have significance for pregnant women. The normal bacteria in women's vaginas sometimes include beta strep. About one women in every five has beta strep living ("colonizing" is the medical term) in her vagina. There is a difference between being colonized by beta strep (many of us are) and infected (sick).

Usually, the presence of group B strep causes no symptoms in women. There are occasional urinary-tract infections in the presence of beta strep and, much more rarely, infections of the placenta that lead to premature rupture of the membranes and premature labor.

In the fifteen to twenty percent of women who have group B strep in their vaginas during labor, about half of the babies will be colonized at birth. But this does not mean that all of these babies become ill. In fact, ninety-eight percent or more do not become infected. When the infection does occur, however, it is serious, as it is fatal in ten percent of cases. Still, it is important to remember that only two babies out of a thousand in the population at large get infected. The problem is that there is no really accurate way to know which two babies out of a thousand those will be.

Certain situations are associated with a higher than usual risk of infection in the baby. These include:

- low birth weight or premature babies
- membranes ruptured for more than eighteen hours before birth
- long labors, especially when there have been multiple vaginal examinations
- interventions such as induction of labor, internal fetal monitors, vacuum extractors, and forceps
- babies whose heart rates are unusually fast during labor
- mothers who develop a fever during labor
- mothers whose vaginal cultures show especially heavy beta strep colonization
- babies who need resuscitation at birth

Several prevention strategies have been developed to cover group B strep. One is to test all pregnant women to find out if they are colonized by group B strep. Theoretically, those with positive cultures could be treated with antibiotics. The problem with this strategy (which has been tried by researchers) is that it didn't work; it did not reduce the number of babies who became ill. Only in the case of women who had bladder infections caused by group B strep was this strategy helpful.

For years, the American College of Obstetricians and Gynecologists (ACOG), the Centers for Disease Control (CDC), and the American College of Nurse Midwives (ACNM) recommended one of two strategies:

1. Forgo screening and give I.V. antibiotics in labor to all women with risk factors such as prematurely ruptured membranes, premature labor, membranes ruptured for eighteen hours or more, newborn group B strep in a previous birth, or fever in labor. (This would include women with epidurals who develop fever in labor, since this fever cannot be distinguished from that which is caused by infection.)
2. Screen everyone between thirty-five to thirty-seven weeks of pregnancy. Offer all colonized women I.V. antibiotics in labor. Prescribe I.V. antibiotics to group B carriers with membranes ruptured for eighteen hours or more or those who develop a fever in labor.

More recently, the ACOG, CDC, ACNM, and American Academy of Pediatrics (AAP) have agreed to abandon the first-mentioned strategy of treating only when risk factors are present and to follow the second course of screening everyone. This new approach means that many, many women will be treated with antibiotics whose babies would never have developed an infection anyway. Even when this approach is taken, some babies who really do need treatment may be missed.

This new protocol is not entirely risk-free itself. The overuse of antibiotics is well known to contribute to the development of strains of resistant bacteria—bacteria that don't die when antibiotics are given. The new protocol is likely to add to this problem. Antibiotics sometimes cause side effects such as yeast or thrush infections in mothers and babies and diarrhea. The CDC estimates that giving all group B colonized women penicillin (the medication of choice) would result in ten maternal deaths per year from severe allergic reaction.

For all of the reasons cited in the previous paragraph, you should know that you still have the option of declining the test or of declining the I.V. antibiotics if you consent to screening and the test is positive.

You can slightly decrease the risk of your baby becoming infected by declining as many interventions as possible (including vaginal examinations, especially when your membranes have ruptured) and by having everyone wash their hands frequently before touching the baby during the newborn period. (Some group B infections develop during the first three months of the life of the newborn.)

Prenatal Rhogam

As part of your prenatal care, you should have a blood test to determine whether your blood type is Rh positive or Rh negative. Eighty-five percent of Caucasians have Rh positive blood, while the remaining fifteen percent have Rh negative blood. If you are Rh positive or if both you and the father of your baby are Rh negative, you have no particular need to understand the details of prenatal Rhogam. But if you are Rh negative and your baby's father is Rh positive, Rh incompatibility problems can become an increasing possibility with each succeeding pregnancy.

Having Rh negative blood is not in itself a problem. But there may be negative consequences if the blood of an Rh negative person is mixed with Rh positive blood. When an Rh negative mother carries an Rh positive baby, there is usually no mixing of their blood during pregnancy. However, sometimes during pregnancy, labor, and birth, a small amount of the baby's blood gets into the mother's bloodstream. When this happens, the baby's blood is recognized as foreign, and the mother's blood usually produces anti-D antibodies to "fight off" the foreign substance. An Rh negative mother's blood is said to be "sensitized" when this process has taken place. Procedures such as amniocentesis, aggressive external version, and episiotomy increase the chances of sensitization.

Sensitization is rare in the case of a first baby, unless there has been a previous pregnancy that ended in abortion or miscarriage, or a mismatched transfusion. But if the anti-D antibodies are present in a mother's bloodstream, the safety of her subsequent Rh positive babies may be compromised because these antibodies can cross the membrane at the placenta (although the blood cannot) and attack the rhesus proteins in the baby's blood. The problems that may result from this incompatibility range from mild jaundice to acute hemolytic disease, which is sometimes fatal to the baby.

Injections of a manufactured blood product called Rhogam in the United States and Anti-D in the United Kingdom are generally given to

Rh negative mothers with Rh positive babies within seventy-two hours after birth or after any traumatic event during pregnancy when the mixture of blood might have taken place. Rhogam is pretty effective at preventing the formation of the antibodies that present a danger to future Rh positive babies. Since Rhogam was developed, there has been a great reduction in the number of babies lost to severe hemolytic disease.

Despite the overall benefits of Rhogam administration, some women have qualms about accepting the product. Its manufacturers list its documented side effects, which include local inflammation, malaise, chills, fever, and, rarely, anaphylaxis. Some women report an irritating body rash following a Rhogam injection. Another issue is that some pharmaceutical companies use a mercury-based preservative in the drug, which some women wish to avoid because of potential toxicity. Another concern is related to the issue of blood-borne infections. In the early days of Rhogam's use, some women did contract hepatitis C and HIV through infected Rhogam. Neither of these viruses is currently a danger, as both are now screened for and rendered harmless through the manufacturers' purification processes, but there is a possibility that there may be as yet unknown viruses that might not be destroyed by current treatments.[18]

If your blood type is Rh-negative, you live in the United States, and your maternity care is closer to the techno-medical model than the midwifery model, it is likely that you will be urged to accept a Rhogam injection at twenty-eight and thirty-four weeks of gestation, regardless of whether your baby is Rh negative or Rh positive. The rationale for this prenatal administration of Rhogam (which is controversial internationally) is that some argue that this is the best means of preventing the few cases of "silent" sensitization that may occur during pregnancy. One study showed a fall in the sensitization rate from 1.12 percent (without routine prenatal Rhogam) to 0.28 percent (with prenatal Rhogam), but critics have pointed out that this fall may be attributable to other factors such as failure to offer Rhogam to women with risk factors during pregnancy.[19] The problem with routine prescription of prenatal Rhogam is that many babies who are Rh negative like their mothers will be exposed to the drug, and there has been no systematic study of the long-term effects of this product in babies.[20]

In my own practice, my partners and I—like many other midwives—do not advise women to accept Rhogam prenatally unless there has been a traumatizing event. If an Rh negative woman has a possibly sensitizing event during pregnancy, she is given information about the possible risks and benefits of Rhogam administration, along with the risks of sensitization, and she then chooses whether or not to accept the Rhogam injection.

The administration of Rhogam within seventy-two hours of the birth of an Rh positive baby to an Rh negative mother is much less controversial than at twenty-eight weeks of pregnancy. About 90 percent of Rh negative women giving birth to an Rh positive baby will not need postnatal Rhogam, because there has been no mixing of their blood and the baby's blood and thus there is no sensitization. Unfortunately, there is no accurate way to determine whether you are among the ten percent who will become sensitized without Rhogam.

The decision about whether or not to accept Rhogam is not always an easy one to make. If the woman has no plans for future pregnancies, she usually refuses the Rhogam. Women who have religious convictions that oppose the administration of blood products will not accept Rhogam. Women who have had medical intervention in birth are more likely to be sensitized than those who have not.

Some women choose a Kleihauer test to find out whether fetal cells have entered their own bloodstream. If the test is negative, they may decide that the chance of sensitization after the birth of an Rh positive baby is low enough to refuse Rhogam injection. However, the Kleihauer test is not always accurate.

Informed Consent

Ethical medical and midwifery care requires that your informed consent be given for whatever treatments or procedures your caregiver recommends that you undergo. Before you agree to any procedure or treatment, you should be given information about the test to help you decide whether you want to have it done. Remember, though, that the information you get about the test from your doctor or midwife, although accurate, may be a bit biased. Before you go ahead with screening, you may want to seek out additional sources of information, such as childbirth-preparation books, the Internet, or a genetic counselor.

What degree of consent will you actually have while you are in labor? Most of us who have experienced it know that one of the last things anyone in labor wants to do is read. Hospitals vary; some ask consent separately for each major procedure that is proposed, while others ask women on admission to give blanket permission to whatever procedures a woman's physician decides are necessary. Wherever you plan to give birth, find out what procedures might be used on you. Inform yourself about what you will and will not accept. U.S. courts have accepted the idea that you give your implied consent to procedures if you have not actively objected to various procedures by simply refusing them, firing your caregiver, or discharging yourself from the hospital against medical advice. Some U.S. hospitals have begun to ask women to sign statements that they do not wish to be informed about the potential hazards of drugs they are asked to take.

Notes

1. Rothman, Barbara Katz. *In Labor: Women and Power in the Birth-place.* New York: W. W. Norton, 1972.
2. Davis-Floyd, Robbie E. *Birth as an American Rite of Passage.* Berkeley: University of California Press, 1992.
3. Davis-Floyd, R. and St. John, G. *From Doctor to Healer: The Transformative Journey.* New Brunswick, N. J.: Rutgers U. Press, 1998.
4. Carter, J. P., et al. Preeclampsia and reproductive performance in a community of vegans. *Southern Medical Journal*, 1980; 80(6): 692–97.
5. Primrose, T., and Higgins, A. A study in human antepartum nutrition. *Journal of Reproductive Medicine*, 1971; 7:257–64.
6. Hamlin, R. H. J. The prevention of eclampsia and pre-eclampsia. *Lancet*, 1952; 1:64.
7. Higgins, A. C. Nutritional status and the outcome of pregnancy. *Journal of The Canadian Dietetic Association*, 1976; 37:17.
8. Burke, B., et al. Nutrition studies during pregnancy. *American Journal of Obstetrics & Gynecology*, 1943; 46:38.
9. Brewer, T. H. Human maternal-fetal nutrition. *Obstetrics & Gynecology*, 1972; 40:868.
10. Speert, Harold. *Obstetrics and Gynecology in America: A History.* Chicago: The American College of Obstetricians and Gynecologists, 1980.
11. Brewer, G. S., with Tom Brewer. *What Every Pregnant Woman*

Should Know: The Truth about Diets and Drugs in Pregnancy. New York: Random House, 1977.

12. Brewer, T. H. Metabolic toxemia of late pregnancy in a county prenatal nutrition education project: A preliminary report. *Journal of Reproductive Medicine*, 1974; 13:175.

13. Stewart, A., Webb, J., Giles, D., and Hewitt, D. Malignant disease in childhood and diagnostic irradiation in utero, *Lancet*, 1956; 2:447.

14. Haire, D. B. In *Encyclopedia of Childbearing: Critical Perspectives*, Ultrasound in obstetrics: A question of safety. Phoenix, AZ: Oryx Press, 1993.

15. Robertson, A. *Empowering Motherhood.* Camperdown, NSW, Australia: ACE Graphics, 1994.

16. Rothman, B. K. *The Tentative Pregnancy: Prenatal Diagnosis and the Future of Motherhood.* New York: Viking, 1986.

17. Rothman, B. K., ed. *The Encyclopedia of Childbearing: A Guide to Prenatal Practices, Birth Alternatives, Infant Care and Parenting Decisions for the '90s.* New York: Henry Holt and Company, 1993.

18. Wickham, S. *Anti-D in Midwifery: Panacea or Paradox?* Oxford: Butterworth-Heinemann, 2001.

19. Maybe, S., et al. Rate of RhD sensitisation before and after implementation of a community based antenatal prophylaxis programme. *British Medical Journal*, 1997; 315:1588.

20. Urbaniak, S. Proceedings of the Consensus Conference on Anti-D Prophylaxis. *British Journal of Obstetrics and Gynaecology*, 1998; 105:18, 24.

6

GOING INTO LABOR

As your estimated due date approaches, your thoughts are likely to be dominated by how best to navigate your journey toward motherhood. Depending upon where you plan to give birth, there is quite a range in the routines that may greet you when you arrive at the hospital or birth center you have chosen. Each hospital, for instance, has its own routines and policies, and you may find dramatic differences between hospital policies within the same geographical area. How do you know which routines are optional and which are not? Just because a policy is routine at a particular hospital does not necessarily mean that it is mandatory or even scientifically based. Which routines are scientifically questionable? If some of the routines at your hospital are unjustified, what alternatives might you negotiate with hospital staff?

In Labor or Not?

The first big decision for North American women in labor usually concerns when to go to the hospital or birth center or, if you are having a home birth, when to call your midwife. Do you hurry to get to your destination as soon as possible, or do you take your time? Obviously, the answer to this depends to some extent upon how long it takes to arrive at the hospital. If this is your first labor, you have no reference point for how intense labor must usually become before birth is imminent. You may lean toward traveling to your birthplace-to-be as early in labor as possible—especially if you are expecting your first baby—since nobody wants to give birth in a car. (These births usually happen without complication, by the way.) But before you decide that you'll go in at the first hint of labor, remember that there is good reason to be cautious about going in too early.

Everyone who works in hospital maternity wards is familiar with this scenario: A first-time mother checks into the hospital with what she feels is strong labor, goes through all the admittance procedures, and by the time she gets to the labor ward or birth room, her labor has virtually stopped. If the admittance process is enough to quell *your* labor, I suggest that you consider going home. It may help to know that labor *often* starts and stops a time or two before it becomes powerful enough to complete the birth process. This situation is most likely to happen in the early or latent phase of labor. If you think you are in labor and it's late in the day, try taking a warm bath, drinking a glass of wine, and going to bed for a while. You may be able to take a nap before labor becomes intense. This is a good thing, as it reduces the likelihood of a stalled labor once you get to the hospital, it conserves your energy, and you may even make some real progress in labor as you doze. Even a well-advanced labor can stall or go more slowly once you travel from your home to your hospital or birth center.

Within the midwifery model, when women's labors start, we midwives phone or visit the mother to assess how things are going. If labor then slows or stops, we generally go home and wait for the next call. We know that normal labors often follow a pattern like this. The woman then resumes her normal daily routine, and she calls her midwife when labor starts again. Four or five false starts are not unusual. Such a pattern is perfectly normal and poses no extra risk to the baby if the water bag has not broken. So why not wait? There is nothing to lose.

Before the use of induction drugs became common, most hospital maternity wards sent women in early labor home if labor was not well established. Laboring women walked the halls if their rushes weren't strong enough to thin or dilate the cervix. Nowadays, many hospital maternity wards discourage you from leaving once you are admitted, even if your labor has effectively stopped. With a wider array of induction drugs now available and little public knowledge of any disadvantages of these drugs, there is less emphasis on sticking to natural methods of labor enhancement. Despite this more casual attitude toward induction drugs, if labor is still in its early stages you may be able to negotiate either walking or going home and returning when you are closer to giving birth. If your labor is slow and you stay, you must deal with the time limit that is often placed on labor—twelve to twenty-four hours in most hospitals.

Sometimes time becomes a factor even in a home birth. Years ago I was traveling through southern California on a tight schedule and found myself in the home of my sister-in-law, Sherry, just as she was going into labor. Having had one hospital birth, she wanted me to attend her at home, so she decided to make a fast change in her previous plans. The only problem was that my schedule allowed me only twenty-four hours at her house before I had to move on to my next appointment. Her labor seemed to intensify in direct proportion to the amount of attention she paid it. Canceling a canasta game she had arranged to play with her neighbors helped. An hour or so later, I had

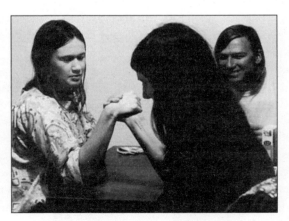

Arm wrestling: an unusual but effective way
to accelerate labor

a wild hunch of something else that might help: I asked Sherry if she would consider arm-wrestling (between rushes) with our friend Margaret. I knew that she would beat Margaret easily, and I was pretty sure that the boost she would get from this victory would help her labor kick in even stronger. That is exactly what happened. My beautiful niece, Christina, was born in the early morning, several hours before I had to leave. We celebrated her birthday with my husband, as it was his too. Contracting the arm muscles during labor distracts women's attention from holding their pelvic and thigh muscles tight to "protect" themselves during labor.

Induction of Labor

One of the choices faced by as many as a third of U.S. women in late pregnancy concerns the artificial induction of labor. There *are* legitimate medical reasons for induction. These include cancer, hypertension, diabetes, kidney disease, a small-for-dates baby, a decrease in the amount of amniotic fluid or an intrauterine death followed by a long wait for labor to begin (we're talking weeks, not days). In these cases, the risks posed by the induction method are more likely to be outweighed by those associated with waiting for the natural process to kick in. Many studies agree that fewer than ten percent of women require labor induction for medical reasons. A consensus meeting organized by the World Health Organization on Appropriate Technology for Birth held in Fortaleza, Brazil, in 1985 recommended that "No geographic region should have rates of induced labor over ten percent."[1]

Obviously, nonmedical reasons to induce labor have increased over the last decade, as working women and obstetricians try to crowd more into already busy schedules and as new drugs have become available. The U.S. induction rate doubled between 1989 and 1998 (from 9 percent to 19.2 percent) and is apparently still rising, although there was no corresponding rise in the size of babies, the length of pregnancies, or the incidence of maternal illnesses requiring induction.[2-4] With so many inductions taking place, a common misconception has arisen that obstetricians are now able to start labor at will, with no disadvantages from the procedures used. Most U.S. working women, with only six weeks of maternity leave to look forward to, are understandably ready to start labor if there are no risks associated with induction. They assume—often wrongly—that their caregiver will inform them of any risks induction might carry.

Disadvantages to the Mother from Induction

Labor (including its onset) involves an extremely complex interplay of hormones that cannot be altered without upsetting the normal physiological pattern. Changing the normal pattern often causes other problems, necessitating more obstetrical interventions. An induced labor is quite a different process from spontaneous labor. Women tend to have harsher, stronger, significantly more painful contractions with chemically induced labors, so one who can cope with a spontaneous labor often finds that she needs pain medication to bear the more-insistent contractions of an induced one. When labor is induced with Pitocin (see p. 210), an intravenous infusion has to be set up. The laboring woman's mobility is automatically restricted in these cases because of the discomfort caused by the I.V. needle in her vein and the tubes that attach her to the I.V. stand. Even though I.V. stands have wheels, they are far from easy to "drive" while in labor. Rarely, but far less rarely than in spontaneous labors, pharmaceutical induction can rupture the uterus. This event calls for emergency cesarean section and, sometimes, hysterectomy. Increased postpartum blood loss is another problem associated with artificial induction of labor.

Disadvantages to the Baby from Induction

The main justification for artificially inducing labor is a reduction in the number of compromised babies. The problem with at least half of the artificial inductions taking place in the United States at present is that the induction method itself can compromise the baby. Oxytocin and prostaglandin inductions are well known to cause longer, more-intense contractions of the uterus, thus interfering with the flow of oxygen-rich blood through the placenta to the fetus. For this reason, continuous fetal monitoring is usually part of the protocol of the induced labor. For the fetal-monitoring machine to record the fetal heartbeat, the mother must lie still in bed. If she wants a little more mobility, she can opt to have an internal scalp electrode needle inserted into the baby's head, but this is painful to the baby, requires breaking the water bag, and can cause infection to both mother and baby.

Another heightened risk to the baby from labor induction is related to the higher incidence of fetal distress in induced labors compared with labors that begin spontaneously: A cesarean is more likely to take place in an induced labor than in one that begins naturally. In one study, the cesarean rate for abnormal fetal heart patterns doubled.[5] The uterine contractions of labor squeeze out the fluid that is naturally in the baby's lungs during pregnancy; with a cesarean, this process is circumvented, and the baby's lungs are more likely to be wet at birth, causing breathing difficulties.

Oxytocin and prostaglandin inductions are both known to increase the passage of meconium during labor, probably because the baby is more stressed than it would be during a labor that began on its own. Several studies of labors have documented high rates of meconium in those induced by the newest prostaglandin, Cytotec (discussed in more detail on p. 211).[6–10] When there is thick meconium in the amniotic fluid during labor, the baby sometimes inhales it with its first breath and has serious breathing problems. Newborn jaundice is another problem encountered more frequently after induction than in natural labors. Whether the baby has meconium aspiration or jaundice, it is likely to spend its first few days in the special-care nursery instead of in its mother's arms.

Have you ever heard of iatrogenic prematurity? The term means *doctor-caused* prematurity and had to be invented because so many premature babies are born after labors were induced or cesarean operations performed according to erroneous "due dates." The myth is that obstetric science is so highly evolved that it is no longer possible to be mistaken about when a baby is due. The reality is that iatrogenic prematurity is far more common than most obstetricians like to admit. Too often, it happens after a "convenience" induction—the kind performed for nonmedical reasons.

Common Induction Methods

The most common medical methods used to induce labor are breaking the waters (amniotomy) and various chemical methods: Pitocin intravenous drip and the administration of various prostaglandins (Cervidil, Prepidil, and Cytotec).

Breaking the Waters

Breaking the waters is a crude but sometimes effective way to start labor when a woman is about to go into labor on her own. This method alone will initiate labor within twenty-four hours in seventy to eighty percent of women. The problem is that the remaining twenty to thirty percent will experience a high incidence of intrauterine infection.[11] Breaking the waters alone does not increase the danger of uterine rupture. However, this method puts a time limit on labor to start and *conclude* in most hospitals because of the heightened risk of infection. Sometimes amniotomy causes the umbilical cord to fall out of the cervix below the baby's head, causing a life-threatening emergency for the baby.

Pitocin Intravenous Drip

Pitocin is a synthetic version of oxytocin, a natural hormone that is released from the mother's pituitary gland in tiny amounts during (not before) labor. Given intravenously, a dose that is far larger than that which is naturally secreted in early labor is increased every few minutes until the desired contraction rate is reached. Pitocin induction is more apt than a spontaneous labor to result in a vacuum-extractor or forceps delivery or a cesarean section because of fetal distress stemming from too strong uterine contractions. Oxytocin doubles the odds of the baby being born in poor condition because the extra-hard contractions it can cause interfere with the flow of oxygen-rich blood from mother to baby. Another hazard of oxytocin induction is an increased incidence of postpartum hemorrhage. Oxytocin, by the way, is also used to strengthen contractions in a slow-moving labor.

Oxytocin induction is often unsuccessful, even when it is combined with amniotomy. This is especially true when the cervix is not yet ripe (soft and thin). Some women undergo attempted Pitocin induction for three or four days without ever going into effective labor.

Obstetricians a generation ago were taught never to leave a mother alone during an oxytocin induction.[12] When there is an overdose (some women are more sensitive to the drug than others) resulting in abnormally strong and lengthy contractions, the intravenous drip can be turned off. Pitocin has a half-life in the body of ten to fifteen minutes.

There is a much higher incidence of uterine rupture in chemically induced labors than in spontaneous labors. Generally, the unscarred uterus does not contract so hard as to destroy itself in naturally occurring labors. With induction, between one and three percent of women have a ruptured uterus. Add the factor of previous cesarean to induction, and the rate rises. Nearly six percent of the women in one study had ruptured uteri after a chemically induced labor.[13]

The Prostaglandins

Prostaglandins are substances that are naturally produced by the body that act to soften the cervix and the lower part of the uterus. Over the last few decades chemists have produced several synthetic versions. The Food and Drug Administration (FDA) approved two formulations in the mid-1990s: Prepidil and Cervidil. Prepidil is a prostaglandin gel, which is applied to the cervix, and Cervidil is a tampon that releases the synthetic prostaglandin. Both drugs are often used in conjunction with oxytocin. Some women experience nausea, vomiting, and diarrhea under the influence of these drugs. In the case of hyperstimulation of the uterus, Prepidil can be wiped away from the cervix, and the Cervidil tampon can be pulled out. However, even with these precautions and the administration of the drug terbutaline to relax the uterus, uterine ruptures do sometimes occur.

The newest addition to the induction tool kit is called Cytotec (generic name: misoprostol). This tiny white pill quickly became the favorite induction agent in many U.S. hospitals during the late 1990s, despite its lack of approval from the FDA for use in pregnant women. Approved by the FDA to prevent ulcers, its use in pregnant women is considered "off-label"—legal but ethically suspect, since no formal, carefully planned research preceded its widespread acceptance into the pharmacopoeia of obstetrics. G. D. Searle, the manufacturer of Cytotec, has stated that it does not plan to seek FDA approval for the drug's use in labor induction.[14] The loophole that allows Cytotec to be used experimentally means there is no strong safeguard against disastrous side effects or unpredictable results.

When a manufacturer applies for FDA approval for a pharmaceutical product for a particular use, its product undergoes extensive testing on large numbers of people. Such testing is designed to discover possible dangerous side effects, as well as ideal dosage sizes and intervals. Lacking any such organized evaluation, Cytotec inductions increased year by year anyway. Although there have been many studies of Cytotec's use to induce labor, "the studies were not sufficiently large to exclude the possibility of uncommon serious adverse effects," according to a 1999 review published in a respected British medical journal.[15]

There is not even a manufacturer's recommended dose for labor induction with Cytotec, which means that ob/gyns prescribing the drug choose their own dosage regimens, often based on factors having nothing to do with the mother's or the baby's safety. One group of ob/gyn researchers decided to place the entire 100-microgram tablet in women's vaginas (the drug was tested in *oral* dosages to prevent ulcers) to induce labor, commenting that they selected 100 micrograms "because of the ease of accurately obtaining such a dose."[16] One assumes that they later gave up the 100-microgram dose for induction after a consensus of researchers decided there had been too many catastrophic uterine ruptures associated with it. While they were correct that it *is* sloppy to cut tablets into halves and quarters, their decision to prescribe the 100-microgram dose at all seems incredibly cavalier—especially given the reports of worrisome maternal or fetal symptoms at half or a quarter of a 100-microgram tablet that had been published prior to this study. [5,9] Incidentally, G. D. Searle has stated that it does not intend to manufacture Cytotec in tablets of less than 100 micrograms. As we shall see in Chapter 11, there have been maternal deaths and other catastrophes associated with even the lowest possible dose of Cytotec.

Having heard from conversations with nurses, midwives, and doctors that Cytotec sometimes has terrible side effects (dead or brain-damaged babies, profuse bleeding, hysterectomies, and ruptured uteri), I decided to count up the adverse effects from all of the published studies I could find. Forty-nine studies yielded a total of 5,439 women who were given Cytotec to induce labor.

- 25 women had ruptured uteri
- 16 babies died
- 2 women had such profuse bleeding that they had emergency hysterectomies
- 2 women died

In several studies, a quarter of the babies went to the neonatal intensive-care unit. Ruptured uteri were especially likely to happen in women who had had previous uterine surgery, such as cesarean section.

After exposés of Cytotec side effects appeared in some magazines, Searle sent out a letter to two hundred thousand health-care providers in 2000 warning them that "Cytotec administration by any route is contraindicated in women who are pregnant because it can cause abortion." The company warned that the off-label use of the drug could result in uterine rupture, hysterectomy, and the death of mothers and babies. The author of a *Mother Jones* exposé learned through a Freedom of Information Act request to the FDA that, in the period between 1998 and 2001, the agency had received reports of thirty cases of uterine rupture in connection with Cytotec use, eight cases in which the fetus died in utero, and two more maternal deaths.[17] In a Silicon Valley weekly newspaper, four more maternal deaths, two near deaths, and a case of infant cerebral palsy—all associated with Cytotec and reported to the FDA—were discussed.[18]

I have already mentioned the CDC's data that show a doubling in induction of labor during the 1990s from about 10 percent to about 20 percent. In that same decade, the CDC documented a significant rise in the frequency of births from Mondays to Fridays. One of the reasons for Cytotec's popularity is apparently its efficacy in helping obstetricians schedule their maternity patients to give birth during daylight hours on weekdays.[19] Sometimes women ask for Cytotec induction because the doctor or midwife of their choice has a few days off work around the time of the estimated due date. Usually unaware of the risks involved, the women choose induction as a way to avoid being attended by a partner of their midwife or doctor. (I know too many who wish they had not been induced and had instead taken their chances with their chosen caregiver's partner.)

Some practitioners have used Cytotec to induce labor in women they fear might not go into natural labor before they reach forty-two weeks of pregnancy (at which time the rules and regulations for midwifery practice in many states require that birth must take place in a hospital if the midwife wants to keep her license). There is good reason to believe that such regulations are counterproductive, since they may cause more problems than they prevent. Here's what I mean. The evidence about the risks of "prolonged pregnancy" (all published before the Cytotec studies of the late 1990s) shows that there is nothing to be gained by chemical induction before 41.5 weeks. Even after 41.5 weeks, the few studies we have show that about five hundred women must be induced in order to prevent one perinatal death. Among five hundred Cytotec inductions, it is quite possible for the perinatal death rate to exceed what it would have been without induction.

There isn't enough good research to prove a basic assumption that underlies all the rules, regulations, and courtroom judgments about how long a pregnancy should be—that there is a specific week of pregnancy that is the best time for all women to give birth. We women aren't exactly calibrated to one another. Among the first fifty births I attended, for instance, six women gave birth after forty-two weeks of pregnancy—with no problems. In times when doctors weren't so apt to induce labor, forty-two weeks was considered a normal—even an optimum—time for many women to start labor. A few days either side of forty-two weeks could be all right too. Induction was seen as potentially risky, so there had to be a good justification to use it. One clearcut indication was in a full-term pregnancy with a decrease in the amount of amniotic fluid or a change in the baby's heart-rate pattern (signs that indicate a deteriorating placenta).

During the 1980s the pendulum swung toward action over expectant waiting, in large part because of physicians' defense strategies in potential malpractice lawsuits. Most doctors are aware that more of their colleagues are sued for not performing a cesarean fast enough and losing a baby than for performing one too soon and causing iatrogenic prematurity or injury to the mother. By the 1990s it wasn't unusual to hear of women having their labors induced at thirty-nine or forty weeks—just in case numerous attempts might be necessary.

I believe that women and their babies would be better served if the forty-two-week limit in state midwifery rules and regulations was changed to forty-three weeks—or, better yet, dropped. There are almost always clear symptoms when a baby is in danger from staying in the womb too long.

Midwifery Model of Care

According to the midwifery model of care, women's bodies can generally be trusted to go into spontaneous labor. We realize that good evidence shows that in the absence of danger signs (a decrease in amniotic fluid and changes in the fetal heart rate, for example), there is only a slight increase in risk when women go two weeks past their estimated due date. About 2.5 per thousand babies born at forty weeks will die in labor or soon after. At forty-two weeks, about 4.5 per thousand babies die. A fourth of these babies are abnormal and would have died no matter when they were born.[20]

Midwives sometimes suggest nonpharmacological ways to initiate labor, as several methods are often effective without being invasive or risky:

Sexual Intercourse

Unfortunately, some childbirth-preparation books still spread the myth that intercourse during pregnancy is harmful. A large collaborative study involving nearly forty thousand women found no association between lovemaking during pregnancy and poor outcome for mother or baby.[22] In fact, human semen is the most concentrated source of prostaglandins, the substance that Cervidil, Prepidil, and Cytotec attempt to mimic, which means that pleasurable intercourse during the last weeks of pregnancy helps the woman's body to go into labor. One researcher found that two to four hours after intercourse, prostaglandin concentrations in the cervical mucus were ten to fifty times higher than normal.[21] My partners and I noticed early in our midwifery practice that women who were sexually active during pregnancy were more likely than those who were not to go into labor around forty weeks. Incidentally, the prostaglandins in semen have never been associated with hyperstimulation of the uterus, more-painful uterine contractions, fetal distress, or ruptured uterus. Women who have had a history of miscarriage or premature birth or who threaten miscarriage should avoid sexual stimulation and arousal until their babies are ready to be born.

Breast Stimulation

Everyone who has breastfed a baby probably has noticed her uterus contracting while she nurses. Nipple stimulation causes the release of oxytocin into the maternal bloodstream, and this oxytocin then stimulates contractions of the uterine muscles. Both manual and oral stimulation are effective at stimulating oxytocin release. If stimulating one nipple only doesn't yield the desired result, stimulate both simultaneously. For cultural reasons, some hospitals prefer stimulation by breast pump or a TENS (transcutaneous electronic nerve stimulation) unit, a device that delivers a low electric current through pads applied to the skin. Manual and oral stimulation do not cause uterine rupture. If, under any circumstance, such stimulation did cause excessively long contractions (I have never seen this), it can easily be stopped, and the contractions will subside. Breast stimulation is especially effective in starting labor at term when it is combined with sexual intercourse. Unless your partner is an abysmally poor lover, this combination is by far the most enjoyable method of induction. See the section "Remember: Birth Is Sexual" in Chapter 7.

Castor Oil

Indigenous peoples all over the globe have used castor oil to induce labor for centuries. Taken orally, castor oil acts as a laxative, and the stimulation of the digestive tract often starts labor at term. No one knows exactly why castor oil works to start labor. When there is little or no money to be made as a result of research, generally little or no research is done. Nobody has figured out how to make an appreciable amount of money from castor oil, so this subject has received virtually no research attention. Nevertheless, castor oil seems to be quite safe. Nearly nine percent of nearly eleven thousand pregnant women in a large birth-center study used it to start labor, with no adverse outcomes.[23] At The Farm Midwifery Center, we recommend beginning a castor-oil induction at breakfast after a full night of sleep. One tablespoon of castor oil is added to scrambled eggs or is mixed with fruit juice to make it more palatable for the woman. If necessary, she takes one more tablespoon one hour after ingesting the first.

Sweeping the Membranes

The practitioner inserts two fingers just inside the cervix and gently separates the bag of waters from the inside of the cervix. Doing this stimulates the production of natural prostaglandins in the cervix. In two studies, sweeping the membranes successfully induced labor in about half of the cases attempted.[24,25] This method does not carry the side effect of hyperstimulating the uterus, nor does it cause fetal distress. If the practitioner isn't careful, it is possible to accidentally rupture the water bag.

Electronic Fetal Monitoring

Electronic fetal monitoring (EFM) was introduced widely during the 1970s, with the assumption that it would make labor safer for the baby. Hospitals began using EFM before there was any evidence to back up this assumption, and EFM became routine in many places. For all its great popularity in hospitals (more than eighty percent of U.S. women labor with EFM), this ubiquitous machine has not been associated with any noticeable lowering of infant mortality. Research done since then shows that intermittent listening with a fetoscope is every bit as good at detecting a baby who is in trouble from lack of oxygen. From the mother's standpoint, intermittent listening is far better—less painful and less likely to lead to ineffective labor and cesarean section.

When the uterus contracts, blood can't flow through the placenta as easily as usual, which means that the baby gets less oxygen. Babies normally tolerate these fluctuations in oxygen levels quite well. Generally, uterine contractions don't last long enough to cause damage from oxygen deprivation. If a baby is oxygen-deprived, the pattern of the heartbeat will usually change. When this happens, the baby needs to be delivered quickly.

Continuous EFM is done in two ways. The most common method involves two receivers held in place by belts around your hips. The second method is done with an electrode attached to the baby's head by a small needle stuck into the baby's scalp, which is kept in place until the baby is born. The electrode is attached to a wire that is introduced into the vagina. The signals from the baby's heart are then recorded on the printout.

Lots of research has shown that continuous EFM used routinely sometimes makes doctors and midwives believe that something is wrong when everything is actually all right. Someone misinterprets the tracings on the printout, orders an emergency cesarean, and a perfectly healthy baby is born, showing no sign of distress. The mother, however, has to recover from major surgery that was mistakenly performed. An unnecessary cesarean section or instrumental delivery is less likely when the baby's heartbeat is intermittently monitored with a Doppler or other type of fetoscope.

Even so, many hospitals require all mothers to have the EFM unit attached for twenty minutes after admission, and many others call for continuous EFM throughout labor. This procedure provides a paper printout of the baby's heart rate to assess the baby's condition. Giving in to EFM simply because policy requires it may mean that you begin your hospital stay in the most painful and least effective position: lying flat on your back. Continuous electronic fetal monitoring may be routine at many hospitals, but there is no good evidence that it should be mandatory. EFM has not:

- reduced infant deaths
- reduced the incidence of cerebral palsy. In fact, what evidence we have shows a slight increase in cerebral palsy among babies who have been electronically monitored[26,27]

One little-mentioned feature of EFM is that laboring women who are being monitored this way often feel that the machine becomes the center of attention in the room instead of them. When the midwife or nurse enters the room, she walks straight to the monitor and examines the tracing, sometimes having little to say to the woman in labor. Sometimes even family members become fascinated with the machine to the exclusion of the woman herself.

The alternative to EFM is intermittent listening every fifteen to thirty minutes (more often during the pushing phase) with some type of fetoscope. Fetoscopes are handheld, so intermittent listening requires more staff and more human attention than is commonly used with EFM. One reason hospitals like EFM is that it helps them cut costs. The printout gives the appearance that each woman is receiving a midwife's or obstetrical nurse's full attention during every minute of labor, but the reality is that EFM makes it possible for one person to "monitor" four or five laboring women simultaneously. Obviously, a caregiver who is providing care for so many women at once cannot spend much time encouraging any one of them during labor.

Routines to Refuse

The Pubic Shave
In certain backward areas some other hospital routines linger on, which you can quite safely refuse, according to strong medical evidence. For

instance, you don't need a pubic shave in order to give birth. Pubic shaving was introduced during the early days of hospital births as a preventive to infection. Studies later found that the rate of infection was actually higher in women who had been shaved, so most institutions abandoned the practice. Everyone who has experienced a pubic shave knows how uncomfortable razor nicks can be and how itchy the area is as the hair grows back.

The Enema
Another routine you may safely refuse is the enema. At one time, this procedure was considered necessary at most hospitals and was administered on arrival. Nowadays it is less common. Two studies found that enemas do not shorten labor or reduce infection rates. If you do not have an enema (occasionally, even if you do), you will poop a little as the baby's head emerges. Don't worry about this, as it is easily cleaned. This said, I have been at births where an enema helped a slow-starting labor get going.

The Involuntary Fast
You may wonder about whether you should eat or drink in labor. Many hospitals place restrictions on eating and drinking once you have been admitted. Some maintain a strict policy of denying anything by mouth. The reasons for this are historical rather than scientific. The fear behind this policy is that if a woman should need a cesarean section under general anesthesia, she might vomit and inhale some of the food into her lungs while she is unconscious from the anesthesia. Those who devised this policy hoped that restricting food and drink during labor would guarantee that there would be nothing to vomit in those rare cases when general anesthesia was used.

However, subsequent research has shown that restricting food and drink after hospital admission does not guarantee an empty stomach. When you are in labor, digestion happens slower than usual, so the food you ate several hours before coming to the hospital is likely to still be in your stomach. In addition, even when your stomach has been "empty" for hours, it will still secrete gastric juices, and these can be vomited and inhaled under general anesthesia. This kind of inhalation can burn the lining of the lungs or cause aspiration pneumonia, a serious disease.

Anesthesiologists in some hospitals give women antacids before general anesthesia in order to reduce acidity; this reduces but does not totally prevent aspiration pneumonia.

General anesthesia was the only kind used during cesarean sections until epidural anesthesia came into use. Women who have epidurals during cesareans do not become nauseous as easily, and even if they do vomit, they are conscious and therefore not in danger of inhaling their stomach contents. In any case, good anesthetic technique can prevent aspiration pneumonia.

Routine Intravenous Infusion

Hospitals that do not permit women to eat and drink during labor generally want all laboring women to be given intravenous sugar water. Studies have demonstrated that routine intravenous fluids are not a completely safe substitute for food and fluids in labor.[28-30] Large volumes of I.V. fluids can cause respiratory distress and seizures in newborns, because they cause low blood sugar and low blood sodium. When these fluids are given too fast for mothers to excrete, women can have convulsions or their lungs can fill as in drowning.

Some hospitals—usually those where midwives have been able to influence policy by presenting the best evidence—allow women to eat and drink at will during labor. No poor outcomes have been reported from this change in policy. Lifting restrictions against drink, in particular, avoids maternal dehydration, weakness during labor, and complications caused by intravenous fluids.

In a large birth-center study, Judith Rooks and colleagues reviewed the charts of 11,814 women who ate and drank at will during labor. Twenty-two percent of the women in the study chose to eat solid foods in labor.[23] There was no reported mortality or morbidity from aspiration pneumonia, even though there were some women who required emergency cesarean sections. Data from The Farm Midwifery Center support these findings. The Netherlands is one country in which obstetrical practice reflects a closer understanding of midwives' perceptions of women's needs during labor. A recent Dutch study found that eighty to eighty-five percent of Dutch obstetricians and midwives leave the decision of eating and drinking in labor to the women themselves, with no apparent harmful effects on women or babies.[31] Another Dutch study compared a group of women who ate during labor with another group who had only clear liquids. The group which had no food had a higher incidence of poor progress in the pushing stage of labor. How good it would be to see this feature of Dutch good sense applied world-wide to obstetric practice in hospitals.

Labor is the only hard work that people do that carries a medical prohibition against eating and drinking. I think that much of the "uterine dysfunction" noted in hospitals can be attributed to low blood-glucose levels caused by fasting for a number of hours. Judith Goldsmith, author of *Childbirth Wisdom from the World's Oldest Societies*, tells us that in most cultures in recorded history, if the mother felt a strong desire for food and drink she was not denied. Depending upon her culture, a woman might be offered a thin porridge, some chicken, goat, or a bowl of rice with an egg.[32] I don't know any midwives attending out-of-hospital births who prohibit eating and drinking during labor. In fact, I think that some women *require* nourishment in labor. *I* always did. I never had a baby in less than twelve hours, and each time, rather late in labor, I needed a tofu salad sandwich and regular gulps of water in order to feel strong and relatively comfortable. In some births I have attended, I know that a few bites of food gave the mother the strength she needed to push her baby out without forceps or a vacuum extractor. In these cases, the woman experienced an almost immediate benefit after taking a little nourishment. Her contractions almost instantly resumed their former vigor, and she gained enough strength to push her baby out when it had previously appeared that she wouldn't be able to do this. No one in our care has suffered from eating or drinking during labor. Occasionally, a woman who has eaten will throw up, but this is not a problem in women who are conscious. Vomiting normally helps the dilation of the cervix, à la Sphincter Law.

Many women never feel hungry in labor, and their labors progress so quickly that eating would be bothersome to them. If labor is progressing well and the mother does not want to eat, I find it best to honor her wishes. She knows what is best for her. On the other hand, many women, particularly those having their first babies, may be in labor far longer than six hours. My partners and I always provide food for laboring women when they express a desire to eat. Usually they want something nourishing that doesn't require chewing—for instance, soup or a bit of sherbet (soybean ice "cream" for vegetarians). Others want a slice of pizza or a hamburger. The strangest request I have encountered was that of a first-time mother who—just before pushing—asked her husband for a jar of peanut butter and proceeded to eat two heaping tablespoonfuls. She then washed the peanut butter down with nearly a quart of raspberry leaf tea and pushed her baby out. I was impressed.

Drinking fluids is more necessary than eating for most women. Many breathe through their mouths enough during the most intense phase of labor that a drink every now and then is a welcome relief. My partners and I like to keep water and electrolyte-balancing drinks available to each woman and let her choose which is most appealing to her. Naturally, the woman who drinks fluids in labor will eventually have to urinate. When women pee at regular intervals during labor, their urethra rarely becomes so swollen that it's necessary to place a catheter to drain the bladder—a situation I have seen happen when women don't drink enough during labor. Besides, getting out of bed to walk to the toilet can be a good way of facilitating the further descent of the baby.

It is also important to remember that the short time limit for unaided delivery that has been imposed upon laboring women in hospitals (usually twelve hours or less) is directly related to the practice of withholding food and drink during labor. When women become hungry after several hours of labor, their labors often become less effective. Intravenous fluids may satisfy fluid requirements but do not prevent women getting weak from hunger. Starving women don't have the endurance required for some labors. Many of the women whose births my partners and I have attended have labored for more than twenty-four hours. All required nourishment to keep up their stamina. Women who drink and eat throughout labor may be able to labor much longer than twenty-four hours, without harm to them or the baby.

Notes

1. Wagner, M. *Pursuing the Birth Machine: The Search for Appropriate Birth Technology.* Camperdown, NSW, Australia: ACE Graphics, 1994.
2. Wing, D. A. Labor induction with misoprostol. *American Journal of Obstetrics and Gynecology,* 1999; 181:339–45.
3. Ventura, S. J., Martin, J.A., Taffel, S. M., Mathews, T. J., and Clarke,

S. C. Advance report of final natality statistics, 1993. Monthly vital statistics report vol. 44. Hyattesville, MD: Public Health Service, 1995; 1–88.

4. ACOG Practice Bulletin No. 10, November 1999: Induction of Labor.

5. Wing, D. A., et al. Misoprostol: An effective agent for cervical ripening and labor induction, *American Journal of Obstetrics & Gynecology*, 1995; 172: 1811–6.

6. Fletcher, H. M., et al. Intravaginal misoprostol as a cervical ripening agent. *British Journal of Obstetrics & Gynaecology*, 1993; 100:641–4.

7. Wing, D. A., et al. A comparison of misoprostol and prostaglandin E2 gel for preinduction cervical ripening and labor induction. *American Journal of Obstetrics & Gynecology*, 1995; 172:1804–10.

8. Mundle, W. R., and Young, D. C. Vaginal misoprostol for induction of labor: A randomized controlled trial. *Obstetrics & Gynecology*, 1996; 88:521–5.

9. Wing, D. A., and Paul, R. H. A comparison of differing dosing regimens of vaginally administered misoprostol for preinduction cervical ripening and labor induction. *American Journal of Obstetrics & Gynecology*, 1996; 175:158–64.

10. Surbek, D. V., et al. A double-blind comparison of the safety and efficacy of intravaginal misoprostol and prostaglandin E2 to induce labor. *American Journal of Obstetrics & Gynecology*, 1997; 177:1018–23.

11. Chard, T. The physiology of labour and its initiation. In *Benefits and Hazards of the New Obstetrics*, ed. T. Chard and M. Richards. London: Heinemann, 1997; 81.

12. Pritchard, J. A., and MacDonald, P. C. *Williams Obstetrics*, 16th ed. New York: Appleton-Century Crofts, 1980.

13. Plaut, M. M., Schwartz, M. L., and Lubarsky, S. L., Uterine rupture associated with the use of misoprostol in the gravid patient with a previous cesarean section. *American Journal of Obstetrics & Gynecology*, 1999; 180:1535–42.

14. Wing, D. A., Lovett, K., and Paul, R. H. Disruption of prior uterine incision following misoprostol for labor induction in women with previous cesarean delivery. *Obstetrics & Gynecology*, 1998; 91:828–30.

15. Hofmeyr, G. J., Gulmezoglu, A. M., and Alfirevic, Z. Misoprostol

for induction of labour: A systematic review. *British Journal of Obstetrics & Gynaecology*, 1999; 106:798–803.

16. Kramer, R. L., Gilson, G. J., et al. A randomized trial of misoprostol and oxytocin for induction of labor: Safety and efficacy. *Obstetrics & Gynecology*, 1997; 89:387–91.

17. Goodman, D. Forced labor: Why are obstetricians speeding deliveries with an ulcer drug that endangers mothers and their babies? *Mother Jones*, January/February 2001.

18. Stein, L. Jagged Little Pill. Metro: Silicon Valley's Weekly Newspaper. www.metroactive.com. March 21–27, 2002.

19. *www.cdc.gov/nchs/birth.* Accessed May 1, 2001.

20. Barrett, J., and Pitman, T. *Pregnancy and Birth: The Best Evidence.* Toronto: Key Porter Books, Ltd., 1999.

21. Toth, M., Rehnstrom, J., and Fuch, A. Prostaglandins E and F in cervical mucus of pregnant women. *American Journal of Perinatology*, 1989; 6:142–4.

22. Kelbanoff, M. A., Nugest, R. P., and Rhoads, G. G. Coitus during pregnancy: Is it safe? *Lancet*, 1984; 20:914–7.

23. Rooks, J. P., Weatherby, N. L., and Ernst, E. K. M. The national birth center study. II: Intrapartum and immediate postpartum and neonatal care. *Journal of Nurse–Midwifery*, 1992; 7:301–30.

24. Berghella, V., Rogers, R. A., and Lescale, K. Stripping of membranes as a safe method to reduce prolonged pregnancies. *Obstetrics & Gynecology*, 1996; 87:927–31.

25. El-Torkey, M., and Grant, J. M. Sweeping of the membranes is an effective method of induction of labour in prolonged pregnancy: A report of a randomized trial. *British Journal of Obstetrics & Gynaecology*, 1992; 99:455–8.

26. Luthy, D. A., Shy, K. K., van Belle, G., et al. A randomized trial of electronic fetal monitoring in preterm labor. *Obstetrics & Gynecology*, 1987; 69:687–95.

27. MacDonald, D., Grant, A., Sheridan-Pereira, M., et al. The Dublin randomized controlled trial of intrapartum fetal heart-rate monitoring. *American Journal of Obstetrics & Gynecology*, 1985; 152:524–39.

28. Hazle, N. Hydration in labor: Is routine intravenous hydration necessary? *Journal of Nurse–Midwifery*, 1986; 31:171–6.

29. Lind, T. Fluid balance during labor: A review. *Journal of Reproductive and Social Medicine*, 1983; 76:870–5.

30. Morton, K., et al. A comparison of the effects of four solutions for the treatment of ketonuria in labor. *British Journal of Obstetrics & Gynaecology*, 1984; 92:473–9.

31. Scheepers, H. C., Essed, G. M., and Brouns, F. Aspects of food and fluid intake during labour: Policies of midwives and obstetricians in the Netherlands. *European Journal of Obstetrics, Gynecology & Reproductive Biology*, 1998; 78:37–40.

32. Goldsmith, J. *Childbirth Wisdom from the World's Oldest Societies*. Brookline, MA: East-West Health Books, 1990.

7

GIVING BIRTH:
MOVE FREELY, LET GRAVITY WORK FOR YOU

Wherever you intend to give birth, it is good to know that most women in labor need to be able to change position and to move around freely. Movement greatly helps cervical dilation during the early part of labor and helps bring the baby into the most advantageous position for passage through the pelvis. Don't be surprised if you feel restless during the first stage of labor. You may want to sit on your partner's lap, a birth stool, a birth ball, or the toilet. If your movement is not hampered by intravenous lines, electronic fetal monitoring, and most forms of epidural anesthesia, you will generally have an easier time assuming the positions that favor cervical dilation and, when that is complete, descent of your baby. EFM causes no pain, but when you move around while yours is attached, the transducer usually quits picking up the sound of the baby's heartbeat, and this generally brings an excited nurse or midwife into the room to find out what is going on. Most kinds of epidural anesthesia temporarily paralyze your lower limbs. Even the

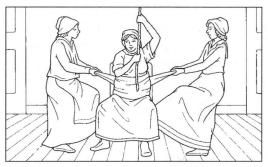

Nineteenth-century birth scene in California:
Pulling the ends of the sheet wrapped around the
mother's hips is another way of applying the
pelvic press (*Source:* Witkowski)

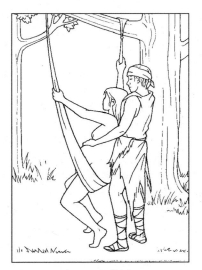

Nineteenth-century birth scene in
San Luis Potosi, Mexico (*Source:*
Engelmann)

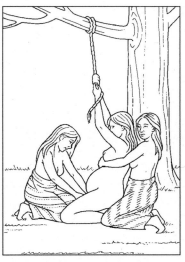

Nineteenth-century birth scene
among the Orinoco Indians
(*Source:* Witkowski)

so-called "walking epidural" is something of a misnomer; nurse–
midwives sometimes call it a "shuffling epidural," since it still greatly
limits most women's movements.

Women in traditional societies all over the world almost always
choose upright positions in labor. This worldwide consensus suggests

that women don't choose to lie down to labor and give birth unless forces within their culture pressure them into doing so. The labor postures common to traditional women's cultures all over the world include sitting, kneeling, standing, squatting, or the hands-and-knees position. Sometimes these postures involve the use of supports of various

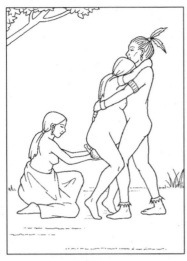

Nineteenth-century birth scene among the Iroquois people (*Source:* Witkowski)

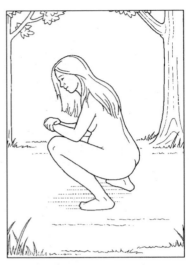

Nineteenth-century birth scene; Tonkawa woman (*Source:* Engelmann)

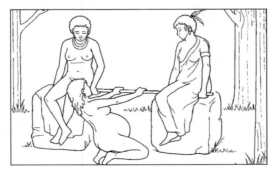

Nineteenth-century birth scene; Tonkawa woman (*Source:* Engelmann)

kinds: ropes for the mother to pull on, birth chairs, stakes pounded into the ground, or the embrace of a husband or female attendant. The list of benefits of upright positions in labor includes:

- better use of gravity
- maximum circulation between mother and baby (no compression caused by the baby's weight on the mother's major blood vessels)
- better alignment of the baby to pass through the pelvis
- stronger rushes
- increased pelvic diameters when squatting or kneeling

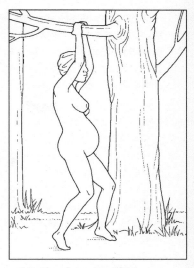

Nineteenth-century African woman in labor (*Source:* Witkowski)

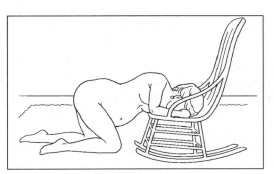

Nineteenth-century Georgia (U.S.A.) woman in labor (*Source:* Engelmann)

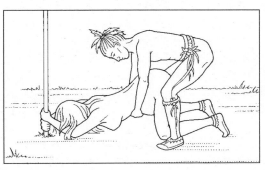

Nineteenth-century Kootenai birth scene (*Source:* Engelmann)

The first recorded instance of a woman lying on her back during labor was of Louise de la Vallière, a mistress of King Louis XIV of France in 1663.[1] The choice of position was probably not hers but her lover's. He wanted to sit behind a curtain and witness the emergence of the baby. As King, he had privileges that did not belong to other men. Previous to that time, it had been taboo for men—including babies' fathers—to be present in the birth room. Less than one hundred fifty years before de la Vallière gave birth, Dr. Wertt from Hamburg was burned at the stake for daring to dress in women's clothes so that he could attend a birth. (Apparently, his cross-dressing was unconvincing to the other attendants at that birth.)

The prohibition against man–midwives in the birth room began to break down with the invention of forceps, which were first used in England and France. Forceps reinforced the fashion of the reclining position in labor, as this is the best position for their use. In 1668, François Mauriceau published a treatise on midwifery that recommended that women lie on their backs for giving birth. This recommendation was made for the benefit of the physician or man–midwife who might want to use forceps, not for the benefit of the laboring woman herself. Two hundred years later, Queen Victoria became the first woman in England to use chloroform while giving birth. This event quickly popularized the use of various forms of anesthesia for labor, which led to a significant number of influential women lying down during labor. By the end of the nineteenth century, birth chairs were rarely used any longer. "Fashionable" ladies expected to lie down to have their babies. Giving birth in a squatting position came to be considered low-class—far from "ladylike." Given this history, it is not an exaggeration to call the supine position an invention of the industrial revolution. It is a male-derived position—one invented for the convenience of the birth attendant. As women often realize when they are caught in the "stranded beetle" position, it can be very hard to work against gravity when pushing a baby out.

Not every woman is willing to go along with the fashion of laboring while lying on her back. In 1882, George Engelmann quoted a letter from one of his physician correspondents, who had attended a wealthy woman in two of her labors.

In her first labor, delivery was retarded without apparent cause. There was nothing like impaction, or inertia, yet the head did not

advance. At every pain she made violent efforts, and would bring her chest forward. I had determined to use the forceps, but just then, in one of the violent pains, she raised herself up in bed and assumed a squatting position, when the most magic effect was produced. It seemed to aid in completing the delivery in the most remarkable manner, as the head advanced rapidly, and she soon expelled the child by what appeared to be one prolonged attack of pain. In subsequent parturition, labor appeared extremely painful and retarded in the same manner; I allowed her to take the same position, as I had remembered her former labor, and she was delivered at once, squatting.[2]

We midwives and the women in our community were free to experiment with whatever positions occurred to us. Before we established our community in rural Tennessee during the period when I began attending births, my husband and I and three hundred others traveled together around the country. We called our group "The Caravan." Most of the women on the Caravan labored in some kind of a sitting position because of the confines of the small campers and buses in which we lived at the time. Once we bought land in Tennessee, our living quarters expanded and so did our options. A few women in labor in those early days hugged trees and found that extremely helpful. We noticed in the first fifty births that some women *must* be upright or on all fours to have a baby. Women often make this choice spontaneously. I remember one particular birth I attended in 1978, years before I saw any drawings of tribal women giving birth. It was at this birth that I realized how important it can be to suggest the upright position for women who have not discovered it for themselves. The mother—I'll call her Kathy—was having her first baby, after having had three miscarriages. I was called in to help after she had labored for two days with slow progress. She was nearly fully dilated, but she was quite tired. So was her husband. Her baby felt pretty large for her size. Once the baby's head was clearly through the cervix, I kept wishing that Kathy could stand up while holding on to something above her head. Pushing while she was leaning back at a forty-five-degree angle was doing little except tiring her further. I had a strong feeling that the combination of gravity and pulling on a rope attached above her might help this baby come. I suggested that we try this. Her husband quickly anchored a soft nylon rope to the ceiling above their bed for her to pull on with her hands as she pushed. Her husband stood behind to steady her as she pushed. The difference this position made was nothing short of remarkable. Down slid the baby's head into view, and Kathy's eight-pound son was soon born in good condition.

When I found George Engelmann's *Labor among Primitive Peoples*, I was delighted but not surprised to find out that women from all around the world had used the same position that we discovered at Kathy's birth. After that, we midwives frequently advised mothers to take an upright posture if their babies were slow in descending. Engelmann wrote:

> *If we wish to obtain an idea of the natural position we must look to the woman who is governed by instinct, not by prudery; and it is only among the savage races that we shall find her at the present day. In this purely animal function instinct will guide the woman more correctly than the varying customs of the times.*

He added:

> *...it was not until I had undertaken this work, and had begun to study the positions assumed by savage and civilized people during labor, that I began to understand that there was a method in the instinctive movements of women in the last stage of labor. I had seen them toss about, and sought to quiet them; I bade them have patience, and lie still upon their backs; but, since entering upon this study, I have learned to look upon their movements in a very different light. I have watched them with interest and profit, and believe that I have learned to understand them.[2]*

Unfortunately, most U.S. physicians have never read Dr. Engelmann's book, which is now available only in rare-books collections in some medical libraries.

Medication for Pain Relief

If you are planning for your first labor and will be giving birth in a hospital, you may have already considered taking some form of pain-relieving medication during labor. Before you decide what you might choose, it is important to know the advantages and disadvantages of the medications that you are likely to be offered (or pressured into taking) during labor. Of course, I'm not talking about anesthesia in its use for cesarean section or other surgery. My focus in this section is really on analgesia—the use of drugs to dull or erase the pain of labor. I am grateful that we have pain medications that are reasonably safe for obstetric use. At the same time, I believe that women giving birth need to be knowledgeable about the hazards that come with the use of painkilling drugs in labor and birth and that generally it is wise to avoid their use when possible.

Tranquilizers

There are no advantages to taking tranquilizers during labor. Tranquilizers (Valium is the most commonly used) are supposed to reduce anxiety and tension, but they cross the placenta and interfere with the baby's ability to breathe, to suck, and to maintain a healthy muscle tension (tranquilized newborns tend to be limp). Tranquilizers, sedatives, and sleeping pills all have negative effects on babies, and they do not reduce pain.

Narcotics

If given in sufficient amounts, narcotics would be effective at significantly reducing labor pain. The problem is that doses high enough to lower pain are not safe for mother or baby, so they are given in lesser amounts. Demerol is the narcotic most commonly used in U.S. maternity wards. Given intravenously or by injection, a relatively safe dose can cause sleepiness, and it often causes nausea, vomiting, and a drop in blood pressure. Don't expect it to significantly relieve pain, however. Some studies have shown long-lasting effects in babies exposed to Demerol, causing them to be irritable, poor at feeding, and sleepy.[3]

Other narcotics in common use include Nubain, fentanyl (Sublimaze), and butorphanol (Stadol). These narcotics don't last as long as Demerol—just an hour or two—but this is preferable as this means less chance that they will depress the baby's breathing at birth.

Antinausea Drugs

When labor itself or a drug such as Demerol, Stadol, fentanyl, or Nubain causes nausea, Trilafon (perphenazine) and Phenergan (promethazine) are often prescribed. However, the antinausea drugs themselves cause dizziness and drowsiness in women.[4] One study found that Phenergan interferes with the ability of the baby's blood to clot.[5]

Inhaled Pain Medications

Nitrous oxide combinations have been used in Britain for many years to dull labor pain, both in hospital and home births. Women inhale the gas through a mask they hold tightly to their nose and mouth during the peak of a contraction. The effects are immediate and short-lived. No obvious side effects have been found in babies. A disadvantage of this method is that it takes a certain amount of effort to show the woman how to use the mask effectively and many women don't like the mask. However, the main disadvantage is that most U.S. hospitals do not offer this method of obstetric analgesia.

Epidural Anesthesia

Epidural anesthesia is the most commonly used method of pharmaceutical pain relief for women who labor and give birth in hospitals. The medication is given by injecting the numbing drug into the lower back just outside the spinal cord through a fine plastic tube, which is left in place in case more pain relief is required. In order for the drug to be given, you must curl forward to increase the space between the bones of the spine. The epidural numbs and weakens the lower part of the body. For most women, it is the most effective form of pain relief. In some U.S. hospitals more than eighty-five percent of women have an epidural during labor. The epidural is not used in birth-center or home births in the United States.

The epidural has some advantages over other forms of obstetric anesthesia:

- It doesn't cause nausea and vomiting, as does general anesthesia, and it leaves the mother conscious.
- Administered correctly, it doesn't cause a spinal headache, as spinal anesthesia sometimes does.
- From the institutional perspective, epidurals have the advantage of keeping women quiet and in one place during labor.

For these reasons, it is the usual choice for cesarean section, when there is time to place it (this takes ten to twenty minutes).

Epidural anesthesia does have several side effects:

- Sometimes it causes a dramatic drop in blood pressure, which can put both mother and baby at risk (the heart rates of both sometimes plummet). For this reason, women who have an epidural must also have an I.V. in place so that the infusion of more fluid can help to return her blood pressure to a less dangerous level.

- In about one women in every five, the epidural causes a fever, which cannot be readily distinguished from that caused by intrauterine infection. Whenever a laboring woman has a fever, her baby will undergo a septic workup, which generally means several needle jabs, sometimes a spinal tap, and nearly always some degree of separation from the mother.

- Epidurals don't always work. Even when the epidural is given correctly, it does not provide pain relief in about three percent of women. About twelve percent of women get some but not complete relief, and about eighty-five percent experience complete relief.

- Sometimes women who thought they wanted an epidural dislike the effect of the drug and complain about feeling detached from what is going on.

- In about two percent of epidurals, the anesthesiologist makes an accidental lumbar puncture, which means that the needle went in too far and punctured the membrane that surrounds the spinal cord. In these cases, an epidural can't be given, and the woman ends up with a severe headache that lasts for days or even weeks.

- Some women experience itching all over their bodies after having an epidural.

- Given too early in labor, the epidural often slows the process of dilation, descent of the baby, and proper positioning of the part of the baby emerging first.

- Epidural labors are more likely to result in cesarean section than natural labors.

- Epidural labors are more likely to result in a forceps delivery or vacuum-extractor delivery than a natural labor.

- The epidural site can become infected, since the skin is punctured.
- Women for whom the epidural gives strong pain relief may be injured by improper positioning by inattentive caregivers, since the injury is not felt by the woman when it is taking place.
- Babies whose mothers have had epidurals sometimes have breathing difficulties and a difficult time establishing breastfeeding.
- Very rarely (one in five thousand cases or so), an epidural can result in a maternal death or permanent paralysis.

There is a lot of variation in epidural rates from hospital to hospital in the United States. Rates tend to be high in those institutions where obstetric anesthesiologists stroll the halls in the daytime, informing women of their working hours and the need to have an epidural before they go home. Many women have told me that they accepted an epidural that they didn't really need at the time, because the anesthesiologist threatened that he was leaving in half an hour and the chance to have pain relief would soon be lost.

General Anesthesia
General anesthesia was once the preferred form of obstetric anesthesia, but it was abandoned, for the most part, when the epidural came on the scene. General anesthesia has a comparatively high hazard of producing breathing difficulties in babies. Sometimes it causes nausea and vomiting in women and, rarely, results in aspiration pneumonia. However, it can be more quickly administered than an epidural, so it is still used when an emergency cesarean is required. General anesthesia does not cause a drop in blood pressure as the epidural does.

Spinal Anesthesia
Spinal anesthesia is similar to epidural anesthesia: An intravenous infusion is first set up, and then a local anesthetic is put in through a needle in the back. The pain relief it provides for cesarean section is as good as an epidural, sometimes better. However, a catheter is not left in place, so the anesthesia can last only so long. The complications caused by spinals are similar to those for epidurals. Spinals sometimes cause a sudden and drastic drop in blood pressure. About one percent of women have a spinal headache after birth.

Suggestions for Maximizing Your Chances of Having an Unmedicated Labor and Birth in the Hospital

Maybe you are sure that you will feel safer about giving birth in a hospital, but you want to maximize your chances of having an unmedicated labor and birth experience. I have some suggestions.

Hire a Doula

If you can find one in your area, doulas are sympathetic and knowledgeable labor companions who typically provide some form of prenatal preparation and stay at your side once labor begins until your baby is born. The doula's job is to make you as comfortable as possible and to reassure your partner as well.

The evidence in favor of doulas comes from more than eleven carefully designed studies: Quite simply, hiring one cuts in half the odds of your having an unnecessary cesarean. It also halves the odds of your having a forceps or vacuum-extractor delivery. That's not all! Having a doula also shortens labor by greatly reducing stress, pain, and anxiety. In the typical U.S. birthing unit, the doula you bring with you may be the only person whose sole responsibility is to make you more comfortable and to help you labor as effectively as possible.

If your baby's father plans to be with you throughout labor, you may wonder if it makes sense for you to hire a doula. The answer is yes. Fathers often have significant fears and anxieties surrounding birthgiving. The calming influence the doula can have on expectant fathers is often as significant as her effect on the laboring woman. Klaus, Klaus, and Kennell, the authors of *Mothering the Mother,* an excellent book about doulas, wisely point out that our society makes demands on first-time fathers that exceed those made upon medical students. Remarking that medical students are *expected* to get pale and sweaty when first exposed to new medical situations, they note there are no consequences when *they* must leave. On the other hand, no such allowances are made for first-time fathers. When they must leave, the mother is left alone and often resents her partner's absence. The dilemma of one first-time father mentioned in *Mothering the Mother*, a physician, is especially poignant. He told the Klauses: " 'With our first baby I was so overcome emotionally that I could not make any rational observations about what was happening, and I truly believed there was imminent danger at every step of labor.' Many physicians' wives face this prospect every time they give birth, since doctors are typically more afraid of labor and birth than the average person. Doulas can be immensely helpful in situations like these."

No matter how dedicated or well prepared a father may be, he'll need to have a bite to eat or go to the bathroom if labor lasts more than a few hours—as is likely. The doula can provide this respite while assuring that the laboring woman gets the continuous attention she needs. Besides, many men are better able to touch the laboring mother in a helpful way if such behavior has already been sanctioned and demonstrated by a doula.

Doulas typically spend time during pregnancy with expectant parents, educating and developing a relationship of trust and respect. Some offer childbirth classes, while others prefer to meet with women or couples individually during the pregnancy to establish a relationship. Doulas are not usually employees of the hospital and so are answerable only to the mother, not to the hospital. Unlike nurses, they stay around when shifts change. Some large hospitals have doulas on staff as well, but their ability to speak freely is sometimes compromised. I would take the trouble to seek out an independent doula whenever possible. Some doulas charge a fee; a few work as volunteers. Note: some hospitals don't allow independent doulas.

In North America, doulas are certified by Doulas of North America (DONA), the International Childbirth Education Association (ICEA), and the Association of Labor Assistants and Childbirth Educators (ALACE). See Chapter 13 for some suggestions of questions to ask when you interview potential doulas.

Your Clothes

Take your own favorite comfortable nightgown with you, so that you don't have to wear the regulation hospital outfit. Wearing your own clothes will remind you that you're not an inmate.

Drink and Pee

Be sure to drink a lot while in labor and to pee every hour or so. Drinking a lot will prevent dehydration as you labor. It also prompts the need to pee, which will send you to the toilet. This is good, because you likely have a conditioned response that causes your pelvic muscles to relax when you sit on the toilet. This will increase pressure against your cervix if you are still dilating or help descent of the baby if you are pushing.

Try Hydrotherapy

I have already mentioned one kind of hydrotherapy—drinking water. The other useful kind is to get into a shower or, better, to immerse yourself in a deep tub of comfortably warm water (if your water bag has not broken). Most women get immediate pain relief from hydrotherapy. Being in water is calming and relaxing. In fact, it is difficult to remain tense while in water. Water helps a woman enter the meditative state that favors effective labor.

Remember: Birth Is Sexual

It is safe to say that the sexual dimension of labor and birth is almost always ignored in U.S. hospitals. The chief reason for this is that doctors had to downplay the sexual nature of birth in order for medical men to be admitted to the birth chambers of women during the eighteenth and nineteenth centuries, when virtually all births were attended by midwives. When birth moved into the hospital in most industrialized countries and under the direct control of doctors, this denial of the sexuality of birth was institutionalized.

In fact, sex is *the* central fact of reproductive behavior from conception to birth. If the sexual aspect of labor and birth is ignored, it will often work against progress in labor. Of course, the converse is also true—the application of sexual energy can make labor more effective and less painful without any use of medication. Dr. Peter Curtis, a British-born faculty member of the Department of Family Medicine at the University of Chapel Hill in North Carolina, provided me with an excellent example of the high stakes that often surround this issue in U.S. hospitals. I met Peter in the early 1980s. Trained in England by both obstetricians and midwives, he was used to women-centered care in hospital and home-birth settings, so he felt comfortable attending the births of women who were motivated to have natural-childbirth experiences. He told me about the young couple who first introduced him to the use of breast stimulation to intensify labor. He was monitoring the woman's labor with her first baby in the home-style room. Unfortunately, her labor pattern was poor, and after several hours of labor her cervical dilation hadn't increased. The senior obstetric nurse had begun to hint to Dr. Curtis that he should start intravenous oxytocin to augment labor. But when he discussed this intention with the couple, they asked him for the chance to first use the breast-stimulation technique they had read about in *Spiritual Midwifery*. He had never heard of this technique himself but could see the logic of it, so he agreed—however, he had no opportunity to tell the obstetric nurse about the change in strategy, as she was dealing with another laboring woman. Curtis tells the rest of the story like this:

"About twenty minutes after this conversation, the obstetric nurse and I went back into the delivery room to find the husband 'latched on' to the patient's breast and sucking enthusiastically, while another friend was busy doing the same on the other side. Standing beside me, the nurse paled visibly, grabbed my arm for support, and looked quite disturbed by this seemingly outrageous behavior. We hurried outside to discuss the matter and compose ourselves, and then returned to check on progress. Surprisingly, labor was now moving along rapidly, showing an active contraction pattern and progressive cervical dilation. Two hours later a healthy baby boy was born without difficulty."[6]

A similar situation a month later persuaded Dr. Curtis that there must be a cause-and-effect relationship between breast stimulation and a more effective labor pattern. He began trying to study how breast stimulation might be used to lower the thirty percent rate of oxytocin augmentation at his hospital. He learned that this method had been used traditionally for centuries to augment labor in ethnic groups from many different areas of the world, and that eighteenth- and nineteenth-century medical texts from France, Germany, and England recommended consensual breast stimulation as a valid method for dealing with prolonged labor.

What he hadn't counted on was the opposition he received from physician colleagues he consulted, "who exhibited a fair amount of cynicism laced with strong opinions about my 'flakiness.'" Several years passed before Dr. Curtis and his research assistants could carry out a clinical trial to test scientifically the effectiveness of breast stimulation. Why? Because several Departments of Obstetrics and Gynecology (including that at Curtis's own hospital) turned down this request because the idea seemed too unorthodox and such a questionable project "would likely tarnish the reputation of the maternity service."[6] Dr. Curtis may have been born and raised in the country that invented Victorianism, but through his efforts to study breast stimulation, he found out that the United States had become more prudish than the British.

If you will give birth in an institution where the medical model is particularly strong, and your labor slows down, you are more likely to be offered intravenous Pitocin to stimulate labor than to be encouraged to do breast stimulation. In those where the midwifery model has some respect, breast stimulation will be suggested before drugs are brought up, as breast stimulation is less invasive than drugs. My advice is to refuse to let the puritanism of others affect your labor any more than necessary. Don't worry about the disapproving looks or pursed lips that manual breast stimulation (or any other touching that reminds staff members of sex) during labor might cause. The benefits outweigh the risks. If you and your partner raise a sexy enough vibration to do your labor some good, you may even succeed in running off unsympathetic help and get a better replacement.

Provisions for Privacy

Labor pain can be significantly reduced in a number of ways that don't require a prescription from a hospital pharmacy. The trend during the 1980s of designing hospital birth rooms to be more like bedrooms was a good one. However, some of the most important features of bedrooms were often omitted—for instance, the ability to prohibit unwanted interruptions or to lower the lights. What is needed for effective labor with lowered levels of stress hormones is a comfortable, dimly lit, cozy space that allows you to access the part of your primitive brain that sets up the process of hormonal ebb and flow and facilitates the smoothest functioning of the normal birth process. We share this need for privacy during labor with virtually all other female mammals.

Explore Touch

Touch and massage can give incredible relief when labor is painful. You probably already know if you are one of the people who would appreciate this form of pain relief. I was greatly helped by thigh massage and by hand pressure against my lower back. I found both heavenly during labor.

Here's a form of touch that you may not know about. Shaking the large muscles of the mother's bottom or thighs is an effective way of helping some women—me, for one—relax during labor. While it may not look comfortable to bystanders, laboring women often appreciate how relaxing it is to be jostled rhythmically. (German-speaking people call this "shaking the apples.")

I attended a labor many years ago for a woman expecting her first child. She was slim, scared, extremely tense, and surprisingly strong. Her fear was very powerful, and I had not yet found a way to effectively calm her. Usually, intense rushes will soften muscle tension in the legs. In spite of the intensity of her rushes, her leg muscles were as hard as oak. The challenge was how to help her relax and soften her legs. Soft pelvic muscles would then follow, allowing her cervix to become yielding and open. I massaged her feet and then her calves during a rush. This type of massage had noticeably helped most of the thirty-five women whose births I had already attended. This strong woman, however, was accumulating tension in her legs faster than I could dissipate it by massage. Each rush seemed more powerful than the one before it, and she was becoming more miserable by the second. I kept on kneading her calves and thighs as I continued to demonstrate the slow, deep abdominal breathing that best facilitates opening up. Her eyes started shifting from side to side in panic. I then applied a technique I had never used, or *thought* of using, at a birth. Stephen at times shook the muscles of my thighs and butt, and I found it relaxing. Using the same technique, I gripped her thigh muscles during a rush and began gently and rhythmically shaking them from side to side. At first she was holding her thigh muscles so rigidly, I could barely get anything to move at all. Then she sighed a little bit, and I continued. It was like watching a crying baby relax while being rocked. As I shook her thighs, she gradually gave in to the rocking rhythm. The muscles of her calves and thighs finally began to relax, and I could tell from warm feelings in the region of my own cervix that hers was probably opening. After about twenty minutes of shaking and deep breathing, her thighs felt soft, hot, and silky like those of a woman about to give birth. Her cervix was fully dilated, and she was finally ready to push her baby out.

I have used this technique for many births since then. Sometimes the woman's partner shakes her bottom up and down or side to side; sometimes we roll the backs of her thighs. I had been using this technique for some years before I found out that it has been documented around the world in traditional cultures.[2]

A few years ago a Florida midwife told me about a U.S. obstetrician who had traveled extensively in rural China. He observed that when a woman was having a long and difficult labor, the midwives would *chung* the mother. *Chung* means that two or three women would shake the laboring woman very vigorously all over her body. The obstetrician observed the use of the method several times. It worked every time he saw it.

The midwife tried the technique herself during a prolonged labor. "We tried everything, including long walks and jeep rides over bumpy roads. Suddenly I remembered the article and told everyone there what *to chung* is. The three of us shook the laboring woman all over as hard and as long as we could while she was standing, leaning over a dresser with her arms braced. I thought it would hurt, since she was having such strong contractions. To our surprise, she said it felt good! We laughed and continued to shake her until our arms were sore. The woman went to full dilation and delivered a healthy boy a few hours later. I feel the shaking did the trick." The fact that so many peoples around the world discovered the same method without communicating with one another strongly indicates the universal value of muscle-shaking during labor.

Let Your Monkey Do It

Let's say you want some advice that might help you give birth, wherever that might be. My shortest answer is: Let your monkey do it. (By the way, this advice works for any physical pursuit that can be short-circuited by the mind, whether it is white-water rafting, dancing well, platform diving, or giving birth.)

Letting the primate in you do the work of labor is a short way of saying not to let your over-busy mind interfere with the ancient wisdom of your body. To give you an idea of what I mean, here are some things monkeys and apes don't do in labor that many women do—and that interfere with labor:

- Monkeys don't think of technology as necessary to birth-giving.
- Monkeys don't obsess about their bodies being inadequate.

- Monkeys don't blame their condition on anyone else.
- Monkeys don't do math about their dilation to speculate how long labor might take. (A typical mind sequence might be: *It has taken me eight hours to get to five centimeters. That means it will take eight more hours to get to ten or full dilation.*)
- Monkeys in labor get into the position that feels best, not the one they're told to assume.
- Monkeys aren't self-conscious about making noise, farting, or pooping during labor. All queens, duchesses, and movie stars poop—every day, if they're healthy.

How can you "let your monkey do it" in a hospital? I believe that it helps to mentally prepare to be a little wild while you're there. Try to behave as much as possible as you would in your own bedroom. Be willing to be unconventional if that might help your labor along.

A young couple told me the story of how they managed to snatch a natural-birth experience from the assembly-line treatment they encountered at their hospital when they had their first baby. They found themselves up against the clock, as their baby was breech, and that made all of the obstetricians at the hospital nervous except their own (who was expert at attending breech deliveries). One obstetrician felt free to walk into the laboring women's birth room and scold her doctor, "You mean she's *still* in labor? When are you going to get her into the operating room?"

The mother said she felt her cervix tighten up every time there was such a disturbance, and there had already been several. Finally, the peer-group pressure convinced her doctor to say that she would have to reach full dilation within an hour's time if she was to avoid a cesarean. Eager to escape any more rude interruptions, she decided to retreat to the tiny bathroom attached to her birth room. She sat on the toilet for the next few rushes. As she relaxed during each one, her legs fell outward and she could feel her cervix dilate. But there was still a problem: The room was so small that, as she relaxed, one of her legs fell against the heating element on the wall. After talking over the situation with her husband, they decided to put on their coats while no one was looking and take a little walk on the grounds outside the hospital. This they did without asking permission. By the time the nurses located the runaways, dilation was complete, and the mother was ready to push. She went back to the birth room and pushed her baby out with no problems, ecstatic that she had been able to beat the system.

Another couple I know underwent an oxytocin induction in the hospital for their first baby because of hypertension. This particular hospital had a policy of routine intravenous infusion and "nothing by mouth" for all laboring women. Hour after hour, this young woman trudged the halls of the maternity ward, pushing her I.V. pole-on-wheels past vending machines and nurses snacking at their station, her uterus periodically contracting and her stomach constantly growling. By the time twenty-eight hours had passed, she was close to full dilation and was willing to keep trying, but her energy was flagging, and her husband wondered how she could keep up her strength without sleep or nourishment. Both had read enough on the Internet to know how poor the evidence is against eating and drinking in labor, so he brought her a sandwich, which she ate while they were alone in the room. With the energy boost she got from eating, she reached full dilation and soon pushed her baby out.

Learning to Love the Primate in You

Many of us have grown up with the idea that being like other primates in any way is somehow shameful or disgraceful. Given that all other primates are known to cope well with labor and birth, while civilized humans often aren't, it seems that we would be wise to emulate other female primates as much as possible. My husband has often commented on the similarities between humans and other primates and finds no dishonor in being related to apes.

For my own part, I have little trouble thinking of myself as a type of ape, since I often used to imagine that I was a horse, a lion, or a dog when I was a young child. I was usually a horse when I was running and a noble-looking dog (a collie or a German shepherd) when I was sitting in the back of my dad's car with my brother and sister, bored on the long trip to visit my rural relatives. In labor with my first baby twenty years later, without thinking about why, I reverted to the old pattern and imagined that I was a mountain lion. Emulating an animal made it easier for me to access that power that I instinctively knew I needed during labor.

I often suggest to pregnant women that they imagine themselves to be a large mammal when they are in labor. Many say it helps them to find the wild woman within and to tap into the ancient knowledge that is the potential of all women.

The Baby Who "Gets Stuck" during Pushing

Sometimes pushing efforts begin, and the baby's head moves down well—to a point—and then descends no farther. Within the medical model, the usual treatment of this situation is a forceps or vacuum-extractor delivery (both forceps and vacuum extractors occasionally injure babies). We midwives have a quite different technique that works

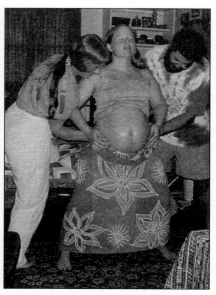

Pelvic press: Stephanie's hips are being pressed by Pamela and Ari

effectively in most cases like these. Instead of affixing an instrument to the baby's head, we take advantage of the flexibility and range of movement of the woman's pelvic bones. The technique, called the "pelvic press," involves putting pressure on the upper part of the woman's hips (the upper iliac crest) while she pushes. This pressure pinches her hipbones closer together at the top while opening them a corresponding amount at the bottom, thus freeing the stuck head. (See also the illustration at the top of page 227.) The first time I ever used this technique (after reading about it in Nan Koehler's book *Artemis Speaks*), it worked well enough to make possible the birth of one of the most difficult presentations—forehead-first.

Brow presentations, as these are called, almost always require cesarean section if the pelvic press is not used. Our brow baby was born without instruments, episiotomy, or injury to his mother's perineum. Forceps and vacuum-extractor deliveries, on the other hand, nearly always involve considerable injury to the woman's perineum, requiring many stitches.

Notes

1. Graham, H. *Eternal Eve*. London: William Heinemann, Ltd., 1950.
2. Engelmann, G. *Labor among Primitive Peoples, 2nd ed.* St. Louis: H.J. Chambers, 1883.
3. Brackbill, Y., et al. Obstetric premedication and infant outcome, *American Journal of Obstetrics & Gynecology*, 1974; 188:347–84.
4. Rosen, M. *Benefits and Hazards of the New Obstetrics*, ed. Chard, T., and Richards, M. London: Heinemann, 1977.
5. Inch, S. *Birthrights*. New York: Random House, Inc., 1982.
6. Curtis, P. *Birth*, June 1999; 26:123–6.

... in the ordinary course of a healthy labour, the mouth of the uterus opens by some secret agency; or at least without any apparent force.

—Dr. William Dewees, 1847

When one sees, for the first time, the maternal soft parts stretched out to a diaphanous thinness by the presenting part of the child, to all appearances just upon the point of cracking open, the impulse to place the hand upon the bulging flesh becomes almost an instinct. We must not, however, forget that these tissues are not only elastic, but living and sentient; and— what is still greater weight—that the process of labour is a strictly physiological act. Nature in all her operations intends to adapt means to ends, and the perineum was certainly not created to be torn, unless shored up by the hand of the physician.

—Dr. William Goodell, 1879

8

FORGOTTEN VAGINAL POWERS AND EPISIOTOMY

Of the first fifty births that Pamela and I attended, forty-three gave birth without episiotomy or laceration. The seven women who needed stitches had only minor tears and no complications from them. This experience so early in my career (I have always counted my partners' and my statistics from the first birth I ever saw, obviously, before I had any training to be a birth attendant) taught me that most women are well equipped to give birth without the slightest injury, given the appropriate help, preparation, atmosphere, and consideration. As my partners and I gained more experience, we learned even better how to help women give birth without damage to the vagina or perineum.

If you feel fearful about being "too small to give birth," here is a meditation that may help you as much as it helped Judy, the woman who inspired it. Even though I had been attending births and respecting women's bottoms for their amazing powers for twenty years, Judy showed me something new and exciting. A first-time mother, she came to our birth center because her baby was in breech position. Several people tried to scare her into having a cesarean by warning her that her baby's head could be caught inside at birth. I told her that in my experience, her baby's large bottom was actually going to prepare the way for his head. Holding my hands in a circle to indicate the size to which her vagina would open gradually (about the size of a large grapefruit), I told her, "You're going to get *huge.*"

One week later, her son's bottom was just coming into view after seventeen hours of labor. Before his butt pushed directly against her perineum, her vagina enlarged and opened to an extent that astounded me. I had seen this phenomenon in women who had already had seven or eight children, but never before in a first-time mother.* Judy's vagina would easily have allowed the passage of a baby considerably bigger than her seven-pound eight-ounce son without a tear.

Some days later when Judy and I were talking about her birth, I told her how surprised I had been to see how open her vagina became without direct pressure on her perineum. (I was still amazed.) Judy said, "I used that mantra you gave me."

"Mantra?" I repeated, uncertain of what she meant.

"I kept thinking while I was pushing, I'm going to get huge. I'm going to get huge!" she said.

The only thing that Judy did differently from other women I have helped in labor was to concentrate on that mantra as she pushed. One thing about a meditation like this is that you can use it without worrying about negative side effects, so it can't hurt you to try it. I thought about this birth for a long time afterward for the lessons it contained and the clear exhibition of a human ability I had never before witnessed. After all, Judy had taught me that a woman could actually increase the size of her vagina during birth by directing her attention in the right way. From that time on, I began to think of new ways to explain women's vaginas to their owners. See what this does for you.

Men take it for granted that their sexual organs can greatly increase

*There is a video record of this occasion, by the way. Judy's is the fifth birth shown on the video *Assisting a Vaginal Breech Birth*. See Resources.

in size and then become small again without being ruined. If obstetricians (and women) could understand that women's genitals have similar abilities, episiotomy and laceration rates in North America might go down overnight. But obstetricians of earlier generations planted the idea (which is still widely held) that nature cheated women when it came to the tissues of the vagina and perineum (give it one good stretch, and it's done for, like a cheap girdle), and a lot of women have bought the idea that their crotches are made of shoddy goods. Of course, no one expects that a man's penis can be pulled and stretched to the size it easily attains during erection and engorgement. Why should we expect women's vaginas to stretch to their full capacity without engorgement?

I like to ask female audiences what happens during a good kiss. What sensations do we feel? Eyes begin to roll, and women get interesting looks on their faces when I ask this. Finally, someone gets the courage to point to her crotch and say, "It gets all tingly." Then we agree: Engorgement happens. Birth is one of the acts that enlarge the vagina. (Sexual foreplay is another.) Probably the great difference between the engorgement experienced by a man and that of a woman is that he can see his, and she can't see hers. But hers is just as real and important as his—especially when she is giving birth. If her tissues aren't well-engorged when the baby's head starts to emerge, her uterus is going to keep pushing the baby's head against them anyway, forcing its way through vaginal tissues that aren't all the way softened and open. Tears happen this way. Ideally, all women would be engorged at the time of birth, because this would mean less stitching. However, a better ambience in the average hospital maternity ward would be a necessary first condition.

There is no doubt that women who have several pregnancies close together will experience some relaxation in pelvic and vaginal muscles if they don't take time to exercise these muscles after giving birth. Kegel's pelvic-strengthening exercises consist of contracting the pelvic muscles for five to ten seconds at a time and working up to eighty squeezes a day. Several ancient cultures recognize the need for pelvic-muscle strengthening after childbirth in the dances that women do. The hula and other hip-swinging dances of the Pacific island nations, Middle Eastern belly dancing, and the rhythmic butt-shaking dances of Africa are all examples of dances that strengthen the pelvic muscles.

Let's say that nature's design *is* that all women have the potential to get as gigantic as Judy did and that, as with male erections, it is easier for this to happen in women when the atmosphere is right. (I've never seen a tear in a woman who was kissing her way through the pushing phase of labor or touching herself as her baby emerged.) It is midwives and other kindly female helpers in constant attendance during labor who carry along the knowledge of what the undisturbed female body/mind is capable of in birth. What actually happens can be so difficult to believe as to seem impossible to the uninitiated. (Remember the words of William Goodell, which I quoted at the beginning of this chapter.)

I'll never forget the words of the thirty-six-year-old mother, hugely pregnant with her first baby, who came in for a visit during the last week of pregnancy. We were talking about the coming birth, and she blurted out her greatest worry—one that is extremely common in women who have had little exposure to the powers and abilities of the female body in giving birth. "I just can't see how anything this big"— she patted her globular belly as she spoke—"can come out of such a small place."

I am reminded of another story that illustrates the emotional difficulty that uninformed women can have in facing the reality of what happens in birth. Some years ago, I was a speaker at a midwifery conference in southern Arkansas. As usual, I showed some videos of women giving birth. Afterward, I had a chance to talk with Mrs. Anna Mary Sykes, a traditional midwife, who was in her seventies at the time.

"I never saw anything like that when I was growing up," she said, her eyes twinkling with amusement. "When I was in labor with my first baby, I didn't even know where my baby was going to come out!"

"Is that right?" I said, half-amazed by her story but knowing that she wasn't exaggerating. She was not a woman who would do that.

"They didn't tell us anything, even when we were getting married," she said. "When I was alone in labor, I looked all over myself. I was trying to find out where that baby was going to come out.

"I had a mirror and was looking all over my body. When I opened my mouth, I thought that must be it. When I saw that little thing in the back [her uvula], I thought that was the baby's big toe. I thought I was

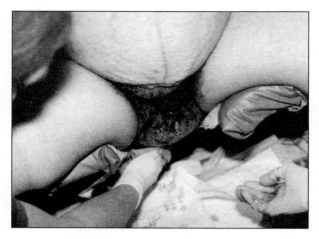

Squatting and crowning

going to have to throw up the baby. It wasn't till the midwife came and washed between my legs that I knew that was where the baby was going to come out!"

Men can't be fooled about their parts the way women can. Men's convexity makes them as obvious as women's concavity makes us mysterious (even to ourselves). I suspect that this is the reason why so many world cultures produce stone figures that depict women's vaginas in the open state, often during the act of giving birth. I have used the figures pictured on pages 49 and 253 at several births and believe that they truly help women better understand what their bodies can do. The first figure (page 49) comes from Mexico, and she has been around for a long time. Notice how serene her facial expression is as her baby's head emerges from her vagina. She has helped me at many a birth. Little girls who grow up looking at her are less likely to permit an obstetrician with scissors to cut them than are women who have never been introduced to the idea that a woman can give birth intact, uninjured, and unafraid.

Historians and archaeologists have long been fascinated about the meaning of the *sheela-na-gig* (page 253) figures of Ireland, Wales, Scotland, England, and other parts of Europe. These medieval stone carvings of naked females exposing their genitals are found high up on the walls of small tower castles built between the fifteenth and seventeenth centuries. (Most *sheela-na-gigs* were destroyed by church fathers during the nineteenth century.) Some say that this is a demonic figure, meant to ward off evil or attack; others suggest that it may represent a fertility goddess. My idea is that this figure was probably meant to reassure young women about the capabilities of their bodies in birth. Ellen Prendergast, in an article written for an Irish historical journal, remarked, "After a lifetime's awareness of such figures I am convinced their significance lies in the sphere of fertility, and that what is depicted . . . is the act of giving birth." Whether Ms. Prendergast and I are right or not, I can testify that a *sheela-na-gig* figure can be a great help at a birth. As you can see, the vulva of the crouching figure is open enough to accommodate her own head. Such a sight is quite encouraging to a woman in labor. I'd like to see a large rendition of a *sheela-na-gig* as part of the décor of birth rooms in maternity units. I have long believed that television could play an important part in teaching women about the true capacities of their bodies. Unfortunately, current puritanical mores allow national television audiences to witness the surgical cut to the uterus during a cesarean but never

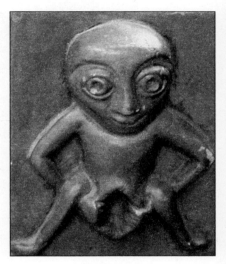

Sheela-na-gig

the natural expansion of the uncut vagina as the baby emerges. The sight of pubic hair is apparently strictly forbidden. There shall be no visible relaxation of a sphincter. These taboos have kept videos of natural births from being aired on national television, when this material is precisely the kind necessary to reduce the great fear and ignorance surrounding the birth process. A few years ago the producer for the Geraldo Rivera show persuaded me to send several of my videos to New York City for possible use on the show (which often featured strippers—male and female—among other subjects). Two days after I sent the videos, the producer called back with her apologies. My videos were "too graphic" for the Geraldo show—however fascinating and helpful they were to the production staff of the show who were of childbearing age. My point? This very strong taboo needs to be broken if we are to really diminish modern women's fear of birth.

Episiotomy: Is It Really Necessary?

Episiotomy, the most common of operations in North America, is a deliberate injury done to avoid what the perpetrator believes would be a worse injury. Strong, consistent evidence tells us how unnecessary routine episiotomy is.

Obstetricians in North America and some other civilized parts of the world have been cutting routine episiotomies—our version of female genital mutilation—on tens of millions of women for over a century, confident in their view that inflicting this trauma on the mother saves her from a serious tear, improves her husband's sex life (nowadays some imply that it helps hers too), saves her from urinary and fecal incontinence, saves her baby from shoulder dystocia, makes their own job of sewing up afterward easier, and prevents oxygen deprivation, mental retardation, and brain injury in the baby. All of these claims were made and widely accepted *without any supporting evidence* by doctors and hospitals all over North America. The trouble (actually, the good thing) is that none of them is true.

By now, plenty of research on this subject has been done and evaluated. Medical science knows that routine episiotomy has *no* benefits and carries many serious disadvantages.

Episiotomies:

- cause pain that sometimes lasts for weeks or months
- increase blood loss
- cause more serious tears because a cut perineum is not as resistant to laceration as an intact one
- often become infected
- are associated with wound breakdown, abscesses, permanent damage to the pelvic-floor muscles, and other complications that do cause incontinence (for example, rectovaginal fistulas—openings between the vagina and the rectum)
- prevent many women from breastfeeding because of the pain they cause

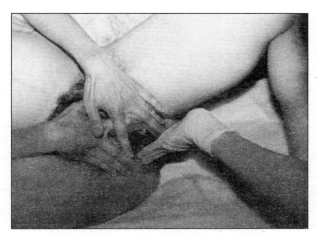

Mother helps me prevent a tear

Rarely, an episiotomy can be justified, as in the case in which a baby about to be born is in distress or when a breech male baby's testicles are the leading part to be born. *A careful review of the evidence shows that an episiotomy rate of over twenty percent cannot be justified on any grounds.*

To date, no nationwide survey has ever been conducted to find out how women feel about the episiotomies they have had.

How can you best avoid an unnecessary episiotomy or a bad laceration?

- You pick a caregiver who has an episiotomy rate lower than twenty percent.
- You pick a caregiver who performs median rather than mediolateral episiotomies (a cut from the bottom of the vagina straight down toward the rectum rather than an oblique cut from the bottom of the vagina toward the buttock). Mediolateral episiotomies are especially painful while healing.
- You push only when the urge comes. Most women like to push two or three times, taking a quick breath between them.
- When the baby's head is about to come out, you slow down your pushing as much as possible.

- Some women like to stimulate their clitoris as the baby emerges. This seems to increase vaginal engorgement, which may explain why I have never observed even the slightest laceration in a woman who used this method of relaxation during birth. Would you be able to discuss this with your doctor or even do it if you knew it was likely to help you? If not, you might benefit from attending a performance of Eve Ensler's theater piece, *Vagina Monologues.*
- If making noise helps you as you push, keep your sound in the lowest register possible, so that it vibrates the lower part of your body. Low, sexy moans are good.

It may help you to know that first babies' heads normally advance toward birth during a push and then recede once that push is over. Women who don't understand this process sometimes think that they are going backward when the baby's head recedes between pushes. I explain then that this process is good, because it helps the vulva gradually attain the size necessary for birth. Circulation to the area increases with the alternate stimuli of pressure, release, pressure, release.

The ignorance exhibited by both the woman who couldn't understand how something as large as a baby could come out of her vagina and Mrs. Sykes, the Arkansas midwife, continues among women today and is perpetuated by the prudishness of North American culture. Even the television channels that air videotapes of childbirth have censored shots of women's vaginas at the moment of birth. On goes the blurry, cubistic filter, obscuring the view of what women most need to see, and lost is the chance for women to reduce their fears about birth. What is gained by this?

As long as women go on accepting episiotomies, doctors will continue to cut them. Only when women take action by forming pressure groups to question this practice or refuse to hire obstetricians with high episiotomy rates will this unnecessary and sometimes dangerous practice change. However, it is important to realize how little real choice many U.S. women have whose maternity care is arranged through a health maintenance organization. Unfortunately, there is so much profit stemming from birth that this personal physiological act has become political.

Notes

1. Graham, I. D. *Episiotomy: Challenging Obstetric Interventions*. Oxford, England: Blackwell Science Ltd., 1997.
2. Prendergast, E. A fertility figure from Tullaroan, *Old KilKenny Review*, 1992.

9

THE THIRD STAGE OF LABOR

Clamping the Umbilical Cord

The time of clamping off the umbilical cord after birth varies a good deal according to where the baby is born. Babies born at home or in birth centers usually have their cords clamped at the time chosen by the parents (usually after the pulsing of the blood vessels in the cord stops). Hospitals, on the other hand, tend to favor cord-clamping at the first opportunity. Those who are critical of the assembly-line approach point out that preempting the physiological process is likely to increase problems such as retained placenta, postpartum hemorrhage, and respiratory distress in babies. Studies have shown that delayed cord-clamping allows between twenty and fifty percent of the baby's blood volume to flow into the baby. Early cord-clamping also results in lower hematocrit or hemoglobin values in the newborn (fewer red blood cells). Midwives agree that premature babies especially benefit from later cord-clamping.

If you plan to give birth in a hospital and want your baby's cord to be clamped later rather than sooner, make sure that you talk this over with your doctor or midwife. The evidence is on your side.

Delivery of the Placenta

Even though your baby is born, you are not quite finished with the birth process. Your body has another job ahead: to expel the placenta, which is no longer necessary to nourish your baby. If you give birth at home or in a birth center, it is likely that the normal process of expelling the placenta will be respected. Usually, this happens within half an hour or so. At The Farm Midwifery Center, our normal practice is to place the newly born baby directly onto his mother's chest with a warm blanket on top. This skin-to-skin contact maintains the baby's body heat and facilitates early communication between mother and baby. We do not vigorously massage the uterus, routinely give oxytocic drugs, or tug on the placenta in order to hurry its expulsion. We have on hand oxytocic drugs to stop hemorrhage whenever we are at a birth, but we use them only three or four times in every hundred births. Instead, we respect the natural process. We do not separate mother and baby. We keep both warm—if possible, in skin-to-skin contact. We have no routines that interfere with the euphoria that is present in the birth room. At some point, we will apply antiseptic to the baby's cord stump and inspect the baby, but all of this can happen at the convenience of the mother and baby. They are doing something more important just by being together. They are falling in love. We enjoy witnessing this process while being conscious not to interrupt it.

If a mother is lying down after birth, has been holding her baby for fifteen or twenty minutes, and the placenta has separated but not yet been expelled, we generally help her into an upright position. Just as upright positions help babies descend, so do they facilitate the expulsion of the placenta in many cases. Breast stimulation also helps.

In many hospitals, there is a greater emphasis on completing this phase of labor within a specific amount of time. Doctors sometimes try to hurry the expulsion of the placenta by pulling on the umbilical cord. But this can tear the cord from the placenta, a situation that may increase blood loss. You may want to negotiate for less intervention while completing this part of labor.

Wherever you give birth, your caregiver should be prepared to deal with postpartum hemorrhage. In hospital settings, about eight to nine percent of women bleed heavily after the birth of the baby or the expulsion of the placenta. The hemorrhage rate in my partners' and my midwifery practice has been consistently lower than 2 percent.

Oxytocin is usually the medication of choice to stop such bleeding in hospitals, birth centers, and in some home-birth practices. Some home-birth midwives rely more heavily on herbs or herbal tinctures, such as shepherd's purse, blue cohosh, or motherwort.

Keeping Your Prize

Your baby is safely born. If you are in your own bedroom or in a birth center, your baby will stay with you as much as you like. If you give birth in a hospital, you may have to negotiate to keep your baby with you continuously after birth. The routines in some institutions push nurses to immediately wash birth fluids off the baby (along with the protective vernix on the baby's skin), weigh and measure the baby, and treat the baby's eyes and cord stump. Persuade your doctor, midwife, or nurse to delay these procedures so that you can have a period of uninterrupted time to relate with your baby. You can also specify that you would like to have the vernix left on your baby's skin.

Choose a hospital that provides for "rooming-in" if you want to keep your baby with you instead of in a nursery. Rooming-in will provide your best chance of getting off to a good start with breastfeeding.

Several routine treatments of the newborn are common in most North American hospitals. One is suctioning of the baby's mouth and nose just after birth. Sometimes parents think that suctioning means their baby is in trouble, when in fact they are witnessing something that is done routinely.

There will be an effort to keep your baby warm. Hospital delivery rooms are normally rather cold places, and wet newborns can quickly lose body heat. The best place your baby can land is on your bare chest, to be covered with a warmed baby blanket. The newborn examination can be done with your baby in your arms. But if your baby needs resuscitation, this will usually need to be done in a warmed area.

Your baby's eyes will be treated with an antibiotic ointment to prevent infection with gonorrhea or chlamydia. Usually this will be tetracycline or erythromycin. Most parents appreciate the chance to look into their baby's eyes for a while before this ointment is applied, as it is gooey enough to slightly interfere with vision for a while.

Vitamin K is given by injection (or orally, at some hospitals) to prevent "hemorrhagic disease of the newborn." This condition is rare, and serious complications from it occur even more rarely. The injectable form of the drug has been shown to lower the risk of hemorrhagic disease of the newborn. Some recent studies suggest that the oral form of vitamin K is not quite as well absorbed as the injected form. The oral form must be given in more than one dose over several days. Vitamin K treatment is based on studies that were done on babies who didn't get much of their mothers' colostrum, which is high in vitamin K. It is quite possible that the risk of this disease is lower in breastfed babies than the available studies suggest.

Remember that you have the right to refuse any treatment or procedure, even when it is routine at the hospital where you give birth.

Avoiding Postpartum Depression

Postpartum depression (PPD) occurs in between three and twenty percent of new mothers. PPD can hit at any time in the year following birth, from a few days' postpartum to several months afterward. PPD can be so debilitating as to severely interfere with caring for your baby or yourself. Symptoms of PPD include feelings of hopelessness, insomnia, lack of appetite, nightmares, new fears and phobias, bizarre thoughts, thoughts of inadequacy, and hostile or suicidal thoughts. In one case out of one thousand, PPD progresses to postpartum psychosis. Most—but not all—cases of PPD and postpartum psychosis can be prevented by providing plenty of help to new mothers during the weeks following birth, but much of this disease is caused by isolation and exhaustion.

Step one to preventing PPD is to find time to sleep after giving birth, no matter how euphoric you feel. Try to sleep as much as you can when your baby sleeps. Consider hiring a postpartum doula if you don't have a friend or family member who will supply meals and do housework for you for the first two weeks or so. Do not feel that you have to accommodate everyone who wants to visit you and your baby. When friends and relatives do come, ask them to keep visits short or to wash dishes, leave food, or do your laundry when they come. Take your time about sending thank-you notes to those who sent cards or gifts. Avoid moving or making big changes in your living situation around the time of birth. Choose to breastfeed. Confide your feelings to your husband or women friends, and if you suspect that you are suffering from PPD, get in touch with a caregiver who is familiar with ways of treating it.

In my community, we have a much lower rate of PPD than is generally reported for our country at large. I believe that the intensive postpartum care that we give and the close communication between mothers lessens the isolation that mothers tend to feel in our society of nuclear families. Mothering is sometimes the loneliest job around, but it shouldn't be.

The Postpartum Doula

In less complicated times than our own, extended families nurtured new mothers for the first few weeks following birth. On The Farm we women take turns caring for each other. Nowadays, with family members scattered far and wide, hordes of new mothers face a loneliness they have never felt before at a time when they carry the responsibility for caring for a new life. Sometimes women are surprised at how low they can feel only a few days after experiencing the joy and excitement of birth. Sleep-deprived, full of hormones, uncertain about their ability to breastfeed, many feel overwhelmed by the responsibilities of mothering.

Maternity care in the Netherlands is designed with a unique recognition of the benefits of mothering mothers during the first eight days following the birth. Special maternity home-care assistants called *kraamverzorgende* are available to new mothers at all economic levels for reasonable hourly rates (partly subsidized by Dutch taxpayers). These assistants attend the birth with the midwife or family doctor, visit the home of the new parents and look after mother and baby, provide health education, clean, prepare meals, walk the dog, baby-sit for toddlers, get the older children off to school, and give breastfeeding support and consultation. While other countries make provision for some of these important services, the Netherlands has the most comprehensive system. This after-birth care is available both to the approximately thirty-five percent of Dutch women who still give birth at home and to those who have their babies in hospitals.

In many areas of the United States, postpartum doulas are providing services similar to the postpartum component of the Dutch maternity home-care assistant. If you hire a doula to help you after childbirth, you may have time for a nap, a bath, some postpartum exercises, and other activities that would be impossible without such help. In addition, you will significantly reduce your chances of experiencing postpartum depression.

See Resources for doula services.

10

BENCHMARKS IN MIDWIFERY

Who sets the benchmark for excellence in maternity care? Who should? Before we answer this question, it's necessary to be sure that we are looking at all the contenders. One of the people who would get my vote is Mrs. Margaret Charles Smith of Eutaw, Alabama. Born in 1906 and orphaned at the age of three weeks, Mrs. Margaret Charles Smith was raised by a woman who was bought as a slave for three dollars and lived to the age of 101. Mrs. Smith still lives in Eutaw, Alabama, the town of five thousand whose childbearing families she served from 1943 until 1981.

According to our national mythology about birth, technology, and what makes childbirth safe, she and the other grand* midwives like her were stopped from working because they were more dangerous care-

---

*The term preferred by the traditional lay midwives of the southeastern United States, also known as "granny midwives." They found the latter term demeaning.

givers than the doctors who replaced them. Public statements by health departments about why it was necessary to get rid of midwives like Mrs. Smith claimed that the midwives' lack of proper education affected their ability to practice safely. Doctors had a hospital-based training in obstetrics, while Mrs. Smith and the other traditional midwives of her generation learned the art and science of midwifery from elder midwives who had never set foot in a hospital.

When she attended her last birth in 1981, Mrs. Smith was still healthy, strong, and sharp of mind, but, like her fellow midwives, she lacked the political clout and the written evidence to support her continued practice. Part of the difficulty the civilized world has in assessing the practice of traditional midwives stems from lack of evidence. Ours is a culture that relies first and foremost upon the written record. I remember the traditional Brazilian midwife who stood before an audience of 2,000 doctors and formally trained midwives and asked in exasperation, "Don't you believe anything that you didn't read about in a book?" Few traditional midwives have been able to record the results of their work.

Mrs. Smith, however, is an exception. Her story is well told in the book about her life, *Listen to Me Good*, which she created with the help of Linda Janet Holmes.[1] In her long career—which would have been far longer if she and the families of the Eutaw area had had anything to say about it—she attended some three thousand births, with very few infant deaths and not a single maternal death. Mrs. Smith kept records of the births she attended, but, sadly, these were lost when her house burned to the ground. I was able to corroborate her figures with two of the physicians—Ruker Staggers and Joe Bethany—who answered her occasional calls for help during the years they worked with her. Both told me they considered it impossible for Mrs. Smith to have concealed a death and that she was a good midwife—in the words of Dr. Bethany, "a legend in her own time." Dr. Staggers used what influence he had to keep her permit to practice current, but in the end he bowed to the pressure of his medical colleagues, who wanted no midwives at all, no matter how good they were.

Mrs. Smith's record is all the more remarkable considering the handicaps (compared to today's home-birth midwives) under which she was working. She and the other grand midwives were not allowed to use blood-pressure cuffs as part of their prenatal care, antihemorrhagic drugs in case of postpartum hemorrhage, or oxygen for the resuscitation of a baby. She had no car, bicycle, or horse, and there was no public transportation available. Most of the families for whom she provided her services earned less than two dollars a day. Many families simply could not afford to pay her for the care she gave them. When she encountered a complication such as chronic high blood pressure in a mother, she was faced with getting her to a doctor or a hospital some twenty miles away. This meant begging a ride. Some families lived in areas far from any passable road.

The women Mrs. Smith cared for had no access to contraceptives when these became available to middle-class women, so she took care of many who had more than ten babies. Many of the women were malnourished and overworked. There were no free prenatal vitamins or iron or calcium tablets for the rural poor at that time. Probably the most shameful aspect of the lack of support she and the other midwives contended with was that if any woman had an outstanding hospital bill from a previous birth, she would not be admitted, even if she was in danger. If there was a way to transport her two hundred miles to Tuskegee, she could get free care, but this was hardly a good option in an emergency, with no ambulance or public transportation system. Mrs. Smith once tried to admit a woman who had high blood pressure and was passing out during labor but was told by a doctor (not Dr. Staggers or Dr. Bethany) to take her home and abandon her. To her eternal credit, she stayed with the woman—who was unconscious—during delivery in the car and for the twelve hours after labor that she continued to be severely ill. Both mother and child survived.

For all of the reasons I have mentioned, Mrs. Smith's record is remarkable—particularly with respect to maternal death. Obstetricians ought to be interested in how she was able to accomplish what she did (without any officially recognized training). See Resources for a video documentary about Mrs. Smith, which aired on public television in 2002.

Another remarkable midwife with a written record is Catharina Schrader. Vrouw (Mrs.) Schrader practiced in what is now the Netherlands from 1693 until 1745 and attended 3,017 births.[2] She recorded notes in her diary about every birth she attended. Some of the births were solely her cases, while others—usually the more-complicated ones—were labors for which other midwives sought her expert help.

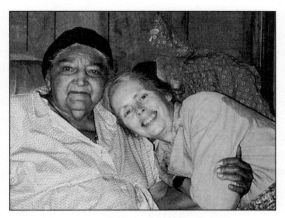

Margaret Charles Smith, midwife, and me

Natural, spontaneous birth took place in ninety-four percent of cases. (The Farm's rate of spontaneous birth is 94.5 percent, incidentally.) Cesarean section was not an option during Vrouw Schrader's time. In cases in which cesarean section would be considered mandatory nowadays, she and other midwives had to do what they could to save women's lives. One such complication is complete placenta previa (the placenta completely covers the cervical opening), which is perilous to both mother and baby. If there is gradual opening of the cervix in these cases (as is usual in normal labors), the mother can bleed to death. It is generally thought that the only way to save mother and baby in these cases is to perform a cesarean section.

Of all those 3,017 cases Schrader recorded, only twenty women died. In six of those, she had been asked to help in other midwives' cases that had already become too grave for anyone to make a difference. There were just fourteen maternal deaths in the 3,017 deliveries (4.6 in one thousand births) for which she had direct responsibility. To put this number into perspective, the maternal mortality rate in the United States in 1935 was 5.9 in one thousand births, even though doctors, forceps, cesarean sections, and hospitals were available to most women who needed them by that time. If Vrouw Schrader had had as high a maternal death rate as the United States in 1935, three or four more women would have died in her care. Just think what she could have accomplished in the twenty-first century!

Professor G. J. Kloosterman of Amsterdam has meticulously analyzed Schrader's data. He notes that the high rate of spontaneous birth in her practice is even more striking when one considers that her practice contained more complicated pregnancies and births than would be expected in a random sampling of the population. For instance, there was a 2.4 percent rate of multiple pregnancy and a two percent rate of complete placenta previa, one of the most dangerous complications that can occur in *any* pregnancy.

Because of the dangers of complete placenta previa, cesarean section has been the method of delivery in these cases throughout the twentieth century. There were ten cases of placenta previa among the births Schrader attended. The first case of placenta previa was number 661, and Vrouw Schrader lost the mother. It is likely that she did not know that such a complication could happen at the time. But she thought about it. She obviously came to the conclusion that she would have to act more quickly if she encountered that situation again. The next case of placenta previa she faced was case number 1,250, and she executed her plan of delivering the woman as soon as possible. Like Louise Bourgeois, the famous French midwife of the previous century, she removed the placenta first, then turned the baby to a feet-first position and pulled him out. Mother and child were both saved in this case, as well as in seven of the other ten cases. The fact that there were only two maternal deaths in ten cases of complete placenta previa in the seventeenth century is remarkable, even phenomenal!

The high rate of spontaneous birth in Schrader's practice is amazing and enlightening. It attests to both her midwifery skills and her knowledge. Not only that, it demonstrates the intrinsic capabilities of the human female in giving birth.

Another midwife who carefully noted all of her attended births in her diary was Martha Ballard, who practiced in Maine from 1785 until 1812. Ballard attended a total of 814 births, with only five maternal deaths. This meant that there was one maternal death for every 198 births.[3] As late as 1930 (when we had doctors, hospitals, and cesarean sections), there was one maternal death for every 150 births in the United States.[4]

A midwife who lived and practiced in Kendal, England, from the 1660s into the 1670s kept detailed records of the 412 births she attended. There was not a single maternal death in her series of births.[5]

Practices with Low Cesarean and Instrumental Delivery Rates (and Low Mortality Rates)

In case you think that the women who gave birth at The Farm Midwifery Center were so special that no one else could achieve cesarean and instrumental delivery rates as low as ours, let me tell you about some other practices with similar outcomes. The first one I heard about was a home-birth midwifery practice in Victoria, Australia, in which Dr. John Stevenson worked with several midwives who had entered midwifery much as I did. Their cesarean rate for 1,190 births attended between 1976 and 1983 was 1.6 percent. The hospital transfer rate was 4.9 percent. As in our practice at The Farm Midwifery Center, breech babies (twenty-three) and twins (thirteen sets) were born at home. When I met Dr. Stevenson and some of the midwives who worked with him, I found him to be a humble, sweet man who had entered medicine later in life than had most of his colleagues. His entry into the home-birth field came from a patient with agoraphobia, who was terrified to have her baby in a hospital. She harassed him into attending her birth at home—against his better judgment, he told me. He was fascinated about how much easier her labor seemed to be than most of those he attended in the hospital. Word soon spread, and his services were in demand.

I was struck by the similarity between their cesarean rate (1.6 percent) and ours (1.4 percent). Dr. Stevenson told me, "If I had looked after less than a hundred home births it could be attributed to sheer good luck, but over more than 1,100 patients in eight years, it has to be something other than just luck." I agreed. Despite the excellent statistics, Dr. Stevenson was de-registered by the Medical Board of Victoria, Australia, in 1984, after being found guilty by that body of "infamous conduct." As is usual in such witch-hunts, the case against Dr. Stevenson focused on the unorthodoxy of his practice, especially his use of unregistered birth helpers he had trained himself. His license to practice medicine was never restored.

In the early 1990s, I read in the *Lancet* about a midwifery service at Vienna's Ignaz Semmelweis Frauenklinik, where Dr. Alfred Rockenschaub served as director between 1965 and 1985. During his tenure, more than 44,500 births took place with a cesarean-section rate that was slightly over one percent and infant-mortality rates below those in Vienna during the same period, where the cesarean rate was more than ten percent.[6] During his tenure at the Semmelweis Women's Clinic, Dr. Rockenschaub was a professor in the midwifery school, where he had considerable influence over midwifery education—if not the respect of most other Austrian obstetricians. These midwives had the primary responsibility for the births that took place at the clinic, as the Austrian maternity-care system (like that of Europe in general) does not have labor and delivery nurses. After he left his position at the clinic in 1985, the cesarean rate there rose sharply. By 1999, nineteen percent of the women of Vienna had their babies by cesarean section. If Dr. Rockenschaub had been able to pass his methods on to enough other obstetricians who saw their value, it is likely that the cesarean rate in Vienna would still be under five percent. Unfortunately, Dr. Rockenschaub's work is barely known in the English-speaking world, because neither of the two editions of his book has been translated from German. If you want to know about Ignaz Semmelweis's life, read Morton Thompson's novel, *The Cry and the Covenant,* which is a fictionalized biography. I recommend it highly, but don't read it while you are pregnant, as the subject matter is quite grim.

Anyone with a scientific bent should find it fascinating that three midwifery practices in the world produced outcomes so similar. There are certain obvious common elements that the three practices share:

- careful psychological preparation during pregnancy
- births attended by midwives able to be constantly with the laboring women
- obstetrical backup provided by physicians able to recognize the abilities of midwives and women
- a philosophy that women are beautifully and admirably designed to give birth

Dr. John O. Williams, Jr. (who is writing his own memoir) was the selfless mentor who provided wonderful support for our midwifery service for its first fifteen years. Incidentally, Drs. Stevenson, Rockenschaub, and I have all been told at one time or another, by doctors who could not imagine that low mortality and morbidity rates are possible with such low cesarean and instrumental delivery rates, that our outcomes are "unbelievable." Still, they are possible. We all did it. We must be doing something right. Others can, too.

Our practice at The Farm Midwifery Center consists of some techniques and procedures that we learned from members of the medical profession and another set of techniques that, for the most part, we "dreamed up" ourselves. The second set of techniques (upright birth postures, pulling on overhead straps or bars while pushing the baby down, breast stimulation to contract the uterus, and the all-fours position for resolving shoulder dystocia, for instance) are all found in cultures where indigenous midwifery survives. Thinking back to the obstetrician I mentioned in the first few pages of this book—the one who wanted me to explain how we achieve our outcomes—I would say that we have tried to use the best that both traditional peoples and the medical world have to offer. Giving birth at home meant that we could be as flexible as possible (in the sense that we didn't have to be governed by idiotic social conventions, institutional habits or furniture), at the same time that we kept up on the medical literature and equipped ourselves with all of the portable technology that is useful for out-of-hospital births (blood-pressure cuffs, antihemorrhage medication, oxygen bottles, suturing supplies, and sterile gloves, for instance).

The work of the late Dr. Galba Alraújo of Ceará, Brazil, is a fascinating and creative example of an alliance forged between the medical profession and traditional midwives. Professor Alraújo saw a way to benefit mothers and babies, medical students, and *parteiras* (Brazil's traditional midwives) at the same time. He required medical students to do a rotation with *parteiras* attending home births so that the students would learn respect for the normal birth process as well as the midwives. His groundbreaking work produced many physicians who are now in the forefront of the "humanization of childbirth" movement that is gathering force in Brazil and other parts of Latin America, where cesarean-section rates in some areas are the highest in the world (more than eighty percent in some areas).

Dr. G. J. Kloosterman followed a similar course in the Netherlands in the 1940s, when he had a great influence on midwifery education. In large part because of him, the system continues to put midwives in charge of normal birth. Dutch women who want specialist care from an obstetrician must pay out of pocket for this. Dutch medical students who go into obstetrics are taught the principles of normal birth before they learn about pathology, which helps them to understand and respect what midwives can do for pregnant and birthing women and to feel comfortable about home birth.

There are many areas of human achievement in which it is easy and obvious to see who sets the benchmark of excellence. I'm thinking of auto racing, basketball, and piano playing, for instance. In these areas, people can't be fooled. Maternity care is something else entirely. If you read up on its history, you'll find that many of the great pioneers (I'm thinking especially of doctors at this moment) were reviled by their colleagues throughout their lives. In the 1840s, about a century before antibiotics became available, Ignaz Semmelweis discovered the contagiousness of childbed fever—a major cause of maternal death in the eighteenth and nineteenth centuries—and thus how to prevent it. Oliver Wendell Holmes attempted to persuade his U.S. colleagues that Semmelweis was right that doctors, not the victims themselves, were causing the disease. Both advised their colleagues to wash their hands after autopsies if they touched women in labor. More than twenty years after Holmes wrote his first paper on how to prevent childbed fever, some doctors were still claiming that the disease was caused by "seduction, remorse, and fretting, and that sepsis arose from the surroundings of the patient's own home" or from "noxious gases" of sewage. Ignaz Semmelweis himself died tragically in a mental asylum from a wound infection caused by a scuffle with an attendant. Some years later, his twenty-five-year-old son committed suicide because he despaired that his father's teachings would ever be accepted. Eventually, of course, they were, but an untold number of lives were lost while doctors remained in denial about the harm they were causing by their closed-mindedness. Even though Semmelweis and Holmes were respectable names by 1910, there were occasional outbreaks of childbed fever in hospitals as late as the 1940s.

Apparently, the women of Vienna during Semmelweis's time knew that the midwives' clinic was a safer place to give birth than the doctors' clinic. If they couldn't get into the midwives' clinic, they would rather give birth in the street than in the doctor's clinic. People then were more able to take their information from one another. Now, because of the mass media, people get their information from television and movies, which generally teach that machines are necessary for safe birth-giving. My hope is that we can find ways to use our mass media to promote public health in maternity-care policy rather than corporate profits.

Notes

1. Smith, Margaret Charles, and Holmes, Linda J. *Listen to Me Good: The Story of an Alabama Midwife.* Columbus: Ohio State University Press, 1995.
2. Marland, H., Kloosterman, G. J., and van Leiberg, M. J. *Mother and Child Were Saved: The Memoirs (1693–1740) of the Frisian Midwife Catharina Schrader.* Bilthoven, the Netherlands: Catharina Schrader Stichting, 1987.
3. Ulrich, Laurel Thatcher. *A Midwife's Tale.* New York: Random House, 1990.
4. Tucker, Beatrice, and Benaron, Harry. Maternal Mortality of the Chicago Maternity Center. *American Journal of Public Health,* January 1937; Volume 27.
5. Tew, Marjorie. *Safer Childbirth? A Critical History of Maternity Care.* London: Chapman and Hall, 1990.
6. Rockenschaub, Alfred. *Gebären ohne Aberglaube.* Vienna: Facultas Universitätsverlag, 2001.

Women are not dying because of diseases we cannot treat. They are dying because societies have yet to make the decision that their lives are worth saving.

—Mahmoud Fathallah

11

WHAT YOU LEAST EXPECT
WHEN YOU'RE EXPECTING

Given good maternity care throughout pregnancy, birth, and the postpartum period, serious injury or death of a mother is an extremely rare event—at least, in wealthy countries. Maternal death in industrialized countries happens so seldom that it is counted by the number of deaths per 100,000 births. That said, there are some disturbing signs indicating that the United States could significantly improve its performance in preventing maternal death.

One warning sign is that there has been no decline in our national maternal death rate since 1982. This is significant, since the rate of maternal death in our country declined every year between the mid-1930s and 1982. In most wealthy countries, maternal death rates continued to decline between 1982 and the present. Unfortunately, we do not have the information necessary to understand exactly why the U.S. rate remains so high. The lack of this vital information partially explains why we have so far made *no* progress in achieving our national goal for reducing maternal deaths set a generation ago. Our Healthy People 2000 goal was 3.3 maternal deaths per 100,000 live births. Obviously, we didn't reach it (although the states of Washington and Massachusetts did) so this is now our Healthy People 2010 goal.

From 1982 to 1996, maternal deaths have occurred at a ratio of about 7.5 deaths per 100,000 live births, with no movement in the right direction.[1] In 2005, the maternal mortality rate was 15.1 deaths per 100,000 births. Maternal death rates are sharply higher for African-American women, who die at four times the rate of the general population of women. Even worse, this difference has increased in recent years (from 3.4 times greater risk of dying than white women in 1987 to 4.1 times greater risk of dying in 1990). Hispanic women have a seventy percent higher risk of death than white women.[1] The problem with all these numbers is that they are gross underestimates.

The federal agency responsible for collecting, analyzing, and publishing statistics of births and deaths in the United States is the Centers for Disease Control and Prevention (CDC). The CDC warned in 1998 that even after substantial improvements had been made in our national reporting system, there is still so much underreporting that the number of actual deaths "is estimated to be 1.3 to three times that reported in vital statistics records."[1] The lower end of this estimate is based on a comprehensive survey of all women of childbearing age in France who died in 1989 (a national U.S. survey of this kind has never been done), which found that the number of women who died was more than double the reported number.[2] CDC officials say that several state surveys have shown that our underreporting problem in 1990 is at least as bad—perhaps worse—than France's. The higher estimate (three times the recorded rate) is based on various state surveys. Michigan, for instance, reported in 2000 that a careful survey demonstrated that its supposed maternal mortality rate of 7.6 deaths per 100,000 births should be revised to 18 per 100,000 births. According to Dr. James W. Gell, who presented the report, "it is likely that other states underestimate maternal mortality as well."[3]

Several factors contribute to the large degree of underreporting of maternal death in our country. For example, researchers often don't have access to all medical records, not all women who die have an autopsy, medical records may be lost, medical records may be sloppy or inaccurate, doctors are rarely trained in the rules or the correct way to complete vital records and may hesitate to report cases to investigators because they have medical/legal concerns. In addition, some deaths occur in early pregnancy before there is any medical record pointing to the woman's pregnancy. According to the CDC, twenty percent of maternal deaths happen in early pregnancy, and some are thus likely to be missed.[4]

My own informal survey of state mortality review committees found that fewer than half the states have maternal-mortality-and-morbidity review committees to analyze the numbers and causes of deaths, injuries, and illnesses so that feedback can be given to hospitals where too many occur. (*Maternal morbidity* refers to all injuries and illnesses directly caused by pregnancy or birth. The CDC estimates that several thousand cases of morbidity take place for every maternal death.) In the rest of the states, there is no collective effort to find out why mothers die. I learned that several states stopped doing maternal mortality review during the 1980s, when obstetricians' fears of malpractice lawsuits were at a high level. In the early and mid-1900s, most states had review committees.[5] Why is there less accountability now than then?

In 2007, the United States ranked forty-first in the world in its rate of maternal death, according to the World Health Organization. Taking into account the CDC's estimate of its underreporting factor, our world ranking would have to be revised if we were accurately reporting the number of deaths.

The CDC estimates that more than half of the maternal deaths that occur every year could be prevented. The knowledge that more than five hundred women could be saved each year should give us the incentive to perfect a system of data collection and standardized review to match those of European countries, which claim that their accuracy in maternal-death reporting is near perfect and all of whose maternal death rates are lower than ours.

Germany and Austria both have highly accurate reporting systems, partly because each has a federal law requiring an autopsy after every death of a woman of childbearing age. Every autopsy generates a record, which can be analyzed in a way that respects confidentiality but provides for self and institutional evaluation and feedback.[3] In the United States, there is no such requirement for autopsy following the death of a woman of childbearing age.

Another group of countries has an accurate reporting system, as well as another enviable feature. Every three years, the Departments of Health of Wales, Scotland, England, and Northern Ireland (the United Kingdom) in conjunction with the Royal College of Obstetricians and Gynaecologists publish a thick book entitled *Saving Mothers' Lives,* covering the three-year period just ended.[6] The book, which is available in bookstores, examines in detail the numbers and causes of deaths. British women who want to lower their risk of dying or sustaining serious injury during birth thus have solid information about the relative frequency of major complications. They can then avoid any elective procedures that carry a higher risk of maternal death or injury.

Equally important, pregnant women in the United Kingdom who are aware of *Saving Mothers' Lives* know that the deaths of about 110 women each year is considered so important by their government that each should be studied and reviewed as part of a strategy of preventing future deaths. It is interesting to note that this national effort began before the women's movement took place in these four countries. (About one-third of the British deaths in the most recent three-year period were considered to have been preventable.) *Saving Mothers' Lives* is made possible by a system of confidential investigations in which there is no risk to the physician, midwife, or hospital from lawsuits from the information gathered. The U.S. states that have mortality review committees also use confidential procedures and have legislation in place that protects this confidentiality from legal discovery. However, the findings of these committees are not made available to the public, as they are in the British system.

Only a system that values women highly and is proud of the work it does toward reducing maternal mortality can publish a book such as *Saving Mothers' Lives* (which has no U.S. equivalent). U.S. women deserve the added security that instituting a system similar to that of the U.K. would provide here. We do a much better job for our people in other areas of public health and safety. Can you imagine, for instance, the U.S. public tolerating a Federal Aviation Administration (FAA) that analyzed the causes of only half of fatal plane crashes?

The CDC is taking one of the first steps necessary to improve our underreporting problem by urging every state to include a check-box on the death certificate that would indicate whether a woman was pregnant within the year before her death. Notice that I said "urging," since the CDC does not have the authority to compel states to provide the information necessary to correctly ascertain the number of maternal deaths. In fact, the CDC does not even have the authority to compel the various states to use the same definitions on death certificates. From 1996 to 1998, 16 states included a question related to the pregnancy status, and by 2003, 21 states had such a question. But, according to the CDC, "In 2003, only four states could capture information consistent with the standard." The UK has no problem with this kind of craziness. All four countries of the UK use the same forms while, when lives are literally at stake, we still haven't got half of the states to cooperate in this gathering of essential public health information. What is our *true* maternal mortality rate?[4]

Much remains to be done to create a system that will equal those of many other industrialized countries. The CDC alone cannot do this important job. Both Congress and the President will have to be involved in the creation of a system that values women's lives and health on a par with other wealthy democracies.

How Aware Are Physicians of the U.S. Maternal-Death-Rate Problem?

Judging by the conversations I have had with many physician friends, U.S. doctors are generally unaware of the stagnant (or possibly rising) U.S. maternal death rate. The lack of a federal mandate for statewide mortality review keeps attention from being focused on this problem. However, in the late 1990s, several obstetrical trade publications ran articles with headlines such as "Maternal mortality: an unsolved problem," "Maternal mortality: no improvement since 1982," "Maternal mortality rate grossly underestimated," and "Pregnancy-related deaths: moving in the wrong direction," with one reference even pointing to a possible rise in the maternal death rate, so it is likely that at least some doctors are aware of our problem.[3,8-11]

In 1997 a number of organizations concerned with maternal health care formed a coalition called Safe Motherhood Initiatives-USA, which by 2001 included as partners the American College of Nurse–Midwives (ACNM), the American College of Obstetricians and Gynecologists (ACOG), the Midwives Alliance of North America (MANA), the March of Dimes, the American Public Health Association (APHA), the National Black Women's Health Project, the National Coalition of Hispanic Health and Human Services Organization, the National Alliance for Hispanic Health, and the National Asian Women's Health Organization. The SMI-USA coalition is part of a broader global Safe Motherhood Initiative, launched in 1987 and led by a unique partnership of international organizations, including the United Nations Children's Fund (UNICEF), the United Nations Population Fund (UNFPA), and the World Health Organization (WHO). These agencies work together to raise awareness, set priorities, stimulate research, mobilize resources, provide technical assistance, and share information according to each organization's mandate. (Unfortunately, the American College of Obstetricians and Gynecologists decided to withdraw from the coalition in 2002.)

SMI-USA presents Model Program Awards to promote Safe Motherhood in the United States through identification and recognition of models of excellence and encouragement of the replication of these models through dissemination.

A second SMI-USA project is the Safe Motherhood Quilt Project, which is a way of honoring and remembering U.S. women who have died from pregnancy-related causes since 1982. The quilt is made up of individually designed blocks, each one devoted to a woman who died.[12] I got the idea for starting it from the AIDS Quilt, after having been told several stories of U.S. women who had died from preventable causes. I hand-stitched the first block while attending a three-day meeting of the Coalition to Improve Maternity Services. During the course of the meeting, about thirty-five childbirth educators, midwives, lactation consultants, science writers, doulas, and physicians trooped by to see what I was making. In that small a group, three of the people at the meeting knew of mothers who had died. I realized then that a quilt could be a way of publicizing the need for legislation to address our underreporting problem, which is the first step toward fixing our maternal death problem. We can't do a good job of preventing unnecessary maternal deaths if we don't have accurate information about how many there are and what causes them. I believe that we need an impartial system of data-gathering, review, audit, and analysis that equals the British system of Confidential Enquiries into Maternal Deaths—one that then makes its findings available to the U.S. public.

Obstetrics is constantly changing, as new technologies, treatments, and drugs are introduced. Some of these innovations—antibiotics and the technology for safe blood transfusions, for instance—have saved countless lives. At the same time, other new drugs and procedures have caused unforeseen harm. Prenatal X rays were used for half a century before a researcher found in the mid-1950s that they significantly increase the number of childhood cancers.[13]

A newly synthesized estrogen product—diethylstilbestrol (DES)—became popular with U.S. doctors during the 1940s and 1950s for preventing miscarriage and was given to about two million women over a period of three decades. The FDA banned DES for use in pregnant women in 1971, after it was found to be the cause of rare vaginal cancers in young women as well as genital abnormalities in both young women and men whose mothers were given the drug.[14] Harm has come to even the third generation in some families exposed to this drug so many decades ago.

The drug thalidomide, introduced in Germany and the U.K. in the 1950s as a sleeping pill, was prescribed to tens of thousands of pregnant women in the first trimester of pregnancy. About twenty-four thousand European babies were born with shortened or misshapen arms and legs and other defects, two-thirds of whom died at birth.[14]

The latter two tragedies caused many reforms to be made in drug regulations around the world, but there are still loopholes in the United States that allow unsafe drugs and treatments to be prescribed or performed on pregnant women.

Cytotec

In Chapter 6 I mentioned Cytotec (misoprostol), the new induction fad that has swept the nation, and discussed side effects that some women have experienced after taking this drug for labor induction. So far, at least seven maternal deaths associated with the use of Cytotec have been documented (either in medical journals or by the Food and Drug Administration—the FDA), and hospital-based nurses, doctors and midwives have told me of additional Cytotec-related deaths that occurred after the medical journal and FDA reports. Five of the seven published deaths were due to amniotic-fluid embolism, which Searle, the manufacturer of Cytotec, does cite as a possible complication, but since the medical journals reported only one of them, this is a complication not generally recognized by U.S. physicians practicing obstetrics. Amniotic-fluid embolism has long been documented and understood to be more likely to occur when the uterus is artificially stimulated to contract, whether by Pitocin or prostaglandins. But this catastrophic complication used to be far more rare than it is nowadays in the United States. I personally know of five amniotic-fluid embolism deaths in women who were given Cytotec to induce labor.

One wonders why the FDA has chosen to keep women and physicians in the dark about the number of amniotic-fluid embolism deaths associated with Cytotec.

Some of the most dangerous maternal complications with Cytotec happened in women who were given a single dose of the smallest amount of the drug ever given (25 micrograms, a quarter of the tiny tablet). Two given the minimum dose a single time had major hemorrhages twelve and thirty hours after taking the drug and required hysterectomies.[15]

From 1990 to 1999, there was a rapid increase in Cytotec induction, including its use on women who had previous cesarean sections. I have seen many hospital protocols for Cytotec induction from that period that never mentioned it might be unwise for use on women with uterine scars. Two studies published in 1999, involving about 250 women with previous cesareans, showed *a twenty-eight-fold increase in uterine rupture in Cytotec induction.* There were three fetal deaths recorded in these studies.[16,17] In November 1999, the American College of Obstetricians and Gynecologists revised its bulletin on Cytotec for labor induction, recommending that it not be used for cervical ripening in women who have had previous cesarean section or major uterine surgery.[18] Now we know that Cytotec should never be used for vaginal birth after cesarean—after almost a decade of use on women who usually had no idea of its dangers. Cytotec is a classic example of why drugs should not be used until they are adequately tested.

Despite all the warnings that have been issued regarding the use of Cytotec, many U.S. doctors and some midwives continue to use it to induce labor. There is no denying its convenience when it comes to starting labor. However, I am certain that many women might have chosen otherwise if they had been fully informed about the possible consequences of taking Cytotec. Women should certainly be fully informed about these risks before taking the drug or any other medication that can be fatal.

I am part of an "e-group" of approximately forty U.S. women who have experienced horrendous complications after labor induction with Cytotec. Several of the women had emergency hysterectomies and nearly died from blood loss. What makes these women angriest is that they were not informed that Cytotec could have the effects it had in their case.

Amniotic-Fluid Embolism

The complication I mentioned above—amniotic-fluid embolism (AFE)—is a rather mysterious one. Once so rare that textbooks estimate its frequency at one in every 50,000 to 80,000 births, it seems to be occurring far more often in recent years—at least in the United States. Chicago writer Deanna Isaacs, whose daughter died of AFE in 1994 after a "routine induction," learned to her surprise—neither she nor her daughter had ever heard of AFE—that the incidence of AFE at the Phoenix hospital where her daughter died is *one in 6,500* births.[19] Isaacs points out in her article that the official U.S. death rate is about one in every five thousand births. If every U.S. hospital had such a high incidence of AFE, we could expect that more than three hundred women would die every year from this complication alone. According to the CDC and the Massachusetts Department of Public Health's Maternal Mortality and Morbidity Review Committee, AFE is now one of the most frequent killers of women in pregnancy and birth in the United States, with more than thirty women dying from this complication every year.[20,21] Of the first forty blocks contributed to the Safe Motherhood Quilt, there were *eleven* deaths from AFE, with all but three cases involving artificial induction or augmentation of labor. During a recent time period in the U.K. (1997 to 1999), there were only two AFE deaths per year in England, Wales, Scotland, and Northern Ireland combined.[22]

AFE kills more than half of the women who are stricken. It almost always happens during or just following labor and, in approximately half of the reported cases, is associated with excessively strong, closely spaced uterine contractions, the kind women may have in labors induced with Pitocin or prostaglandins such as Cytotec, Cervidil, and

Prepidil. Pathologists believe that the condition is more likely to occur when a considerable amount of amniotic fluid (mixed with skin cells, vernix, and fetal hair) is forced into the maternal bloodstream, causing immediate cardiac arrest. However, U.S. obstetrician Steven Clark—now the reigning U.S. guru on AFE—isn't so sure. For two decades he has advanced the theory that some particularly sensitive women can't tolerate amniotic fluid in their bloodstream, while others can—just as most people can be stung by a bee without a severe allergic reaction, while a small number die from it. Despite the plethora of articles documenting the association between AFE and chemically augmented labors, Clark downplays the connection. His campaign to chip away at the pathologists' understanding of AFE has effectively fragmented the U.S. consensus that augmented labors may lead to AFE. The latest edition of *Williams Obstetrics*—one of the two most influential obstetrics textbooks—no longer mentions this association at all.[23] No longer do most U.S. obstetricians think it necessary to remain at the hospital while a mother in their care undergoes an artificially induced or augmented labor. If the outcome is bad and there is a lawsuit, the obstetrician will not usually be blamed by a judge or jury. Who is looking after the mothers?

In an interview with Deanna Isaacs, Clark said: "The frightening thing about this [AFE] is that if [you're pregnant and] you've got the [genetic] mismatch, you're going down...And there's not a cotton-pickin' thing, as of yet, that we can do, unfortunately, to predict it." Isaacs, who interviewed many obstetricians in several countries following her daughter's death, remarked in her comprehensive and exhaustively researched article published in 1998 that she is unconvinced about Clark's genetic theory. She wrote: "In the end, AFE may prove not to be the result of a rare allergy. There's plenty of evidence in the medical literature to suggest that a significant volume of amniotic fluid (especially the fluid of a woman in labor) carrying meconium, vernix, or other chemical or particulate material is toxic if it gets into the woman's bloodstream. It hardly seems necessary to postulate an unusual allergic sensitivity or 'genetic mismatch' to explain the havoc such fluid can raise."[19]

Commenting on her realization that Clark was campaigning to "rewrite" the existing obstetrical doctrine on AFE—to undo the connection between induction and the deadly complication—she said:

"Clark himself provided what looks like evidence to the contrary when he reported that 50 percent of the patients in the cases he reviewed for his 1995 study had been given oxytocin during labor."[19]

Could it be that the frequency of AFE is rising as the number of induced labors increases? My educated hunch is yes. Until we have better research available, it would seem wise to avoid chemical induction of labor whenever possible. Labor is less likely to be induced in the case of home or birth-center birth, but if you plan an out-of-hospital birth, I urge you to interview your midwife and ask her explicitly about her induction policy. My advice is to avoid hiring someone who dabbles in the medical model by using oxytocic (Pitocin) or prostaglandin drugs (Cytotec) for labor induction or augmentation.

A New Technique for Suturing the Uterus after Cesarean

Another fashion of the last decade or so is not a pharmaceutical product but rather a new surgical method. A new surgical technique for stitching the uterus after cesarean surgery has come into vogue in the United States. Sometimes called "the Misgav-Ladach method," the technique calls for stitching the uterine incision in one layer instead of the traditional two layers. For most obstetricians in the English-speaking industrialized world, the two-layer method of closure has been the standard of care for some seventy-five years. Most of our statistics for uterine rupture and certain placental abnormalities (which happen more frequently after a previous cesarean section) are based upon the traditional way of sewing up the uterus.

At an annual conference of the National Association of Childbearing Centers in 1999, Dr. Kurt Benirschke, a renowned pathologist and textbook author, warned that the new fashion of single-layer closure (and, possibly, the change during the same time period from suturing with silk to suturing with removable catgut) was a probable cause of a dramatic increase in the incidence of life-threatening placental problems he had observed in recent years. He remarked that he had encountered about ten cases of *placenta percreta* per year for three consecutive years at a San Diego metropolitan hospital—an extraordinarily high incidence for what has previously been known as an extremely rare complication (one in 12,500 births).[24] Before moving to San Diego, where single-layer suturing had become the preferred method, he had never before in a long career encountered this complication. Women with placenta percreta are in grave danger of bleeding to death, because the placenta has grown over the uterine scar and through the bare uterine connective tissue (with no regeneration of the muscle layer in that area), sometimes into other organs such as the bladder. (In normal cases, the placenta embeds itself in a lining within the uterus, but not into the uterine muscle or connective tissue itself.)

Dr. Benirschke is not the only professional to notice the increasing incidence of placenta percreta in the United States. Dr. Rebecca Baergen, a New York City pathologist, told me that she sees "one placenta percreta a month" at the hospital where she works. There appear to be other possible problems with single-layer suturing. A Montreal study of 2,142 women compared the new method with the old and found a four-times-higher risk of uterine rupture with the single-layer method.[25] The authors of the study concluded: "Considering the widespread use of single-layer closure and its apparent impact on later uterine rupture, it is urgent and important for others to investigate this relationship. Given comparable short-term morbidity with single-layer and double-layer closure, surgeons should consider using a double-layer closure technique for women who may experience a subsequent trial of labor." The publication of this study in its most preliminary form was enough for the chairman of Maternal Fetal Medicine at Yale–New Haven Hospital Center to announce that single-layer closure of the uterus should be abandoned until there is more convincing evidence of its safety. Obstetricians have informed me of four cases of maternal death that are directly attributable to single-layer suturing. In three cases, death came in the next pregnancy; in one, there was bleeding at the incision site after the surgery.

During a recent Internet chat-room discussion among obstetricians, gynecologists, and general surgeons doing gynecology from many parts of the world, a U.S. obstetrician remarked that a small rural hospital that referred to his large teaching hospital suddenly began sending them problem cases of bleeding and failure of healing. These cases mystified him and his colleagues at the larger hospital until the rural hospital informed them of their change in technique to single-layer closure. When they changed back to double-layer closure, there was "no further trouble" with bleeding problems and failure of the incision to heal.

Aware of all this, I began asking physician friends about the new suturing method and learned that it is now taught in many U.S. medical schools, in preference to the traditional method. Many obstetricians have not had much experience in suturing the uterus in layers, and money-conscious health maintenance organizations (HMOs) clearly prefer surgeons who sew up in five minutes to those who require ten or more. Repairing the uterus in layers takes longer.

One thing is abundantly clear. The reasons have nothing to do with solid evidence, for almost no studies have been done to assess the safety of single-layer uterine suturing. The Cochrane Database of Systematic Reviews 2000 found only two studies meeting their criteria for evaluating surgical procedures and drugs, and these studies involved just 382 women who had had a single-layer closure. Both studies found that the new method saves four to five minutes per operation, but neither study was large enough to use as evidence for its safety—especially on a question so important as maternal death.[26]

At the same time that the research community in medical schools ignored the trend toward single-layer suturing, two widely read giveaway (i.e., marketing) publications, *Contemporary Ob/Gyn* and *OBG Management,* discussed the new method in glowing terms. One concentrated on method, while the other claimed that single-layer suturing prevents blood loss, promotes better wound healing, and causes less pain.[27,28] By failing to study the outcomes of the next pregnancy, each article completely ignored the possibility of harm to the women involved.

I know many good doctors who have sutured the uterus in one layer. Most of them are busy people, who generally have little time to spend in medical libraries carefully parsing articles. Most have not necessarily been taught to distinguish between clever marketing and science, as critical reading is not a skill that is well taught in many medical schools. How likely is it that critical reading of this kind is encouraged at medical schools where residents are pressured to stitch the uterus in an experimental way, without women's knowledge or consent?

Practically speaking, it is not really hard to guess why the new cesarean technique so quickly came into vogue in the United States during the 1990s. Policy decisions here often hinge more on economic factors than what is best for public health. Most of the few studies that have measured any outcome following single-layer closure have agreed that less suture material is required, operating-room time is significantly reduced, and there is sometimes a shorter hospital stay for the woman with single-layer closure. All of these factors at least point to cost savings for HMOs and hospitals, if not greater safety for women undergoing cesarean surgery.

My recommendation to pregnant women—at least in the United States—is to specify that if you should need a cesarean, you want your uterus to be closed in two layers. If you have already had a cesarean and are pregnant again, make sure that your placenta is not overlying your previous uterine scar before you attempt a vaginal birth after cesarean.

The good news is that a British research group—the National Perinatal Epidemiology Unit in Oxford—is coordinating a multicenter trial of cesarean surgery techniques that plans to address this relatively unstudied issue.

Cesarean Section by Choice: The Untold Story

Dr. Brenda Sylvester's* choice for the birth of her second baby was really made by the way her first baby arrived. Even though she had prepared for a vaginal birth by taking Lamaze classes, her firstborn turned breech in the seventh month and all attempts at external version failed. Certain there was no obstetrician in the metropolitan-area hospitals who would attend a vaginal breech birth for any mother, let alone a fellow physician having her first child, Dr. Sylvester planned for the inevitable cesarean. She came through the experience satisfied that she had made the best decision possible for her baby. The surgery hadn't been a picnic, but she hadn't expected one.

Two and a half years later, with a positive pregnancy test once again in hand, she already knew that she would have a second cesarean. She realized that a vaginal birth after cesarean (VBAC) was a possibility with the OB practice that employed nurse–midwives, but she wasn't sure she wanted to take the chance. She believed a cesarean to be safer than a trial labor. In her early thirties, she was very healthy and had experienced no complications in her pregnancy. Her surgery was performed by one of the respected and highly experienced doctors of a group of obstetricians and midwives. After the delivery of a healthy,

*A pseudonym.

full-term baby boy, residents (doctors-in-training) were put in charge of her postoperative care. If any complications developed, it was their responsibility to notify the attending physician.

On the day after surgery, the nurses who took care of Dr. Sylvester on the postpartum floor were worried when they couldn't hear bowel sounds. Besides, she had more complaints of abdominal pain than they liked, and her temperature was slightly elevated. Several times they tried to alert the residents about these problems but were told not to worry, that *they* had heard bowel sounds and were in touch with the attending physician. Three days after the surgery, Dr. Sylvester's blood test showed a slightly elevated white count, and more tests were done. Within twenty-four hours, she was in septic shock and placed on life support. Three days later, she died of overwhelming infection brought on by a nicked bowel in surgery that hadn't been caught by the physicians and residents taking care of her. All of the nurses on the floor were furious, because they knew that this death could have been avoided if their warnings had been heeded. What made them even sadder was that Dr. Sylvester's family remained unaware that the nurses had tried fruitlessly to alert the attending physician to her condition at a time when something could possibly have been done to save her life. None of them could afford to "spill the beans," so they kept their silence and their jobs. One of them, however, told me.

Most Americans are unaware that women ever die from cesarean operations, particularly when those surgeries are scheduled, rather than emergencies. Only rarely is a tragedy like this covered by the news media. Most maternal deaths in the United States are kept secret from the general public. Few people have any way of knowing that most maternal deaths take place in hospitals or that unnecessary surgery can actually cause a death. The twenty-first century began with the revelation from the Institute of Medicine of the National Academies of Science that roughly one hundred thousand people die from medical mistakes in the U.S. every year. Some of them—too many—are pregnant women.

Women can hardly make truly informed decisions when some of the most relevant information is not available to them. How many know, for example, that cesarean section (including the scheduled kind) involves the following risks to women?

- increase in hemorrhage requiring transfusion
- hysterectomy for uncontrollable hemorrhage
- accidental cutting of the bowel, leading to peritonitis, possible colostomy, or death
- accidental cutting of the uterine artery
- surgical trauma to bladder and ureters
- increased postpartum infection, scar breakdown
- scar pain, numbness
- long-term severe back pain following epidural block
- increased pulmonary embolism
- anesthesia mishaps, including paralysis and death

When cesarean is elective with no emergency present, the woman's chance of dying from the procedure itself is nearly three times that of nonsurgical birth.[28]

Cesareans involve risks for babies as well. If the cesarean is an emergency, the risks to the baby of doing the operation will likely be outweighed by the risks to the baby of not doing it. But if the cesarean is not medically necessary and the baby is not in trouble, the risks to the baby from doing the surgery mean that the baby is put in unnecessary danger.

Dangers to the baby in these cases include:

- accidental fetal laceration, which occurs in nearly two percent of all cesareans; in breech presentations, the incidence rises to six percent.[29]
- respiratory distress, a major cause of neonatal mortality; it is greatly reduced if the woman is allowed to go into labor prior to the cesarean section. Most women who choose cesarean, however, do not labor at all, since scheduling the surgery is often a high priority for them and their obstetricians.[30,31]
- accidental prematurity because the cesarean was performed too early. Even repeated ultrasound scans do not rule out this possibility.

Risks to women from cesarean section are not limited to the current pregnancy but extend to future pregnancies as well because of scarring of the uterus. These risks include:

- decreased fertility.
- abdominal adhesions leading to bowel obstruction. This risk can happen irrespective of future pregnancy and can be fatal. See http://www.nancylim.org.[32] I know two women who suffered life-threatening bowel obstructions twenty-five years after their cesareans. One, a good friend of mine, died from these complications.
- increased tubal pregnancy.
- increased placenta previa (the placenta lies over the cervical opening).
- increased placenta accreta (the placenta attaches too deeply into the uterine wall to separate normally; profuse and often fatal hemorrhage is the result).
- increased placental abruptio (the placenta is prematurely separated from the uterus, cutting off the baby's only source of oxygen).
- increased uterine rupture.

The great Dutch obstetrician and professor G. J. Kloosterman made the following observation in 1984: "In no way can we improve a normal pregnancy and labour in a healthy woman; we can only change it, but not for the better."[33] This statement is still true, despite the ever-increasing rate of obstetrical meddling that goes on.

Cesareans and, more rarely, chemical inductions of labor are sometimes necessary to the safety of mother or baby. At the same time, we need to recognize that cesarean surgery significantly increases the risk of death of a woman. This risk may be higher if new surgical techniques are widely introduced before they are adequately monitored for their relative safety.

Please understand that my wish is not to frighten but to inform. In this chapter, I have kept in mind the words of too many women who have told me, "I wish I had known this when I was still pregnant."

Over the past thirty years, I have watched as wave after wave of medical fads have washed over the institution of modern childbirth. But one thing, unfortunately, hasn't changed: The push to discover a panacea to cure the pain and inconvenience of childbirth drives many doctors and midwives to experiment—or at least to convince women that such a panacea is now available—and the women are usually the last to know.

Notes

1. Maternal mortality—United States, 1982–1996. *The Morbidity and Mortality Weekly Report*, 1998; 47:34, 705–7.
2. Bouvier-Colle, M. H., Varnoux, N., Costes, P., and Hatton, F. Reasons for the underreporting of maternal mortality in France, as indicated by a survey of all deaths among women of childbearing age. *International Journal of Epidemiology*, 2001; 20: 717–21.
3. Maternal mortality rate grossly underestimated. *Ob/Gyn News*, January 11, 2000.
4. Donna L. Hoyert, "Maternal Mortality and Related Concepts", National Center for Health Statistics, Vital and Health Statistics Series 3, no. 33 (February 2007)
5. *Strategies to Reduce Pregnancy-Related Deaths: From Identification and Review to Action*, Centers for Disease Control and Prevention, 2001.
6. *Why Mothers Die 1997–1999: The Confidential Enquiries into Maternal Deaths in the United Kingdom*. London: Royal College of Obstetricians and Gynaecologists Press, 2001.
7. Hall, M. H., and Bewley, S. Maternal mortality and mode of delivery. *Lancet*, 1999; 354:776.
8. Pregnancy-related deaths: Moving in the wrong direction. *OBG Management*, January 1998.
9. Maternal mortality: No improvement since 1982. *ACOG Today*, August 1999.
10. Maternal mortality: An unsolved problem. *Contemporary Ob/Gyn*, September 1999.
11. McCarthy, B. U.S. maternal death rates are on the rise. *Lancet*, 1996; 348:394.
12. www.rememberthemothers.org
13. Stewart, A., Webb, J., Giles, D., and Jewitt, D. Malignant disease in childhood and diagnostic irradiation in utero. *Lancet*, 1956; 2:447–9.
14. Katz Rothman, B. *Encyclopedia of Childbearing: Critical Perspectives*. Phoenix, AZ: The Oryx Press, 1993.
15. Wing, D., and Paul, R. H. A comparison of differing dosing regimens of vaginally administered misoprostol for preinduction cervical ripening and labor induction. *American Journal of Obstetrics and Gynecology*, 1996; 175:158–64.

16. Plaut, M. M., Schwartz, M. L., and Lubarsky, S. L. Uterine rupture associated with the use of misoprostol in the gravid patient with a previous cesarean section. *American Journal of Obstetrics and Gynecology,* 1999; 180:1535–42.

17. Blanchette, H. A., Nayak, S., and Erasmus, S. Comparisons of the safety and efficacy of intravaginal misoprostol (prostaglandin E1) with those of dinoprostone (prostaglandin E2) for cervical ripening and induction of labor in a community hospital. *American Journal of Obstetrics and Gynecology,* 1999; 180:1551.

18. Induction of labor with misoprostol. *ACOG Committee Opinion,* November 1999.

19. Isaacs, D. Code Blue Birth. *The Chicago Reader,* May 15, 1998. Available at *www.inamay.com.*

20. *Maternal Mortality and Morbidity Review in Massachusetts: A Bulletin for Health Care Professionals,* Number 1, May 2000.

21. Berg, C. J., Atrash, H. K., Koonin, L. M., and Tucker, L. Pregnancy-related mortality in the United States, 1987–1990. *Obstetrics & Gynecology,* 1996; 88:161–7.

22. *Why Mothers Die 1997–1999: The Confidential Enquiries into Maternal Deaths in the United Kingdom.* London: Royal College of Obstetricians and Gynaecologists Press, 2001.

23. Cunningham, F. G., Gant, N. F., et al. *Williams Obstetrics,* 21st ed. New York: McGraw-Hill Medical Publishing Division, 2001.

24. Gabbe, S. G., Niebyl, J. R., and Simpson, J. L. *Obstetrics: Normal & Problem Pregnancies,* 2nd ed. New York: Churchill Livingstone, 1991.

25. Bujold, E., Bujold, C., Hamilton, E. F., and Gauthier, R. J. The impact of a single-layer or double-layer closure on uterine rupture. *American Journal of Obstetrics and Gynecology,* 2002; 186:1326–30.

26. The Cochrane Database of Systematic Reviews, The Cochrane Library, 2000.

27. Bivins, J. A., Jr., and Gallup, D. G. C/S closure techniques: Which work best? *OBG Management,* April 2000, 98–108.

28. Chez, R. A., and Stark, M. The Misgav Ladach method of cesarean section. *Contemporary Ob/Gyn,* June 1998, 81–88.

29. Smith, J., Hernandez, C., and Wax, J. Fetal laceration injury at cesarean delivery. *Obstetrics & Gynecology,* 1997; 90:344–6.

28. Hall, M. and Bewley, S. Maternal mortality and mode of delivery. *Lancet*, 1999; 354:776.

30. Lomas, J. and Enkin, M. Variations in operative delivery rates. In *Effective Care in Pregnancy and Childbirth*, eds. Chalmers, I., Enkin, M., and Keirse, M. Oxford University Press, 1989.

31. Cohen, M., and Carson, B. S. Respiratory morbidity benefit of awaiting onset of labour after elective caesarean section. *Obstetrics & Gynecology*, 1985; 65:818–824.

32. See a website dedicated to the memory of one such woman: *www.nancylim.org*.

33. Kloosterman, G. J. Lecture to the Second Annual Conference of the Midwives' Alliance of North America, Toronto, Ontario, Canada, May 1984.

Actions or policies that coerce patients to undergo either a trial of labor or a repeat cesarean delivery interfere with patient autonomy and the informed consent process.

—ACOG Practice Patterns, August 1995

12

VAGINAL BIRTH AFTER CESAREAN (VBAC)

For over a generation, more than one-fifth of U.S. women have had their babies by cesarean surgery. With such a high rate of surgical birth, the question of how to give birth after a previous cesarean comes up for tens of thousands of women every year. If you are one of them, you have probably already noticed that there is a lot of confusing, even contradictory, information circulating about vaginal birth after cesarean (VBAC).

The medical evidence about VBAC is actually clearer than some recent medical and media interpretations of it would suggest. Cesarean surgery is just as risky as any other major abdominal surgery for the mother—a considerably higher risk for her than vaginal birth. With repeat cesarean she has three times the chance of dying and roughly five to ten times the risk of suffering complications such as infection; dangerous blood loss; transfusion; complications from anesthesia; injuries to the bladder, intestines, or urethra; and future bowel obstructions, hysterectomy, ectopic pregnancies, infertility, and dangerous placental complications. The more cesareans a woman has, the more the risks to her increase. Most of the above complications involve weeks of recovery, inconvenience, emotional trauma, and expense—at the least. According to Marsden Wagner, a neonatologist and perinatal scientist who worked for WHO for fifteen years, if women lose the option of VBAC, we can expect there to be at least twelve maternal deaths every year in the United States because of unnecessary cesarean section, not to mention thousands of cases of injury and illness.

VBAC, on the other hand, is safe when other risk factors, such as Cytotec or other prostaglandin induction, aren't added. The risk of uterine rupture in a woman with a previous transverse lower-uterine incision (the safest location on the uterus for incision) has always been and remains about 0.5 percent.

Changes in VBAC Policy

For most of the twentieth century, North American doctors automatically scheduled repeat cesareans for those women who had a previous cesarean, because they feared that the scar on the woman's uterus might rupture during labor. (European physicians have, for the most part, long understood that VBACs are safe for most women.) Many U.S. doctors assumed that these women had their first cesarean because of some physical defect, which was likely to still exist in a subsequent pregnancy. Neither of these assumptions turned out to be true.

In the 1970s, during the peak years of the North American homebirth movement, another campaign quickly took hold of the nation. While most women who had a previous cesarean still followed their doctors' advice about having a repeat cesarean, a few skeptics and assertive women argued with their doctors and won their cooperation to try for a vaginal birth. When they succeeded in giving birth vaginally, they wrote books and started organizations that challenged obstetricians' long-held assumptions about VBAC, uterine rupture, and women's capabilities. In the early 1980s, one of the books, Nancy Wainer Cohen's *Silent Knife,* was covered on the front page of *The Wall Street Journal*, which dubbed it "the bible (of cesarean prevention)." When many other women followed this lead and a handful of doctors became hardworking advocates of VBAC, North American statistics on VBAC began to appear for the first time. The results were encouraging and reassuring. When women who tried VBAC were compared with those who had repeat cesarean, researchers consistently found that:

- VBAC trials were safer for mothers (with transverse lower-uterine incisions) and as safe for babies as repeat cesareans.
- Nearly eighty percent of women who tried VBAC were able to give birth vaginally.

By 1988, when the U.S. national cesarean rate reached twenty-five percent, the American College of Obstetricians and Gynecologists (ACOG) added its voice to the chorus calling for women's right to choose vaginal birth in most pregnancies following a cesarean section. The rate of VBAC increased significantly between 1970, when only two percent of U.S. women tried VBAC, and 1996, when twenty-eight percent of women with prior cesareans gave birth vaginally. (Since 1996, the VBAC rate has dropped precipitously, for reasons that I explain below.) By 1995, the cesarean rate had dropped to about twenty-one percent, largely because of the increasing number of VBACs.[1]

ACOG has published bulletins on VBAC since the late 1980s. In 1995, ACOG's VBAC bulletin recommended limiting repeat cesarean births to those that were medically necessary. Obstetricians should counsel and encourage women to try to give birth vaginally, it said, as this would lead to shorter hospital stays, fewer transfusions, fewer postpartum fevers, and a savings of more than four thousand dollars per birth.[2] Not only would this course of action be better for women, said ACOG, it would not cause any greater risk for their babies. ACOG also recommended that women with two or more previous cesareans with no contraindications who want VBAC should not be discouraged from trying for a vaginal birth, that women with large babies should not be automatically exempted from trying a VBAC, and that VBACs should not be limited to the largest hospitals. All of the above recommendations were supported by published evidence cited in the references to the bulletin.

Despite the 1995 ACOG recommendations and the evidence supporting them, some physicians continued to prefer the convenience of scheduled cesarean section and the lowered medico-legal risk they face in maintaining the status quo. A sampling of obstetricians' responses to the question "Should we rethink the criteria for VBAC?" published in a widely read magazine for obstetricians included the following:

- "Medico-legal risk = multimillion-dollar lawsuit: only one lawsuit ruins your life and your family's future." [Notice that the focus of this doctor's concern is not the woman having the baby but his family's and his own welfare.]
- "The risks to mother and newborn with VBAC are far greater than has been reported. Cesarean section by competent obstetrical surgeons is just another way to deliver babies."
- "I have directly observed bad cases involving uterine/bladder ruptures, especially when epidurals and uterotonics [oxytocin and prostaglandins] are used!"
- "It is primary C/S [first cesarean section], not VBAC, that puts women at risk.... Why is primary C/S done more between 10 A.M. and 6 P.M.?" [This response from an obstetrician who obviously thinks too many cesareans are performed points to the convenience factor.][3]

As far back as 1985, *The New England Journal of Medicine* published an opinion piece written by two young obstetricians proposing that *all* women should give birth by cesarean. Since there was (and still is) no evidence to support this preposterous and outrageous proposal, the doctors based their arguments on their admittedly "very crude hypothetical estimations and a tortuous line of reasoning." One of the most noteworthy passages was this colossal What If: "We probably would not vary our procedures [section every woman] if the cost of saving a baby's life were the loss of a mother's. But what if it were a question of two babies saved per mother lost, or five, or ten, or (as our calculations roughly suggest) as many as 36 or 360?"[4] If it seems that these good doctors might have been pulling numbers out of a hat much as a magician pulls out a rabbit, that's close. According to obstetrician Bruce Flamm, who has written extensively about VBAC for two decades, he and several colleagues were at first convinced that the *NEJM* article was a satire.[5] Unfortunately, it wasn't. In the summer of 2000, one of the two authors of the article resurfaced with the idea that women should choose cesarean section for the good of their babies, this time aiming her message at childbearing women who read—of all the possible choices!—*Self* magazine.

In 1998, ACOG abruptly reversed its 1995 position of encouraging VBAC by issuing a new, quite different bulletin on the subject.[6] Still another version of this document was published in 1999.[7] The newest ACOG bulletin withdraws the organization's 1995 recommendation that "repeat cesarean births should not be done routinely, but rather for a specific indication" and strongly recommends that a physician capable of performing an emergency cesarean be "immediately available" when women are laboring for a VBAC. The same guidelines specify that anesthesia and staff for emergency cesarean be available in all hospitals where women are allowed to have VBAC.[8] Comparatively few U.S. hospitals are able to offer round-the-clock emergency services to the degree stated in these documents, so increasing numbers of pregnant women who wish to have VBAC are reporting that their caregivers have been scheduling them for repeat cesareans since the publication of the 1998 and 1999 ACOG Bulletins. In many areas of the country, those who choose to give birth in a hospital can no longer have a VBAC.

ACOG's new bulletins state that it is controversial to allow VBAC for women with breech babies, twins or other multiple gestations, post-term pregnancy (a definition that for some doctors seems to mean the day after the estimated due date, instead of the former forty-two weeks), and babies expected to be larger than usual. All of the above recommendations for restrictions on women "allowed" to give birth vaginally after cesarean have no basis whatsoever in evidence. Whereas the 1995 ACOG bulletin reads like a scientific article meant to persuade, the 1998 and 1999 bulletins are full of unfounded assertions and heavy implications. For example, "Reports indicate that maternal and infant complications also are associated with an unsuccessful trial of labor. Increasingly, these adverse events during trial of labor have led to malpractice suits." No references are provided for the statement about maternal and infant complications, because no studies support it. The statement about malpractice suits, however, is given three citations. Incidentally, ACOG's fear of litigation (never mentioned in the 1995 bulletin) is made obvious in the recommendation that obstetricians should "counsel patient regarding benefits and risks of VBAC" without suggesting a similar need to counsel her regarding the benefits and risks of repeat cesarean.

ACOG's 1999 recommendation that VBAC should occur only in hospitals equipped to respond to emergencies with physicians immediately available has just as little evidence to support it. There are no studies showing any improvement in maternal or infant death rates related to the characteristics of hospitals or the availability of physicians, which is possibly why the latest ACOG bulletins on VBAC fail to cite one. Anyone who has given birth in a U.S. hospital since 1990 probably already knows that physicians are only rarely "immediately available throughout active labor." Usually, they are across town in their offices, as the United States and Canada are the only countries to employ obstetrician–gynecologist–surgeons to provide prenatal care to healthy pregnant women. The best evidence in the world says that midwives ought to be doing this work, and in the countries with the lowest maternal and infant death rates, midwives attend births and provide prenatal care for eighty percent of childbearing women.

Sadly, the newest ACOG recommendations effectively close the door to VBAC to most women. For them it might as well be 1970, when few U.S. physicians conceded that women facing repeat cesarean ought to have a choice in the matter. At least one California hospital requires women to sign an informed-consent form before they can have a vaginal birth.[9] Some doctors think that requiring such consent forms will lead more women to choose cesareans, since the dreaded phrase *uterine rupture* won't appear in the consent form for cesarean surgery and the unpleasant fact of increased maternal death, injury, and illness can be glossed over by an accomplished wordsmith.[10] Instead of interpreting the latest medical studies for what they actually reveal, ACOG has made VBAC the scapegoat for the reported increase in uterine ruptures. Blaming VBAC keeps ACOG from admitting that the evidence shows that the real cause of the rise in ruptures is almost certainly the aggressive labor-induction policies that have doubled the induction rate in only a decade—not the still comparatively low VBAC rate. Meanwhile, we in the United States are entering into a new era of forced repeat cesareans for women.

Media-Driven Obstetric Policy

With so little medical evidence to back ACOG's recent revision of its VBAC policy recommendations, it is hard not to conclude that the radical changes in the document were driven by other factors. As I have explained above, the fear of malpractice suit is a big one. The way that the mass media interpret medical studies (and confuse opinion with research) is another. Obstetrician Bruce Flamm agrees that ACOG's withdrawal of support for VBAC stems from a couple of anti-VBAC opinion pieces—not research studies—published in *NEJM*.[11,12]

One of the most influential editorials, which attracted sustained national attention, appeared in 1999. Written by three Boston physicians, it took the Department of Health and Human Services (DHHS) to task for its Healthy People 2000 goal of reducing the national cesarean surgery rate from twenty-one percent to fifteen percent. (The World Health Organization says that the rate should not exceed ten to fifteen percent.) First paragraph, sentence three of the editorial reads: "The advantages of a safe vaginal delivery over a cesarean delivery are clear: a vaginal delivery is associated with lower maternal and neonatal morbidity, and it costs less." The authors might have omitted the word *safe* in the first part of the sentence, because plenty of evidence tells us that it would still be true without the qualifier. The sentence that follows is the kicker: "We contend that these advantages apply only to safe vaginal deliveries and that reducing the rate of cesarean delivery *may* [emphasis mine] lead to higher costs and more complications for mothers and their babies."

The authors then go on for four pages, pointing to the tripling of uterine rupture in Massachusetts between 1985 and 1995, without ever considering that recent changes in practice might be responsible rather than some previously undiscovered weakness that suddenly turned up in Massachusetts women's bodies. Please note the evidence I discussed in Chapter 11 that could well have caused the sudden increase in uterine ruptures noticed in Massachusetts and the other states mentioned in the editorial (Pennsylvania, New York, and Florida). Most of the increased rupture rates took place during the period when obstetricians were inducing more and more labors with oxytocin, Cytotec, and other prostaglandins and when many were switching to one-layer suturing (associated with four times the rupture rate in VBAC as the traditional method). Nowhere in the editorial do the authors mention that unequivocal evidence points to the heightened risk of maternal death, injury, and illness from cesarean over vaginal birth or to the gross underreporting of deaths. Instead, they accused the DHHS of promoting a goal "that *may* [emphasis mine] have a detrimental effect on maternal and infant health."

No wonder there is so much confusion about VBAC in women's minds! In a November 1999 Committee Opinion on Cytotec, ACOG rightly, if belatedly, recommended that Cytotec should not be used on women who had previous uterine surgery, including cesarean.[13] ACOG, however, was not prepared to recommend against the use of other prostaglandins and oxytocin for induction of VBAC labor in its 1999 bulletin on VBAC. Instead, it deemed *close monitoring* sufficient in such inductions. The problem here is that there is evidence—not totally conclusive but strongly suggestive—that using oxytocin with VBAC *does* increase the chance for uterine rupture.[14] We already know that prostaglandin gels and tampons can cause severe uterine rupture. Conservative practice would mean adherence to the basic rule of medical practice enunciated by Hippocrates: *First do no harm.*

VBAC at The Farm Midwifery Center

My partners and I at The Farm Midwifery Center (FMC) have been attending out-of-hospital vaginal births after cesarean for almost twenty years. More than ninety-eight percent of the 115 women who tried for a VBAC with us managed to give birth vaginally. Only two women required transport to the hospital during labor because we suspected dehiscence (thinning or separation of the previous scar) and, possibly, an impending rupture. Each had her baby by cesarean, and neither had a ruptured uterus. All of the babies whose mothers attempted VBAC with us had good outcomes. We know some Amish women who had a cesarean for their first baby and then had twelve or thirteen VBACs with no problems. My partners and I believe that our good outcomes are partly due to the fact that none of the women's labors was induced or augmented with oxytocics or prostaglandins.

We know that in the event of an emergency, we can telephone our regional hospital, describe the emergency, and start on our way to the hospital, knowing that the staff is preparing itself and the operating room for our client's arrival. Our decision-to-incision time is less than that of many hospitals.

We have been able to provide out-of-hospital care for the vast majority of women who wanted VBACs with us. The following list of conditions covers those we do not feel comfortable about attending in an out-of-hospital setting:

- women whose placenta overlies a previous uterine scar
- women who have had three or more previous cesareans (if they have not already had a vaginal birth since)
- women who had previous classical incisions (if they have not already had a vaginal birth since)

We have attended the hospital VBAC of a woman who had four previous cesareans, and then we attended her next out-of-hospital birth. We at the FMC will continue to attend VBACs as long as women want them. We must first make sure that we rule out a placenta implanted over a previous uterine scar. If we discover a case of placenta accreta (increta or percreta) by ultrasound (we never have), we will arrange for further care with the most highly skilled obstetrician we can find.

Another home-birth practice with a high rate of success in VBAC is that of Dr. Mayer Eisenstein of Chicago. In twenty-seven years of practice and more than fourteen thousand home births, there have been more than one thousand VBACs. More than ninety percent of the women who attempted to give birth vaginally were able to do so.[15]

It would be possible to develop a system throughout the United States in which VBAC women could labor at home, in birth centers, or in small hospitals, closely attended by midwives and family members. Such a system would require close working relationships and good communications among all of the caregivers involved.

Maximizing Your Chance to Have a VBAC

Probably the strongest action you can take to improve your chance of having a VBAC is to pick a caregiver who has a VBAC rate of seventy percent or more. There are lots of practitioners out there who have achieved such rates. Some may have become nervous since the ACOG recommendations changed, but there are plenty of obstetricians and midwives who realize that the evidence hasn't changed and who have a commitment to providing women with the kind of care they desire. In short, hire someone to help you who believes in VBAC.

Avoid labor induction and augmentation. If there is pressure for you to dilate more quickly, try to get into water or walk the halls and arrange for some privacy. Refuse a routine I.V., and make sure that you are well-fed before you get to the hospital (if that's where you are going). Try to find one where drinking and eating is allowed in labor. Finally, keep vaginal exams to a minimum. Skilled practitioners can usually closely estimate dilation by your breathing and your body language. If there is any pressure on you to have an epidural, try to resist it. (There are instances in later labor where one can help, but epidurals should not be used early in VBAC labors, in my opinion.)

Last, spend your pregnancy loving your uterus and your baby. I mean this literally. Positive energy makes a good birth outcome more likely, so go for it.

Notes

1. ACOG Practice Bulletin No. 5, July 1999: Vaginal Birth after Previous Cesarean Delivery.
2. ACOG Practice Patterns Number 1, August 1995: Vaginal Birth after Previous Cesarean Birth.
3. Leveno, K. J., and Socol, M. L. Should we rethink the criteria for VBAC? *Contemporary Ob/Gyn*, March 1999.
4. Feldman, G. B., and Freiman, J. A. Prophylactic cesarean section at term? *New England Journal of Medicine*, 1985; 312:1264–7.
5. Flamm, B. L. *Birth after Cesarean: The Medical Facts*. New York: Prentice-Hall Press, 1990.
6. ACOG Practice Patterns No. 1, August 1998: Vaginal Birth after Previous Cesarean Birth.
7. ACOG Practice Bulletin No. 5, July 1999: Vaginal Birth after Previous Cesarean Delivery.
8. Ibid.
9. *Ob-Gyn Malpractice Prevention*, August 2000.
10. *Ob-Gyn Malpractice Prevention*, November 2001.
11. Sachs, B. P., et al. The risks of lowering the cesarean-delivery rate. *New England Journal of Medicine*, 1999; 340:54–7.

12. Green, M. F. Vaginal delivery after cesarean section: Is the risk acceptable? *New England Journal of Medicine*, 2001; 345(1):54–5.

13. ACOG Committee Opinion No. 228, November 1999: Induction of Labor with Misoprostol.

14. Chauhan, S. P., et al. Cesarean section for suspected fetal distress: Does the decision–incision time make a difference? *Journal of Reproductive Medicine*, 1997; 14:347–52.

15. Eisenstein, Mayer. *Safer Medicine: Towards Clinical Scientific Evidence-Based Medicine*. Chicago: CMI Press, 2000.

13

CHOOSING A CAREGIVER

One of the greatest influences on what happens to you during labor (especially as this relates to medical interventions, procedures, and medications) depends upon whom you choose to be your caregiver. In North America there are three separate professions that provide maternity care: midwives, family doctors, and obstetricians.

Midwives are specialists in normal pregnancy and birth. Midwifery care is individualized and focuses on minimizing the use of obstetrical intervention when possible. Midwives provide all the prenatal care healthy women need. The midwifery ideal is to work with each woman and her family to identify her unique physical, social, and emotional needs. Midwifery care is associated with fewer episiotomies, fewer forceps and vacuum-extractor deliveries, fewer epidurals, and fewer cesarean sections. Midwives are trained to identify the small percentage of births in which complications develop and to refer these to obstetricians.

In the United States, there are three basic categories of midwives. Certified nurse–midwives (CNMs) are registered nurses and have completed additional postgraduate training at an institution accredited by the American College of Nurse–Midwives (ACNM). Direct-entry midwives are those who did not become registered nurses as a step toward midwifery training. There are two varieties of certified direct-entry midwives in the United States: certified professional midwives (who are certified by the North American Registry of Midwives) and certified midwives, who are certified by the ACC, the credentialing arm of the American College of Nurse–Midwives. In several states, another variety of direct-entry midwife is licensed to practice; usually these midwives are called "licensed midwives." Not all midwives are certified or licensed.

Most of the home births in the United States are attended by some variety of direct-entry midwife, with approximately eight percent of home births being attended by certified nurse–midwives. Birth centers are staffed by all varieties of midwives. The bulk of certified nurse–midwives work in hospitals.

About thirty percent of family doctors practicing in the United States provide maternity care. These general practitioners tend to be somewhat more prevalent in rural areas. Many do not have surgical privileges and, like midwives, must refer to an obstetrician if a cesarean becomes necessary. It would be a mistake, though, to consider care by family doctors or midwives inferior to that offered by obstetricians simply on the grounds that obstetricians need not refer care to a family physician or to a midwife if no complications develop during a course of labor. Several studies have found that family doctors tend to have lower rates of obstetrical intervention than obstetricians.[1-3]

Some family physicians practice more within a midwifery mode because part of their residency training involved teaching by certified nurse–midwives. Other family doctors practice much like obstetricians, since in many states most receive the bulk of their obstetric training from obstetricians.

Obstetricians are doctors who have specialized in obstetrics. Their medical training is focused on detecting and treating the pathological problems of pregnancy, sometimes labor and birth. As surgeons, they perform cesarean sections and forceps and vacuum-extractor births. In

North America, for historical reasons, they far outnumber midwives and family physicians who provide maternity care. In part because of their numbers and long-held dominance over the other two professions, they design most of the hospital maternity-department rules and routines. They usually determine the role played by family doctors in maternity care.

Obstetricians are trained to detect pathology. When they detect it, their training focuses on intervention and treatment. Looked at from a world perspective, the role of obstetricians in North America is unusual, since in North America, obstetricians serve as caregivers for healthy pregnant women, as well as for women who are ill or high-risk. When obstetricians provide maternity care for healthy women, they often apply interventions that are appropriate for complicated pregnancies to all women. In most countries, obstetricians focus on providing care to women who are ill or who have developed a complication.

Interviewing a Caregiver

As I've mentioned before, it is not possible to determine solely by licensure, certification, gender, profession, or outward appearance the philosophy of practice of any given practitioner. Not all midwives work within the midwifery model of care; not all doctors work entirely within the limits of the medical model of care. Women are not necessarily more sensitive than men when it comes to providing maternity care.

What I'm saying here is that you need to be a smart shopper. One of the best ways to educate yourself about the care possibilities in your area is to interview several practitioners. Notice how you feel during and after your talks with them. Keep in mind that some practitioners may tailor their answers to match what they think are your prejudices. You might ask, for instance: What is your practice concerning episiotomy on first-time mothers? How often does this happen?

Respect your own intuition. If you get "good" answers from a given practitioner but you just don't feel comfortable with that person, you will probably be wise to continue looking for a good match.

What follows is a list of specific questions that you might ask.

Home-Birth Midwife

- How, when, and where did you receive your midwifery education?
- Are you certified or licensed?
- What physician collaboration or backup do you have?
- Do you maintain statistics from your practice? May I see them?
- How many women are due within a month of my due date?
- Do you work with a partner? If so, what are her qualifications?
- What is your plan if someone else is in labor when I am?
- Do you use pharmaceutical products to induce labor?
- What prenatal tests do you require?
- What are your recommendations about my diet during pregnancy? (You should be wary of anyone who recommends a weight gain of less than twenty-five or thirty pounds. If you are overweight, you should not be encouraged to lose weight or to avoid gaining beyond a certain number of pounds. Watch out for practitioners who recommend salt restriction.)
- Do you carry an oxygen tank to births?
- What methods do you suggest to alleviate labor pain?
- Is your certification in neonatal resuscitation up to date?
- To what hospital do you transport if this becomes necessary? Who will go with me?
- How often will you make postpartum visits?
- Do you participate in regular peer review?

Hospital-Based Midwife

- How many women do you have to care for at once?
- Who will care for me if you aren't at work when I go into labor?
- What prenatal tests do you do routinely?
- What procedures do you do routinely for women in labor?
- Are you open to my having a doula, in addition to my husband/partner?
- May I drink and eat during labor?
- Can I have intermittent monitoring rather than EFM?
- What methods do you suggest to alleviate labor pain?
- Are there tubs or showers at the hospital? Is it likely that I can use one?
- Is there a time limit on labor?
- Can you put my baby on my chest (skin-to-skin contact) after birth?

- Will you wait to clamp the umbilical cord until it has stopped pulsating?
- What kind of postpartum care do you do?

Obstetrician or Family-Practice Doctor
- How likely is it that you'll be present when I give birth?
- If not, who will be there instead?
- Can I meet all of your partners?
- What is your policy on ultrasound?
- What forms of pain relief do you recommend?
- How many women in your practice give birth without pharmacological pain relief?
- What do you think about doulas?
- How often am I likely to see you while I'm in labor?
- What prenatal tests do you do routinely?
- What labor procedures do you do routinely?
- What methods do you suggest to alleviate labor pain?
- Can my baby's heart rate be intermittently monitored by the nurses?
- Do you perform episiotomies routinely? How often do women in your care give birth without episiotomy?
- Can I drink and eat in labor?
- If I go into labor, check in to the hospital, and my labor slows down before I get very far, can I go home?
- What is your induction rate? What methods do you use?
- Can I walk around in labor?
- Is there a time limit for labor? How long can I push?
- Can I choose the position for giving birth? Can I give birth on my hands and knees if I like that position?
- What is your cesarean rate?
- This may seem a personal question, but [if female] can I ask if you ever gave birth vaginally?
- This may seem a personal question, but [if male and a father] can I ask if any of your children were born vaginally?
- What is your forceps and vacuum-extraction rate?
- Will you cut the umbilical cord after it quits pulsating?
- Can you put my baby on my chest (skin-to-skin contact) after birth?

Doula

- What training have you had?
- Do you have any other responsibilities that might keep you from being available when I'm in labor?
- Can you provide references?
- How many clients have you already worked with?
- Can you tell me the range of situations that you've worked with?

Remember that a postpartum doula's job is to care for you so that you can focus on your baby's care. She may do housework or cooking. You want a mature person who will truly listen to you, someone who will be calm even if you are feeling overwhelmed and stressed.

If any of the above questions provokes resentment, sarcasm, hostility, scare tactics, or vague or patronizing answers, keep shopping. You would likely not put up with such treatment in a restaurant, and finding the right caregiver for you during pregnancy and birth is a far more important decision to make than where you eat a meal.

Notes

1. MacDonald, S. E., Voaklander, K., and Birtwhistle, R. V. A comparison of family physicians' and obstetricians' intrapartum management of low-risk pregnancies. *Journal of Family Practice*, 1993; 37(5):457–62.
2. Hueston, W. J., Applegate, J. A., Mansfield, C. J., King, D. E., and McClaflin, R. R. Practice variations between family physicians and obstetricians in the management of low-risk pregnancies. *Journal of Family Practice*, 1995; 40(4):345–51.
3. Rosenblatt, R. A., Dobie, S. A., Hart, L. G., Baldwin, L. M., Schneeweiss, R., Gould D., Raine, T. R., Jenkins, L., Benedetti, T. J., Fordyce, M., Pirani, M. K., and Perrin, E. B. Interspecialty differences in obstetric care. *Journal of the American Public Health Association*, 1997; 87:344–51.

_14_

A Vision for Midwifery and Mothers in the Twenty-first Century

As I prepared to write this last chapter, my telephone rang. On the other end of the line was a woman calling for her Amish neighbors. When an Amish couple or midwife decides that they need the help of the midwives at The Farm, a typical scenario is for the Amish husband to go to the closest "English" neighbor for telephone service. ("English" in Amish usage means those of us who aren't Amish.) He relays his message to the neighbor, who then calls us as he heads back home to his wife. As you can well imagine, this system does not provide for much detail—given the constraints of Amish men talking to "English" neighbors who are not midwives. This time the call was about a labor already in progress, one that my partners and I had not been booked to attend.

"I tried everyone else's line first," the neighbor explained, "but you're the only one of the midwives I could reach."

"Amos Y's wife has been in labor since midnight last night," she said. "She's having a hard time, and the mother-in-law wants you to come."

"I don't know this woman," I said. "What number of baby is this for her?"

"Number seven," she said.

I felt my dilemma full force. I had my publisher's deadline to meet, but I am a midwife. When push comes to shove, the writer always has to give in to the midwife. Grabbing my birth kit, I told the neighbor to get the message to the family that I would come as quickly as possible. I set out on my twenty-five-mile journey just as the sun was sinking low on the horizon. If at all possible, I wanted to reach my destination before it was completely dark.

Finding Amish houses that you've never been to is not easy, especially the day after it has rained for three days straight and flooded everything in the area worse than anyone living can remember. You know there is going to be a lot of mud between you and your destination, because almost all of the Amish live on gravel roads, way off even the county roads. You know there will be no porch light. As I drove, I was aware of the many possibilities that might lie ahead. I thought of the prayer of the gunner on Horatio Hornblower's ship, who, each time they entered combat, said, "Dear Lord, make us truly grateful for what it is that we are about to receive."

Just as the last bit of light vanished in the western sky, I stepped onto the porch of the family's two-story wooden farmhouse and wiped my muddy feet on the blue denim rag rug before the door. Amos greeted me there. He led me into the kitchen. The kerosene lantern he carried provided the only light in the room. He escorted me over to his wife, Emma, who was sitting in a hickory rocking chair with a brown polyester blanket wrapped around her. I was happy to see that she was alert and in good labor. I had never met her or Amos before, but the "mother-in-law" turned out to be an Amish midwife whom I know quite well. She had been with Emma since the wee hours of the morning, and she wasn't sure what was holding up the birth. I knew that she would have recognized any dangerous positioning of the baby (a shoulder or transverse presentation, for instance). Watching Emma go through a couple of heavy-duty rushes let me know that her uterus still had plenty of power.

A vaginal exam told me that Emma's cervix was quite thin and open (though almost out of my reach) and that the baby's head was still relatively high for this stage of labor. I discussed with her the possibility of my carefully breaking the water bag. She agreed, and I put a slow leak in the bag. As the clear amniotic fluid dribbled out, the baby's head began to push directly against her cervix, helping it to open during the next few rushes. Within a few minutes, the baby's head was emerging. Slowly came the forehead, the eyes, the nose, the enormously fat cheeks, and the chin—but no neck. Emma's attempts to push out the baby's body were fruitless, because the baby's shoulders were tightly impacted.

"I need you to turn over on your hands and knees," I told her (an action I had suggested earlier might be necessary).

"I can't!" she said. I knew that the long dress she was wearing wasn't going to make the move any easier (it is usual for Amish women in labor to wear their day clothes).

"You'll be able to do it," I said. Over she rolled, and with a great effort of will and some help from Amos, she pulled herself onto her hands and knees. She gave a great push, which produced one shoulder, then the other. I gently inserted my fingers under the baby's arms and tugged her chubby body out. She weighed in at ten pounds, more than a pound larger than her largest sibling. No tear, no episiotomy, and no postbirth healing for either mother or baby. Two hours later, I left for home under a starry winter sky and a moon nearly full, grateful for what I had received.

Back now in the twenty-first century with my laptop, electricity, and telephone nearby, I have a little more to say about the maternity care I would like to be in place when my grandchildren and yours need care. I'm visualizing that I'm at a smorgasbord of the world's best ideas. I may have missed some great ones (I haven't been everywhere yet), but the following list sums up the features I think we in the United States need the most:

- *more* midwives, gradually, until we reach a proportion of midwives-to-obstetricians that works to empower—rather than create illusions for—pregnant and birth-giving women. Such a system will eventually have considerably more midwives than obstetricians.
- a national system for collecting data about maternal death and injury equal in reliability and accuracy to the system of Confidential Enquiries in the United Kingdom.

- independent community-based boards predominantly composed of public members but including midwives and other health professionals are placed throughout the country, to assure public accountability.
- a national health-insurance system as good as that of the Netherlands, Denmark, Finland, Sweden, Norway, Canada, and Japan.
- postpartum care for ten days for all women, like that available in the Netherlands, which is partially subsidized by the government (see Chapter 9).
- a revolution in obstetrical education so that midwives teach medical students normal birth before they are exposed to birth pathology.
- the need for multiple educational routes into the practice and profession of midwifery is recognized.
- every medical student who will eventually provide maternity care learns to dress a newborn baby without making him or her cry.
- the art of vaginal breech birth is maintained and transmitted in the next generation of midwifery and obstetrical caregivers.
- rarely use machines for what humans can do far better.
- every mother gets to choose where she gives birth.
- vaginal birth after cesarean is an option for women in all regions of the country.
- no woman is compelled to have surgery under court order.
- every hospital becomes Mother-Friendly, as designated by the Coalition for Improving Maternity Services (CIMS).
- advertising of pharmaceutical products to the general public is forbidden.
- postpartum psychosis is recognized as a disease and a public-health problem.
- nine months' paid maternity (or paternity) leave, depending upon what works best for each family.
- on-site day care.

The Dutch still put the rest of the world to shame when it comes to maintaining a system that views home birth as a normal, socially acceptable event. Only in Holland is it likely that the mayor of a town will be photographed congratulating the parents of a special baby in his parents' own bedroom. My friend, Dutch midwife Mary Zwart's

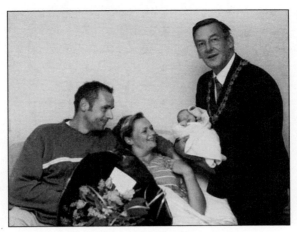

The Lord Mayor of Harderwijk, the Netherlands, welcomes the 40,000th inhabitant of the city in his parents' bedroom, his birthplace

grandmother, Marie Striekwold-Ebben, passed along this piece of wisdom: "Even if you don't have much money, keep in mind that the bedroom is the most important room in the house. Love and sadness are shared under the sheets, and you hope that your children will come into the world in your bedroom and that you will leave the world there." Naturally, Mary grew up knowing that it is all right to receive guests there. Speaking again of her grandmother's thoughts on the importance of the bedroom, she added another of her grandmother's wise sayings: "If there's a quarrel, it will be made up under the blankets."

Maybe one of these days a New Year's baby's birth will be honored in a U.S. couple's bedroom. I am going to continue working toward that goal.

One thing is certain: That goal cannot be realized as long as most U.S. women remain convinced that their bodies are poorly made to give birth. If I have persuaded you of nothing else in this book, I hope that one message will stay with you. Your body is not a lemon!

GLOSSARY

Abdominal adhesions

The growth of scar tissue in the abdomen, which causes surfaces of organs to adhere to each other.

Acidosis

Condition that increases the acidity of body fluids. It is associated with respiratory distress.

Adrenaline

Hormone whose effect produces increased heart rate, blood pressure, and blood sugar, contraction of skin blood vessels, and increase in muscle blood flow.

Afterpains

Pains from uterine contractions after birth.

Amniotic-fluid embolism

Dangerous, often-fatal maternal complication around the time of labor, in which amniotic fluid is forced into the mother's bloodstream.

Aspiration pneumonia

Pneumonia caused by the inhalation of vomited contents of the stomach.

Braxton-Hicks contractions

Painless contractions that occur during pregnancy.

Chung

Chinese word for gently shaking a woman in labor to relax her. Also called "apple-shaking" in German.

Colostomy

Operation to create an opening in the abdominal wall that leads to the colon.

Cord entanglement

Condition when the umbilical cord is wrapped around the baby.

Diuretic

Drugs that increase the flow of urine.

Doula

An experienced woman who helps other women around the time of birth. This is U.S. usage; the word actually means "slave" in Greek. Oh, well.

Eclampsia

Serious metabolic illness of pregnancy, which is associated with poor nutrition and inadequate expansion of maternal blood volume. It is often lethal.

Endorphins	Neurohormones that numb pain and produce euphoria.
Epidural	Local anesthetic injected into the nerves coming out of the spinal column in the lower back area to numb labor pain.
Episiotomy	A surgical cut in the perineal muscles, measured in degrees to enlarge the vaginal opening.
Fetal bradycardia	Slowing of the unborn baby's heart rate.
Forceps	Large spoon-shaped metal tongs that are inserted into the vagina and cupped around the head of the baby, which is then delivered by pulling on the handles.
Grand multipara	Woman who has had more than five babies.
Hysterectomy	Surgical removal of the uterus.
Iatrogenic prematurity	Premature birth caused by induced labor or scheduled cesarean before the baby has reached an appropriate gestational age to be born.
Intubation	Insertion of a tube into the airway to use in resuscitation.
Kraamverzorgende	Dutch term for maternity home-care assistant.
Malpresentation	Presentations other than vertex at birth.
Morbidity	Disease or injury.
Neocortex	The "thinking" part of the brain.
Oxytocin	Hormone secreted during labor that causes uterine contractions. Synthetic oxytocin is given intravenously to stimulate labor in hospitals and, sometimes, by injection to stop a postpartum hemorrhage.
Pelvimetry	Art of measuring the bones of the pelvis.
Perineum	The band of muscle between the vagina and the anus.
Peritonitis	Infection of the abdominal cavity.
Pitocin	Synthetic oxytocin.

Preeclampsia	Milder form of eclampsia, a metabolic disease of pregnancy. [See Eclampsia.]
Prostaglandins	Substances that stimulate smooth muscles, such as those of the cervix.
Pubic bone	Front part of the pelvis.
Pulmonary embolism	Obstruction of blood vessels in the lungs.
Placental abruption	Premature separation of the placenta from the uterine wall.
Placenta accreta	The placenta implants deeply into the uterine wall.
Placenta increta	The placenta implants even more deeply into the uterine wall.
Placenta percreta	The placenta grows through the placental wall, sometimes into surrounding organs. A complication caused by previous damage to the uterus.
Placenta previa	The placenta implants over the cervical opening, exposing mother and baby to extreme danger when the cervix begins to dilate.
Relaxin	Hormone of pregnancy, which relaxes the ligaments.
Rooming-in	Hospital practice of keeping mother and baby together.
Sacrum	Wedge-shaped pelvic bone, which makes up part of the spine.
Shoulder dystocia	Stuck shoulders after birth of the baby's head.
Stadol	Narcotic-like analgesic used to dull labor pain.
Toxemia	Eclampsia and preeclampsia.
Urethra	Tube leading from the bladder to the outside of the body.
Vacuum extractor	Device that attaches to the head of the fetus.
Vertex	Baby is born headfirst.

THE FARM: OUTCOMES OF 2,028 PREGNANCIES:
1970–2000

Births completed at home	95.1%
Transports	4.9%
Emergency transports	1.3%
First-time mothers	44.7%
Multigravidas	55.3%
Grand multiparas	5.4% (72% of the grand multips were Amish)
Cesareans	1.4% (61% were first-time mothers)
Forceps deliveries	0.5%
Vacuum-extractor deliveries	0.05%
Vaginal births after cesarean	5.4% (108 attempted; 106 completed vaginal birth)
Postpartum hemorrhage	1.8%
Precipitous births	8.9%
Inductions	5.4%
Castor oil	4.9%
Swept membranes	0.5%
Ate & drank in labor	29.1%
Drank clear fluids	49.9%
Meconium staining	10.6%
Postpartum depression	1%
Intact perineum	68.8%
1st degree	19.1%
2nd degree	11.5%
3rd degree	0.3%
4th degree	0.1%
Preeclampsia	0.39%
Prematurity	2.9% (less than 37 weeks)
Occiput anterior	93.4%
Occiput posterior	2.2%
Frank breech	2.1%
Footling breech	0.7%
Complete breech	0.1%
Face presentations	0.5% (all but 1 were vaginally born)
Brow presentations	0.2% (2 were cesarean deliveries/ 2 were vaginally born)

Twins	15 sets; all vaginally born
Initiation of breastfeeding	99%
Continued breastfeeding among the women of The Farm	100%; 4–5 women supplemented

Lethal anomalies	5 (0.2%)
Maternal mortality	0
Neonatal mortality excluding lethal anomalies	8/2028 (0.39%)*

4 of these deaths occurred during labor.

2 placental abruptions (1 during the last ten minutes of an otherwise straightforward frank breech labor; the other in a first-time mother transported to hospital because of protracted labor).

2 prolapsed cords (1 of these involved a mother whose legs were paralyzed from polio, whose cord prolapsed at the first sign of labor).

4 of these deaths occurred during the first week of life:

1 crib death

1 premie who died from hyaline membrane disease after hospital delivery in 1972

2 deaths from probable infection

* Although the Farm Midwifery Center functions in some ways like a birth center, we have counted our statistics differently from the standard way birth centers do. Birth centers normally "risk out" all breeches, twins, premature labors, and grand multiparas, and postdates pregnancies so such births are not reflected in their statistics. Our statistics reflect the outcomes of *every* mother who is given prenatal care by the Farm midwives, whether they planned a home birth attended by us or a hospital birth attended by physicians near The Farm.

Organizations

Doula UK
PO Box 26678
London
N14 4WB
United Kingdom
(+44) 0871 433 3103
www.doula.org.uk

Independent Midwives Association
PO Box 539
Abingdon
OX14 9DF
United Kingdom
(+44) 0845 4600 105
www.independentmidwives.org.uk

La Leche League (Great Britain)
PO Box 29
West Bridgford
Nottingham
NG2 7NP
United Kingdom
(+44) 0845 456 1855
www.laleche.org.uk

Maternity Alliance
45 Beech Street
London EC2P 2LX
United Kingdom
(+44) (0171) 588 8582
www.maternityalliance.org.uk

Multiple Births Foundation
Hammersmith House Level 4
Queen Charlotte's & Chelsea Hospital
Du Cane Road
London W12 0HS
United Kingdom
(+44) (020) 8383 3519
Email: *info@multiplebirths.org.uk*
www.multiplebirths.org.uk

National Childbirth Trust
Alexandra House
Oldham Terrace
London W3 6NH
United Kingdom
(+44) 0870 444 8707
www.nct.org.uk

Royal College of Midwives
15 Mansfield Street
London W1G 9NH
United Kingdom
(+44) (020) 7312 3535
www.rcm.org.uk

Tamba (Twins and Multiple Births Association)
2 The Willows
Gardner Road
Guildford
GU1 4PG
United Kingdom
(+1) 01483 304 442
www.tamba.org.uk

ICEA
PO Box 20048
Minneapolis, MN 55420
USA
(+1) (612) 854 8660
www.icea.org

International Cesarean Awareness Network (ICAN)
1304 Kingsdale Ave.
Redondo Beach, CA 90278
USA
(+1) (310) 542 5368
www.childbirth.org/section/ICAN.html

Lamaze International
2025 M Street, Suite 800
Washington, DC 20036
USA
(+1) (202) 367 1128
www.lamaze.org

Postpartum Support International
PO Box 60931
Santa Barbara, CA 93160
USA
(+1) (805) 967 7636
www.postpartum.net

American College of Nurse-Midwives (ACNM)
818 Conneticut Ave. NW, Suite 900
Washington, DC 20006
USA
(+1) (202) 728 9860
www.midwife.org

Midwives Alliance of North America (MANA)
4805 Lawrenceville Hwy.
Suite 116-279
Lilburn, GA 30047
USA
(+1) (888) 923 6262
Email: *info@mana.org*
www.mana.org

Australian Nursing and Midwifery Council
PO Box 873
Dickson ACT 2602
Australia
(+61) (02) 6257 7960
www.anmc.org.au

Birth International
PO Box 366
Camperdown
NSW 1450
Australia
(+61) (02) 9564 2322
Email: ozinfo@birthinternational.com
www.birthinternational.com

NSWMA (New South Wales Midwifery Association)
PO Box 62
GLEBE NSW 2037
Australia
(+61) (02) 9281 9522
www.nswmidwives.com.au

Pregnancy, Birth and Beyond
27 Hart Street
Dundas NSW 2117
Australia
(+61) (02) 9873 1750
www.pregnancy.com.au

Books

A Guide to Effective Care in Pregnancy and Childbirth
Murray Enkin, Marc J.N.C. Keirse, et al.

A Perfect Start
Christine and Peter Hill

After the Baby's Birth: A Complete Guide for Postpartum Women
Robin Lim

Baby Catcher: Chronicles of a Modern Midwife
Peggy Vincent

Birth as an American Rite of Passage
Robbie Davis-Floyd

Birth and Beyond
Dr Yehudi Gordon

Birthing from Within
Pam England, CNM

Birth in Four Cultures, 4th ed.
Brigitte Jordan

Birth Skills
Juju Sundin and Sarah Murdoch

Childbirth and Authoritative Knowledge
Edited by Robbie Davis-Floyd and Carolyn Sargent

Childbirth Unmasked
Margaret Jowitt

Childbirth Without Fear, 5th ed.
Grantly Dick-Read
Read this fifth edition if you can; it includes the author's account of
the difficulties he faced in presenting his message.

Diary of a Midwife: The Power of Positive Childbearing
Juliana van Olphen-Fehr

The Five Standards for Safe Childbearing
David Stewart, Ph.D.

In Labor: Women and Power in the Birthplace
Barbara Katz Rothman

Metabolic Toxemia of Late Pregnancy
Thomas H. Brewer
www.ebook.kalico.net
The Brewer Pregnancy Hotline (802) 388-0276

Mother and Baby Health
Dr Yehudi Gordon with Harriet Sharkey, Andy Raffles
and Felicity Fine

Mothering the Mother
Marshall Klaus, M.D., John Kennell, M.D., and Phyllis Klaus

Natural Health after Birth
Aviva Jill Romm

The Natural Pregnancy Book
Aviva Jill Romm

Obstetric Myths Versus Research Realities
Henci Goer

Pursuing the Birth Machine
Marsden Wagner

The Thinking Woman's Guide to a Better Birth
Henci Goer

The Tentative Pregnancy
Barbara Katz Rothman

For a policy statement about midwifery, see: *Charting a Course for the 21st Century: The Future of Midwifery.* A Joint Report of the Pew Health Professions Commission and the University of California, San Francisco Center for the Health Professions (*www.pewtrust.org*).

INDEX

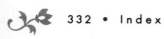

Staengl, Anita, 43–44
Staggers, Ruker, 265
Stephens, Lois, 79–81
Stevenson, John, 269
Stockham, Alice B., 154
Striekwold-Ebben, Marie, 315
Stuck babies
brow presentation, 97, 246
shoulder dystocia, 98–99, 102–104, 106, 109–110
Sweeping the membranes, 216
Sykes, Anna Mary, 251–252

T

Techno-medical model of care, 185–187
the Three Ps, 167–169
toxemia/nutrition connection and, 188
See also caregivers; hospital births; induction of labor; prenatal screening
Television and film, 3, 164–165, 253–254, 272
TENS (transcutaneous electronic nerve stimulation), 216
Thalidomide, 280
Thompson, Morton, 270
Three Ps, Law of, 167–169
Throat and mouth relaxation, 178–180
Topf, Sue and Chris, 92–95
Touch and massage, 241–243
Toxemia. *See* metabolic toxemia of late pregnancy
Trainor, Kim, 19–23
Tranquilizers, 233
Transcutaneous electronic nerve stimulation (TENS), 216
Trilafon (perphenazine), 233–234
Trust, relaxation and, 180–181

U

Ultrasound scanning, 191–193
Umbilical cord, clamping, 258–259
United Kingdom, maternal mortality, 276–277
Upright positions, *227, 227–232, 228, 229*
Uterine rupture
induced labor and, 208, 210–211, 212, 281
single-layer suturing of cesarean sections and, 285
vaginal birth after cesarean (VBAC) and, 295, 297, 299, 300–301
Uterus, changes during pregnancy and labor, 143–147

V

Vacuum-extractor deliveries
epidural anesthesia and, 165, 235
induced labor and, 210
Vaginal birth after cesarean (VBAC), 294–303
changing policy regarding, 295–299
at The Farm Midwifery Center, 301–302
New England Journal of Medicine editorial, 300–301
risks of cesarean surgery, 294–295
successful, improving chances of, 302–303
uterine rupture and, 281, 297, 299, 300–301
Vaginal enlargement (engorgement), 149, 248–254
Vaginal tearing (laceration), 248, 256. *See also* episiotomies
Vallière, Louise de la, 230
Van de Castle, Kathryn B., 23–26
VBAC. *See* vaginal birth after cesarean
Viavant, Suzy Jenkins, 76–79
Vitamin K, 261

INA MAY GASKIN is the author of the internationally renowned book *Spiritual Midwifery*. In 1970 she co-founded The Farm community in Summertown, Tennessee, with her husband, Stephen, and 250 other young people and brought worldwide attention to natural birthing. She is also the founder and director of The Farm Midwifery Center, located on The Farm. To date, the midwifery center has handled more than 2,200 births. In 1994 the *American Journal of Public Health* published the center's statistics, noting its low morbidity and mortality rates and its low rates of medical intervention in birth.

Over the past three decades Ina May has lectured at midwifery conferences and medical schools around the world. In 1997 she received the ASPO/Lamaze Irwin Chabon Award and the Tennessee Perinatal Association Recognition Award. In 1999 a birthing technique popularized and taught by Ina May—which she learned from indigenous Mayan midwives in the highlands of Guatemala—was officially recognized in obstetrical literature. The "Gaskin maneuver" is the first midwifery or obstetrical technique named after a woman. Ina May is a co-founder and past president of the Midwives Alliance of North America (MANA). She represents MANA at the Safe Motherhood Initiatives–USA coalition meetings and initiated the Safe Motherhood Quilt project in order to bring public awareness to the problem of avoidable maternal mortality. She is one of the creators of the consensus document of the Coalition to Improve Maternity Services (CIMS) and its Ten Steps to Mother-Friendly Birth Services. In 2002 she became a Visiting Fellow at Morse College, Yale University.

She received her masters in English from Northern Illinois University in 1962, served in the Peace Corps from 1963 to 1965, and is a certified professional midwife. She continues to live on The Farm with her husband, Stephen.